D1374667

Current orthopaedic practice

A concise guide for postgraduate exams

Sanjeev Agarwal

tfm Publishing Limited
Castle Hill Barns
Harley
Shrewsbury
SY5 6LX
UK

Tel: +44 (0)1952 510061
Fax: +44 (0)1952 510192
E-mail: info@tfmpublishing.com
Web site: www.tfmpublishing.com

Design and layout: Nikki Bramhill BSc (Hons) Dip Law
First Edition   © September 2012

ISBN 978 1 903378 59 5

The entire contents of *Current orthopaedic practice – a concise guide for postgraduate exams* is copyright tfm Publishing Ltd. Apart from any fair dealing for the purposes of research or private study, or criticism or review, as permitted under the Copyright, Designs and Patents Act 1988, this publication may not be reproduced, stored in a retrieval system or transmitted in any form or by any means, electronic, digital, mechanical, photocopying, recording or otherwise, without the prior written permission of the publisher.

Neither the author nor the publisher can accept responsibility for any injury or damage to persons or property occasioned through the implementation of any ideas or use of any product described herein. Neither can they accept any responsibility for errors, omissions or misrepresentations, howsoever caused.

Whilst every care is taken by the author and the publisher to ensure that all information and data in this book are as accurate as possible at the time of going to press, it is recommended that readers seek independent verification of advice on drug or other product usage, surgical techniques and clinical processes prior to their use.

The author and publisher gratefully acknowledge the permission granted to reproduce the copyright material where applicable in this book. Every effort has been made to trace copyright holders and to obtain their permission for the use of copyright material. The publisher apologizes for any errors or omissions and would be grateful if notified of any corrections that should be incorporated in future reprints or editions of this book.

Printed by Gutenberg Press Ltd., Gudja Road, Tarxien, PLA 19, Malta.

Tel: +356 21897037; Fax: +356 21800069.

Contents

Contributors

Mr Sanjeev Agarwal FRCS Orth
Consultant Orthopaedic Surgeon, University Hospital of Wales, Cardiff, UK

Mr Robert Ashford FRCS Orth
Consultant Orthopaedic and Musculoskeletal Tumour Surgeon, East Midlands Sarcoma Service, University Hospital of Leicester, Leicester, UK

Mr Venkateswaran Balachandran FRCS Orth
Consultant Orthopaedic Surgeon, Mid Yorkshire NHS Trust, Wakefield, UK

Dr Jyoti Bansal MRCP FRCR
Consultant in Radiology, Cardiff and Vale NHS Trust, Cardiff, UK

Ms Eleanor Clare Carpenter FRCS Orth MD
Consultant Orthopaedic Surgeon, University Hospital of Wales, Cardiff, UK

Mr Iqroop Chopra FRCS (SN)
Consultant Spinal Surgeon, University Hospital of Wales, Cardiff, UK

Dr Sharon M. Jones BM MD FRCP
Consultant Rheumatologist, University Hospital of Wales, Cardiff, UK

Mr Suraj Joshy FRCS Orth
Consultant in Paediatric Orthopaedics, Royal Manchester Children's Hospital, Manchester, UK

Dr Sridhar Kamath FRCR
Consultant in Musculoskeletal Radiology, University Hospital of Wales, Cardiff, UK

Mr Andy Logan FRCS Orth
Consultant Hand Surgeon, University Hospital of Wales, Cardiff, UK

Mr Khitish Mohanty FRCS Orth
Consultant Orthopaedic Surgeon, University Hospital of Wales, Cardiff, UK

Mr Anthony Perera FRCS Orth
Consultant Orthopaedic Foot and Ankle Surgeon, University Hospital of Wales, Cardiff, UK

Foreword

Current Orthopaedic Practice is designed as a useful addition to the textbooks that are used by orthopaedic trainees preparing for the Intercollegiate Examination in Trauma and Orthopaedic Surgery. It covers the main areas of clinical orthopaedic practice.

Each chapter has a similar layout and uses simple diagrams to help clarify information presented in the text. The chapters cover the regions of the body but in addition there are sections dealing with topics such as arthroplasty, bone and soft tissue tumours, infections, non-unions and imaging – all things that are commonly asked in the examination.

The book is usefully divided into 'bite'-sized sections which means that the trainee who is waiting for an operating list to start or for the anaesthetist to anaesthetise the next patient can comfortably read and learn a particular topic. Of special value however are the highlighted notes. These provide the most relevant references and also give an indication of the outcomes as reported in the referenced paper. This information is invaluable to those taking the examination since most candidates will be asked something about the literature in either the clinical or viva sections of the examination. Being able to comment knowledgeably on the published literature is a guaranteed way of impressing the examiners!

I have no doubt that this text will be valuable to all orthopaedic trainees irrespective of their year of training.

Mr David Stanley MBBS BSc FRCS
Chairman of the Intercollegiate Specialty Board in
Trauma and Orthopaedic Surgery

Foreword *continued*

The FRCS (Tr & Orth) examination presents a considerable hurdle for trainees, most of whom will devote about a year to revising and preparing for this essential summative part of the curriculum. This final preparation should consolidate, and build on, knowledge, skills and experience that have been accumulated over the previous years of higher surgical training.

The standard of the examination is high, requiring a good depth of knowledge across the breadth of the syllabus. This high standard not only helps to ensure that future patients are treated by orthopaedic surgeons who have an excellent grasp of their subject matter, it also makes success in the examination an achievement to be proud of.

Candidates may be unsuccessful in the examination for a number of different reasons, including insufficient depth or breadth of knowledge, lack of clinical experience and lack of logical and organised thought processes. There are no 'tricks' to passing; the only real 'secret' of success is thorough preparation. Good sources of knowledge, such as this book, are a key component of this preparation.

Putting together a textbook is not a light undertaking. Much hard work is involved with little reward for the authors other than the satisfaction of knowing that they have helped to make the topics more understandable and, hopefully, interesting. The authors of this book are to be congratulated on producing a book that is very readable. The focus on key relevant papers is a particularly strong feature; knowledge of the orthopaedic literature can be an important factor in scoring highly in the oral sections of the examination, demonstrating an evidence-based approach to the practice of orthopaedics, but all too frequently the evidence provided by candidates to support their opinions is at the 'someone told me' or 'I read it somewhere' level.

This book should not, however, be seen solely as a revision text; it will prove useful reading for orthopaedic trainees at all levels and also for more senior surgeons helping trainees to prepare for the examination.

Mr Kevin P Sherman MA FRCS MEd PhD
Consultant Orthopaedic Surgeon

Formerly Examiner and member of the
written paper committee FRCS (Tr & Orth)

Formerly Charnley Orthopaedic Tutor
Royal College of Surgeons of England and
Chair of the Orthopaedic Regional Specialty Training Committee and
Regional Specialty Advisor in Orthopaedics (Yorkshire)

Abbreviations

3D	three-dimensional
AAOS	American Academy of Orthopedic Surgeons
ABC	aneurysmal bone cyst
ABCD	airway, breathing, circulation and disability
ABER	abduction, external rotation
AC	acromioclavicular
ACI	autologous chondrocyte implantation
ACJ	acromioclavicular joint
ACL	anterior cruciate ligament
ADI	atlantodens interval
AFO	ankle-foot orthosis
ALPSA	anterior labral periosteal sleeve avulsion
ALVAL	aseptic, lymphocytic, vasculitis-associated lesions
AP	anteroposterior
AR	autosomal recessive
AS	ankylosing spondylitis
ATLS	Advanced Trauma Life Support
AVN	avascular necrosis
BMP	bone morphogenetic protein
CDM	cisplatin, doxorubicin and methotrexate
CMCJ	carpometacarpal joint
CMF	chondromyxoid fibroma
CMTD	Charcot-Marie-Tooth disease
CNB	core needle biopsy
CRP	C-reactive protein
CT	computed tomography
DANA	Designed after Natural Anatomy
DASH	Disability of Arm, Shoulder and Hand (score)
DDH	developmental dysplasia of the hip
DIPJ	distal interphalangeal joint
DMAA	distal metatarsal articular angle
DMD	Duchenne muscular dystrophy
ECRB	extensor carpi radialis brevis
ECU	extensor carpi ulnaris
EDB	extensor digitorum brevis

EDC	extensor digitorum communis
EHL	extensor hallucis longus
ELISA	enzyme-linked immunosorbent assay
ER	external rotation
ESR	erythrocyte sedimentation rate
EULAR	European League against Rheumatism
EURAMOS	European and American Osteosarcoma Study
FABER	flexion, abduction and external rotation
FAI	femoroacetabular impingement
FCR	flexor carpi radialis
FCU	flexor carpi ulnaris
FDG	[18F]-2-fluoro-2-deoxy-D-glucose
FDL	flexor digitorum longus
FDP	flexor digitorum profundus
FDS	flexor digitorum superficialis
FHL	flexor hallucis longus
GCT	giant cell tumour
HA	hydroxyapatite ceramic
HAGL	humeral avulsion of the glenohumeral ligament
HLA	human leukocyte antigen
HO	heterotopic ossification
HTO	high tibial osteotomy
Ig	immunoglobulin
IPJ	interphalangeal joint
IR	internal rotation
ITB	iliotibial band
JIA	juvenile idiopathic arthritis
K-wire	Kirschner wire
LCL	lateral collateral ligament
LCP	Legg-Calvé-Perthes
LDH	lactate dehydrogenase
LHRH	luteinising hormone-releasing hormone
LISS	less invasive stabilisation system
MACI	matrix-associated autologous chondrocyte implantation
MCL	medial collateral ligament
MCPJ	metacarpophalangeal joint
MESS	Mangled Extremity Severity Score
MHE	multiple hereditary exostoses
MR	magnetic resonance
MRI	magnetic resonance imaging
MT	metatarsal
MTPJ	metatarsophalangeal joint
NICE	National Institute for Heath and Clinical Excellence
NSAID	non-steroidal anti-inflammatory drug
ORIF	open reduction and internal fixation
PADI	posterior atlas and dens interval
PASG	pneumatic antishock garment
PCA	porous-coated anatomic

PCL	posterior cruciate ligament
PE	pulmonary embolism
PET	positron emission tomography
PF	patellofemoral
PGE$_2$	prostaglandin E$_2$
PHV	peak height velocity
PIPJ	proximal interphalangeal joint
PL	palmaris longus
PLC	posterolateral corner
PMMA	polymethyl methacrylate
PROSTALAC	prosthesis with antibiotic-loaded acrylic cement
PSA	prostate-specific antigen
RCT	randomised controlled trial
RF	radiofrequency
RF	rheumatoid factor
rhBMP	recombinant human bone morphogenetic protein
ROM	range of motion
RVAD	rib-vertebral angle difference
SCFE	slipped capital femoral epiphysis
SGHL	superior glenohumeral ligament
SI	sacroiliac
SLAP	superior labral anterior and posterior
SLE	systemic lupus erythematosus
SLR	straight leg raise
SONK	spontaneous osteonecrosis of the knee
SpA	spondyloarthropathy
SPECT	single-photon emission computed tomography
SPLATT	split anterior tibial tendon transfer
STIR	short tau inversion recovery
TAR	thrombocytopenia with absent radius
TE	echo time
TG	trochlear groove
THR	total hip replacement
TKR	total knee replacement
TMCJ	trapeziometacarpal joint
TNF	tumour necrosis factor
TR	repetition time
TRAP	tartrate-resistant acid phosphatase
TSR	total shoulder replacement
TT	tibial tubercle
UBC	unicameral bone cyst
UCBL	University of California Biomechanics Laboratory
UKR	unicompartmental knee replacement
VAI	vincristine, actinomycin-D and ifosfamide
VATER	vertebrae, anal malformations, trachea, oesophagus anomalies and renal syndrome
VMO	vastus medialis obliquus
VTE	venous thromboembolism
WCC	white cell count

Acknowledgements

I am deeply indebted to the contributors of this book, who set time aside from their busy schedules and clinical practices to make this project possible. Each is an expert in their chosen fields and their experience and knowledge has greatly enriched this book.

I owe a special thanks to some fantastic people, with whom I had a chance to work with, and gain knowledge and skills over the years. These are Steve Godsiff, Richard Power, Stuart Birtwistle, David McDonald, Kevin Sherman, Stuart Calder, Brian Scott, Roger Hackney, Peter Giannoudis, Mark Andrews, Andrew North, Peter Milner and Keshav Singhal in the UK; Professor U.S. Mishra and Professor U.K. Jain in India; and Andrew Freiberg, Harry Rubash and Professor Bill Harris at the Massachusetts General Hospital in Boston, USA.

The medical students, house officers, registrars and fellows who work in our orthopaedic department are a constant stimulus for academic interaction. They will surely be pushing the boundaries of surgical innovation in years to come.

I am thankful to Nikki Bramhill, Director of tfm publishing Ltd, for her professionalism and expertise throughout this project; and to Catherine Mary Booth for her thorough proofreading and astute comments on the manuscript.

Mr Sanjeev Agarwal FRCS Orth
Consultant Orthopaedic Surgeon
University Hospital of Wales, Cardiff, UK

Dedication

To my parents – Dr Ramesh Chandra and Dr Padam K. Agarwal for making me what I am

To my wife – Jyoti for her love and support

To my children – Suyash and Harshita for making it all worthwhile

Chapter 1 Arthroplasty

Total hip replacement

Total hip replacement (THR) is one of the most successful operative procedures in orthopaedic surgery.

Indications

The indications for THR are as follows:

- To relieve hip pain that is unresponsive to non-operative measures.
- To improve function.

The vast majority of hip replacements are performed because of osteoarthritis. Other indications include rheumatoid arthritis, post-traumatic arthritis, avascular necrosis, dysplastic hip in skeletally mature patients, failed fracture fixations and tumours.

There is an increasing trend towards THR in active patients of 50-80 years with displaced femoral neck fractures.

Contraindications

Contraindications to THR include the following:

- Active infection in the hip.
- Relative contraindications include poor abductor function, medical condition or mobility, an immature skeleton and progressive neurologic disease.

Note

Blomfeldt R, Törnkvist H, Ponzer S, *et al*. Comparison of internal fixation with total hip replacement for displaced femoral neck fractures. Randomised, controlled trial performed at four years. *J Bone Joint Surg Am* 2005; 87: 1680-8. **This study looked at 102 patients with a femoral neck fracture. All were older than 70 years and had intact cognitive function. At 4 years, the mortality rate was 25% in both the internal fixation and THR groups. The THR group had a 4% complication and 4% reoperation rate. The fixation group had a 42% complication rate and 47% reoperation rate. Hip function was better in the THR group.**

Assessment and investigations

Pre-operative assessment should include the following:

- A detailed history and examination to confirm that the hip joint is the source of pain.
- Full blood count, electrolytes and urine analysis to check for urinary tract infection.
- Nasal and perineal swabs for MRSA.
- Cross-matching (or autodonation) of blood.
- Electrocardiogram.
- Chest X-ray, if medically indicated.
- X-ray of: the anteroposterior (AP) view of the pelvis; an AP view of the hip performed in 20°

of internal rotation for templating; and a lateral view of the hip. At some centres, a shoot-through lateral view of the hip is also taken.

Other investigations:

- Lateral C-spine flexion and extension views for patients with rheumatoid arthritis affecting C-spine stability.
- Spirometry for patients with reduced pulmonary function.
- Cardiac assessment – echocardiography.
- Vascular assessment in patients with vascular compromise.

Informed consent

The procedure should be explained to the patient, along with all the risks of surgery. These are described later in the section on complications.

Cemented femoral component design

In the early days of THR, femoral prostheses were made out of cast stainless steel. This was not strong enough to sustain prolonged physiological loading and incidences of stem fracture led to development of cold-forged implants.

Titanium stems in cement transfer more load to the cement as the titanium is less stiff, leading to early cement fatigue and failure. Hence, cemented femoral components are made of stiffer materials – cobalt chrome or stainless steel.

A broad medial border on the prosthesis reduces the load on the cement. Hence, the diamond-shaped Muller prosthesis, which had a narrow medial border, is no longer used. The Thompson prosthesis used in hemiarthroplasty is also diamond-shaped in cross-section and has a narrow medial border. Femoral components should have a broad medial border to reduce cement strain, and a broader lateral border (e.g., C stem) to load the cement in compression (Figure 1.1).

Tapered stems (e.g., the Exeter system) help to transfer the load to cement evenly. Cement is stronger in compression. The flanged Charnley stem is broader laterally and helps to load the cement in compression. The C stem (DePuy) is thicker laterally and thinner medially – known as the third taper – which loads the medial cement mantle.

Offset

The offset of the stem is the perpendicular distance between the centre of the prosthetic femoral head and the longitudinal axis of the femoral stem (Figure 1.2). A high offset produces higher stress in the femoral stem and can lead to failure of the cement or metal. The advantage of a high offset, however, is that less force is required by the abductors because of an elongated lever arm. The offset of the prosthesis selected should normally reproduce the original offset of the patient.

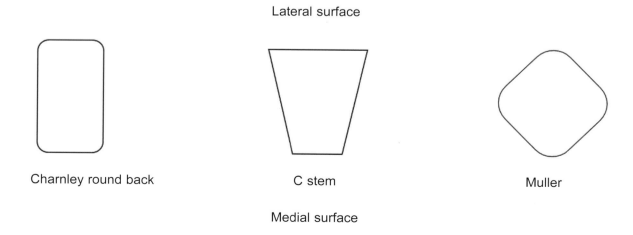

Lateral surface

Charnley round back   C stem   Muller

Medial surface

Figure 1.1. Diagrammatic cross-section of femoral stems to illustrate differences in design.

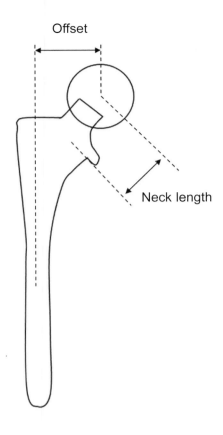

Figure 1.2. The offset and neck length of femoral components.

Most femoral prostheses have a high-offset option. For instance, the Charnley stem provides an offset of 40 or 45mm. In systems in which a range of stem sizes are available, the offset increases with increasing stem size. Increasing the neck length also results in a higher offset.

Implanting a femoral stem in varus alignment increases the offset. However, this is disadvantageous in cemented stems as it leads to an inadequate cement mantle in zones 3 and 7 and may lead to early failure. A cementless stem implanted in varus will be undersized and have less contact with the endosteum.

Offset can be altered during surgery by the following:

- Using a high-offset stem – this will increase offset without increasing leg length.
- Using a longer neck length – this will add to offset as well as leg length.
- Using an offset liner with a cementless socket. The centre of rotation is more laterally placed in offset compared to standard liners.
- Lateral placement of the acetabular component.

Cementing techniques

A summary of cementing techniques is presented in Table 1.1.

Table 1.1. Development of cementing techniques.

First generation	Second generation	Third generation
Finger packing	Cement gun	Vacuum mixing
Cast stem	Pulse lavage	Pressurisation
	Canal brush and dry	Precoated stems
	Cement restrictor	Rough surface finish
	Forged stem	Centraliser
	Broad round medial border	
	Collared stem	

Fourth-generation techniques involve using a proximal centraliser in addition to a distal centraliser. The centraliser cuts through the cement as the stem is inserted and this may have a detrimental effect on the cementation. This has to be balanced against the benefit of having a centraliser to achieve a circumferential cement mantle.

Vacuum mixing and porosity reduction may help to strengthen cement. Vacuum mixing reduces pores and voids. However, pore-free cement may shrink and this can compromise the strength of the cement bond *in vivo*. The benefits are debatable.

A varus or valgus positioning of the femoral stem by more than 5° is related to increased stress in the cement mantle and a higher failure rate.

'Creep' is the deformation of bone cement under constant load and is time-dependent. The viscoelastic nature of cement is responsible for creep. Creep leads to stress relaxation, which is the change in stress due to constant strain. As a result of stress relaxation, tensile stress in the cement reduces and this improves longevity.

Surface finish

The roughness of surface finish is described as R_a (average roughness). This is the average of all variations from the central line of the roughness profile. Rough surfaces adhere well to cement and prevent subsidence, while the bonding of a smooth polished stem to cement is weaker. If loose within a cement mantle, a rough stem generates greater wear debris.

Fixation

Fixation of cemented femoral components can be described under two mechanisms: 'composite beam' or 'sliding taper'. In the composite beam mechanism, the stem is not intended to subside and a collar is useful to prevent subsidence. The stem is matt-finished or grit-blasted to allow a good interface between the metal and cement.

In the sliding taper mechanism (e.g., Exeter stem), the stem is polished and tapered and is intended to subside to a stable position. Such a stem is described as a 'collarless polished tapered' stem. A non-polished stem that subsides within the cement mantle will produce a large amount of debris and lead to early failure.

The Exeter stem has a smooth finish. In 1980 the surface was changed to a matt finish, resulting in a high failure rate. The surface finish was changed back to smooth in 1988 and the results have been excellent.

A precoated stem has a layer of polymethyl methacrylate, which substantially improves the cement-metal interface strength when the stem is implanted. These stems have a rough surface finish (R_a 30-60 microinches) and are not designed to subside. Instead, the composite beam principle is the method of fixation.

Collar

A collar is desirable if subsidence is not intended. A collar pressurises the proximal cement and prevents subsidence of the stem in the event of loosening.

Centralisers

A circumferential cement mantle of 2mm should be present. Centralisers were introduced in third-generation cementing techniques to keep the stem central within the cement mantle. Distal centralisers are used more often than proximal centralisers. Problems with centralisers include voids around the centraliser, failure of the interface and impingement of the centraliser against the cortex.

A thin cement mantle leads to fatigue failure of the cement and loosening of the component. Poor cementing – Barrack type C or D and a mantle less than 2mm – is correlated with early failure.

Note

Chambers IR, Fender D, McCaskie AW, *et al. Radiological features predictive of aseptic loosening in cemented Charnley femoral stems. J Bone Joint Surg Br* 2001; 83: 838-42. **In this study, inadequate cementing had an odds ratio of 9.5 for risk of loosening and failure.**

Grades of femoral cementing

Grades of femoral cementing are presented in Table 1.2.

Table 1.2. Grades of femoral cementing.	
Type A	Complete filling of the femoral canal with no distinguishable border between cement and bone ('white out')
Type B	Near complete filling with some demarcation between cement and bone Radiolucency at the cement-bone interface is <50%
Type C1	More than 50% lucency at the cement-bone interface
Type C2	The cement mantle is <1mm or the prosthesis is in contact with the bone
Type D	Gross deficiency or large voids

Note

Barrack RL, Mulroy RD, Harris WH. Improved cementing techniques and femoral component loosening in young patients with hip arthroplasty. A 12-year radiographic review. *J Bone Joint Surg Br* 1992; 74: 385-9.

Cemented acetabular component design

All-polyethylene acetabular cups are used in preference to metal-backed cemented cups as a thicker polyethylene can be used. The outer surface of the cup has grooves for interlocking with the cement.

Flanged cups allow better pressurisation of the cement mantle around the acetabular component compared with non-flanged cups. The Ogee Charnley cup has a flange that can be cut to the required size so as to pressurise the cement. 'Ogee' is an architectural term used to describe the shape of the flange. The aim is to pressurise the cement so as to achieve a good cement-bone interface.

The minimum thickness of polyethylene recommended for an all-polyethylene cup is 8mm. For cemented cups, the limit is 5mm. With thinner cups, the stress transfer to acetabular bone is not uniform and may lead to failure.

A thicker polyethylene reduces the stress transmitted to the cement mantle.

Cementless femoral component design

The femoral component design should provide adequate primary stability to resist physiologic loads until biologic ingrowth or ongrowth occurs and provides long-term stability. It should prevent axial subsidence, mediolateral and AP displacement, and rotation in all three axes.

Good contact with bone will facilitate biologic integration. A wide range of sizes are available to achieve a good fit with the femur. Some implants have a collar for additional axial stability. Some revision implants allow the matching of different metaphyseal components to different diaphyseal stems to gain maximum contact.

Micromotion should be less than 50µm. Over this limit, fibrous tissue forms in the implant-bone interface.

The surface of the stem may be coated for ongrowth with ceramics such as hydroxyapatite (HA) or tricalcium phosphate. These are osteoconductive and bone growth takes place right up to the surface of the implant, providing stable fixation. The thickness of the coating is between 50 and 100µm. The ideal pore size is 100-400µm.

Bone ingrowth surfaces may have an additional coating of HA to further enhance integration. HA reduces the time to reach final shear strength by 50%. Cortical bone provides predictable bone ingrowth.

Examples of coatings for bone ingrowth include a porous coating of titanium wire mesh, cobalt chrome or titanium beads, or plasma spray.

Some earlier designs (e.g., Harris-Galante, Omniflex) had a patch-porous coating instead of circumferential porous coating. This resulted in some areas that were not bonded to bone. These areas acted as conduits through which wear particles could reach the distal part of the stem (Figure 1.3), leading to stem loosening and failure.

The extent of coating may be proximal only or extensive. Proximal porous-coated stems depend on good metaphyseal contact and demonstrate good fixation, as do extensively coated stems. Extensively coated stems such as the Furlong (JRI, London, UK) and the Corail (DePuy Orthopaedics, Warsaw, IN, USA) may result in distal load transfer through the tip of the stem and proximal stress shielding due to reduced forces on the femur proximal to the load-bearing tip of the stem.

Proximally coated stems usually have coating in the proximal part of the femoral component, with grit blasting of the stem distal to the coating. Grit blasting encourages ongrowth. The removal of proximally coated stems at revision surgery is considered to be easier than that of extensively coated stems.

Cobalt chrome cementless stems (e.g., porous-coated anatomic [PCA]; Howmedica; Stryker, Rutherford, NJ, USA) are commonly coated with sintered beads, while titanium stems (e.g., Zimmer; VerSys, Warsaw, IN, USA) have wire mesh. Furlong and Corail have an HA coating.

Implants may be shaped as follows:

- Metaphyseal filling wedge-shaped – these gain stability on the metaphysis.
- Wedge-shaped and relatively flattened AP – to gain stability in the metaphysis.
- Tapered stems fixing at the diaphyseal-metaphyseal junction.
- Distally fixing cylindrical stems with flutes or porous coating.

Modular implants allow matching different stems and proximal components but introduce a risk of failure at the modular junction and corrosion. A common combination is a cobalt chrome head over a titanium stem (titanium is not used to make femoral heads because of poor wear characteristics; femoral heads are instead made of cobalt chrome or ceramics), which leads to galvanic corrosion, fretting and third-body wear. Clinically significant problems as a direct result of modularity are not common.

Fully coated implants may cause stress shielding proximally and are difficult to remove if revision is required. Proximal porous coating is adequate when a metaphyseal fit is aimed for. For stems achieving diaphyseal fixation, the stem must be coated to allow bone integration.

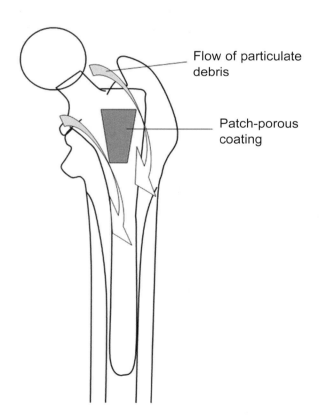

Flow of particulate debris

Patch-porous coating

Figure 1.3. Route for particulate debris in femoral stems with patch-porous coating.

Thigh pain in cementless femoral stems may be due to the following:

- A loose stem.
- Fibrous tissue at the implant-bone interface.
- A stiff femoral component with micromotion between the implant and bone when the femur is loaded. This can be minimised by extending the coating to the tip of the stem, which allows osseointegration and reduces the micromotion.
- Stress concentration at the tip of a well-fixed stem. The tip of the stem can be tapered to reduce the stress concentration at the tip. Alternatives are a stem design with flutes or hollow stems to reduce the stiffness.

Cementless acetabular component design

The principles of biological integration with a cementless acetabular component design are similar to those with femoral components.

The most commonly used acetabular components are hemispherical cups. The implants are HA coated (e.g., Furlong) or porous coated – which can be titanium mesh (e.g., Harris-Galante, Trilogy; Zimmer) or beads (PCA).

A press fit of 1-2mm generally gives adequate primary stability. A press fit by 2mm implies the cup is 2mm bigger than the last reamer used. A larger press fit is associated with a higher rate of intraoperative fracture of the acetabulum while impacting the cup and should be avoided. A minimum thickness of 6mm for the polyethylene insert should be allowed in metal-backed acetabular components.

Screws are optional and may be used to augment primary stability. Screw holes may act as passage routes for the wear debris to the pelvic bone and screws may contribute to wear debris through corrosion and fretting.

The safe quadrant for screw insertion has been described by Wasielewski et al. A line is drawn from the anterior superior iliac spine to the centre of the acetabulum. Another line is drawn perpendicular to this line through the centre of the acetabulum, thus dividing the cup into four quadrants. Screws in the posterosuperior quadrant are relatively safe (Figure 1.4).

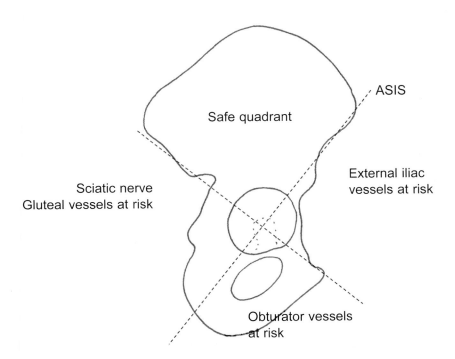

Figure 1.4. The safe quadrant for insertion of screws in cementless cups.

Note

Wasielewski RC, Cooperstein LA, Kruger MP, Rubash HE. Acetabular anatomy and the transacetabular fixation of screws in total hip arthroplasty. *J Bone Joint Surg Am* 1990; 72: 501-8. **This anatomical and radiographic study aimed to determine the safe quadrant for placement of screws in cementless acetabular component insertion.**

Concerns with metal-backed cementless cups are backside wear, dissociation of the liner from the metal backing and osteolysis.

Threaded cups have been abandoned due to a higher failure rate, possibly resulting from increased stresses at the point of contact of the threads.

Effect of head size

In his concept of low-friction arthroplasty in the early 1960s, Sir John Charnley used a 22mm head (22.225mm), which reduced the moment arm on the head. As a result, the distance the head had to move for a certain degree of movement of the leg was reduced. This head size gave a reduced frictional torque and generated less wear particles. The low-friction torque led to the nomenclature 'low-friction arthroplasty'.

Over the years, various head sizes have been used. The introduction of the highly cross-linked polyethylene, which had a significantly lower wear rate in joint simulators, and the use of ceramic articulations and metal-on-metal implants have enabled the use of bigger head sizes while keeping a low wear rate.

A larger head size allows a greater arc of movement and is more stable (Figure 1.5), but generates more wear particles due to greater volumetric wear. For the same arc of movement, a point on the surface of a larger head covers a longer distance against the polyethylene compared to small heads (Figure 1.6). Hence, the volume of wear particles and volumetric wear are greater.

In modular cementless cups, a polyethylene thickness of less than 5mm is associated with a higher risk of catastrophic wear.

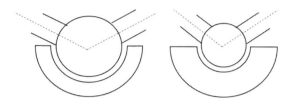

Figure 1.5. Differing arcs of movement with different head sizes.

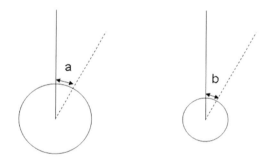

Distance a > b

Figure 1.6. The excursion of a point on the head is greater in a larger head for the same arc of movement.

Stability in hip replacement

The following factors determine stability in hip replacements:

- Implant design-related factors:
  - head size: biomechanically, a larger head should be more stable. However, clinical studies have not shown a significant difference;

- acetabular component size: a larger acetabulum has a lower risk of impingement;
- skirted modular femoral head: a skirt on the femoral head (seen in long-neck versions) predisposes to impingement and dislocation (Figure 1.7);
- elevated lip liners for acetabulum: elevated lip liners can lead to impingement on the opposite side (Figure 1.7). The elevated lip is placed posterosuperiorly when the hip is replaced through a posterior approach to reduce risk of posterior dislocation. However, the combination of an elevated lip and an excessively anteverted cup can lead to anterior dislocation;
- reduced offset: predisposes to impingement.

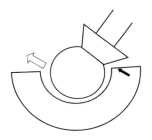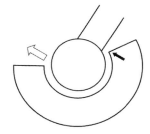

Figure 1.7. The effect of skirted heads (left) and elevated lip liners (right) on impingement.

- Surgical factors:
  - approach: the posterior approach has been blamed for a higher dislocation rate, but an enhanced repair reduces the dislocation rate comparable to a direct lateral approach;
  - component malposition: retroverted acetabular components predispose to posterior dislocation and excess anteversion predisposes to anterior dislocation. A more vertical cup alignment may also predispose to dislocation. Femoral anteversion over 15° can be a factor. The combined anteversion of the femoral component and the acetabular component should not exceed 30°;

- abductor muscle dysfunction;
- trochanteric non-union leading to a higher dislocation rate;
- surgeon's experience;
- secondary impingement: osteophytes and retained excess cement may lever out the head. Impingement of the greater trochanter against the ilium can lead to dislocation.

- Patient-related factors:
  - non-compliance;
  - previous surgery: revision hip surgery has twice the dislocation rate of primary surgery;
  - arthroplasty for femoral neck fractures;
  - poor muscular balance or neuromuscular diseases. In addition, patients with psychiatric disorders may not be able to comply with postoperative instructions or precautions;
  - infection: leads to effusion and dislocation.

Note

Berry DJ, von Knoch M, Schleck CD, Harmsen WS. Effect of femoral head diameter and operative approach on risk of dislocation after primary total hip arthroplasty. *J Bone Joint Surg Am* 2005; 87: 2456-63. This study looked at 21,047 hips over 30 years. The risk of dislocation was 2% in the first year, 3% at 5 years and 6% at 20 years. A larger femoral head diameter was associated with a lower dislocation rate.

Note

Pellicci PM, Bostrom M, Poss R. Posterior approach to total hip replacement using enhanced posterior soft tissue repair. *Clin Orthop Relat Res* 1998; 355: 224-8. A dislocation rate of 6.2% was reduced to 0.8% in 124 hips with enhanced repair.

The direction of dislocation is commonly posterior, even in a hip replacement that has been performed from a direct lateral approach. Patient compliance may be an important factor in outcomes, as some studies have shown no difference in the position of the acetabular component between patients experiencing a dislocation and those with a stable prosthesis.

Management of a dislocated hip replacement

First dislocation
A first dislocation should be managed as follows:

- The history of events leading to dislocation is elicited and the patient's neurological status is checked.
- Adequate and effective pain relief is administered.
- X-rays of the pelvis in the AP view and the hip in the lateral view are obtained to assess the direction of the dislocation, the type and position of components, and whether there are signs of impingement or trochanteric problems.
- Rule out infection, checking the erythrocyte sedimentation rate (ESR) and C-reactive protein (CRP) levels. Aspiration of the hip is not required unless inflammatory markers are elevated with no other systemic cause.
- Perform reduction under anaesthetic. Assess stability in flexion (internal rotation) and extension (external rotation). Assess telescoping for laxity of abductors. The position of components can be more accurately checked with the image intensifier.

Two-thirds of patients who suffer a hip dislocation do so only once. The rest, however, may experience recurrent dislocations.

Recurrent dislocation
In addition to relocation of the hip as described, patients with more than three episodes of dislocation should be considered for revision surgery. The aims of surgery for recurrent dislocation are as follows:

- Identify the cause preoperatively, if possible.
- If infection is present, manage according to infection guidelines.
- Remove any cause for impingement (e.g., cement, osteophytes).
- Correct malalignment of components.
- Use a larger head size.
- Consider elevated lip liners.

- Restore offset and the neck length.
- Consider constrained liners. The constrained liners may predispose to loosening because the restrictions on head movement are transmitted to the implant-bone interface as a shear force.
- Revise to a bipolar hemiarthroplasty; a larger head is more stable. Postoperative pain is a problem.
- If all fails, or if the patient is medically unfit for major reconstruction, consider excision arthroplasty.

Note

Ekelund A. Trochanteric osteotomy for recurrent dislocation of total hip arthroplasty. *J Arthroplasty* 1993; 8: 629-32. **In this study, 17 out of 21 patients had no further dislocation. The authors found that trochanteric osteotomy is indicated when no cause for recurrent dislocation can be found.**

Note

Goetz DD, Capello WN, Callaghan JJ, *et al.* Salvage of recurrently dislocating total hip prosthesis with use of a constrained acetabular component. A retrospective analysis of fifty-six cases. *J Bone Joint Surg Am* 1998; 80: 502-9. **Only two patients experienced a further dislocation after a minimum of 3 years' follow-up.**

Note

Parvizi J, Morrey BF. Bipolar hip arthroplasty as a salvage treatment for instability of the hip. *J Bone Joint Surg Am* 2000; 82: 1132-9. **The records of 27 patients who had undergone bipolar hip replacement as a salvage procedure for the treatment of recurrent instability of the hip after THR were reviewed, with a mean follow-up of 5 years. Bipolar replacement prevented redislocation in 22 hips (81%).**

Note

Goetz DD, Bremner BR, Callaghan JJ, *et al*. Salvage of a recurrently dislocation total hip prosthesis with use of a constrained acetabular component. A concise follow-up of a previous report. *J Bone Joint Surg Am* 2004; 86: 2419-23. **This study looked at 55 patients with a 10.2-year follow-up. Overall, 7% experienced a subsequent dislocation, 4% underwent revision for aseptic loosening, and one hip was revised for osteolysis.**

Hip replacement in dysplastic hips

Hip replacement is needed in dysplastic hips with secondary osteoarthritis. The degree of dysplasia is classified by the Crowe method.

Note

Crowe JF, Mani VJ, Ranawat CS. Total hip replacement in congenital dislocation and dysplasia of the hip. *J Bone Joint Surg Am* 1979; 61: 15-23.

The junction of the head and neck of the femur on the medial aspect is identified. A horizontal line is drawn along the inferior border of the teardrop. The proximal migration of the junction point is assessed in relation to the inter-teardrop line. The femoral head diameter is 20% of the vertical height of the pelvis on the AP radiograph. The proximal migration is measured in relation to the femoral head diameter, or 20% of the vertical pelvic height.

Grading of hip dysplasia is shown in Table 1.3.

Technical problems encountered in the dysplastic hip include anteversion of the acetabulum, deficient anterior and superior support, an oblong and shallow acetabulum, and formation of a false acetabulum with a high hip centre. On the femoral side, the femoral head is hypoplastic, the femoral neck is short and anteverted, and the femoral canal is narrow.

Table 1.3. Grading of hip dysplasia.	
Grade	**Degree of proximal subluxation**
I	<50%
II	50-75%
III	75-100%
IV	>100%

The sciatic nerve is congenitally short, and a leg length discrepancy of up to 2.5cm can be corrected without significant stretching of the nerve. An effort is made to restore the hip centre. If the hip is shortened such that further lengthening would compromise the sciatic nerve, a subtrochanteric osteotomy to shorten the femur should be considered.

Note

Nagoya S, Kaya M, Sasaki M, *et al*. Cementless total hip replacement with subtrochanteric femoral shortening for severe developmental dysplasia of the hip. *J Bone Joint Surg Br* 2009; 91: 1142-7. **Twenty patients with Crowe dysplasia grade IV underwent an 8.1-year follow-up. All of the patients had a subtrochanteric osteotomy, with an acetabulum placed at the anatomical site.**

Complications in total hip replacement

Infection

Infections can be inadvertently introduced at the time of surgery and may spread through the bloodstream. A study from the Royal Orthopaedic Hospital, Birmingham, in 10,735 patients having primary hip or knee replacement, reported infection rates of 0.57% in hips and 0.86% in knees.

Note

Phillips JE, Crane TP, Noy M, *et al*. The incidence of deep prosthetic infections in a specialist orthopaedic hospital: a 15-year prospective survey. *J Bone Joint Surg Br* 2006; 88: 943-8. This study from the Royal Orthopaedic Hospital, Birmingham, looked at 10,735 patients having primary hip or knee replacement. The infection rate was 0.57% in hips and 0.86% in knees. The most common organism was coagulase-negative *Staphylococcus*. Overall, 72% of patients were sensitive to routine antimicrobial prophylaxis. A total of 29% of infections were diagnosed within 3 months, 35% between 3 months and 1 year and 36% after 1 year from surgery. Most were detected acutely and treated aggressively, and infection was eradicated in 96%.

Early postoperative infection occurs within 4 weeks of surgery, while infections after 4 weeks are classified as late chronic infections. Acute haematogenous infection occurs as a late event with acute onset. Late haematogenous spread may develop following dental, gynaecological, abdominal or urologic procedures.

Prevention

Infection can be prevented with the following:

- Preoperative antibiotics given 30 minutes before incision (commonly cefuroxime or cefazolin, Augmentin or Teicoplanin), followed by two further doses at 8 and 16 hours postoperatively. The rationale for postoperative antibiotic therapy is debatable, and some studies suggest that a single dose before the start of surgery is the most effective measure.
- Vertical laminar air flow.
- Antibiotic-loaded cement – the use of gentamicin with bone cement has been shown to reduce the infection rate. Adding 2g gentamicin to 40g cement powder does not significantly compromise the mechanical strength of the cement.

Laminar air flow and perioperative intravenous antibiotics are considered mandatory for hip replacement.

Diagnosis

Clinical suspicion of an infection should be raised by the presentation of pain at rest. Infections may also present with dislocation of the hip. This is thought to be due to distension of the pseudocapsule due to infection.

Investigation

The ESR and CRP level are commonly used blood parameters in investigating infection. The ESR returns to normal 6 months after hip replacement, while the CRP level normalises in 2-3 weeks.

In a study of 202 revision hip procedures, an ESR over 30mm/h had a sensitivity of 0.82 and specificity of 0.85 for the diagnosis of infection, while a CRP level over 10mg/L had a sensitivity of 0.96 and specificity of 0.92. At least one of these two markers was elevated in all patients with infection.

Note

Spangehl MJ, Masri BA, O'Connell JX, Duncan CP. Prospective analysis of preoperative and intraoperative investigations for the diagnosis of infection at the sites of two hundred and two revision total hip arthroplasties. *J Bone Joint Surg Am* 1999; 81: 672-83.

The white blood cell count has poor sensitivity and specificity for hip infections. It may be elevated in only 15-26% of infected hip arthroplasties.

In a prospective study of 78 patients, the combination of a CRP level greater than 3.2mg/L and an interleukin-6 level greater than 12pg/mL identified all patients with a deep infection. Procalcitonin (>0.3ng/mL) and tumour necrosis factor (TNF)-α levels greater than 40ng/mL were very specific for infection (0.98 and 0.94, respectively), but had low sensitivities (0.33 and 0.43).

Note

Bottner F, Wegner A, Winkelmann W, *et al.* Interleukin-6, procalcitonin and TNF-alpha: markers of peri-prosthetic infection following total joint replacement. *J Bone Joint Surg Br* 2007; 89: 94-9.

On X-ray, irregular endosteal scalloping, a lacy periosteal reaction, early loosening and rapidly progressive radiolucent lines indicate infection. Radiological signs are a late feature in infection.

On radionuclide imaging, a Tc-99m scan may be positive in aseptic loosening. An indium-111 leukocyte scan has a high sensitivity but poor specificity for infection. The specificity can be improved by combining the scan with sulphur colloid imaging.

Preoperative joint aspiration has a sensitivity of 92% and specificity of 97% for infection in the hip. It also identifies the organism and helps determine sensitivity to antibiotics prior to revision surgery. However, Barrack and Harris reported a 13% false-positive rate for infection in 270 consecutive aspiration procedures before revision hip replacement.

Note

Barrack RL, Harris WH. The value of aspiration of the hip joint before revision total hip arthroplasty. *J Bone Joint Surg Am* 1993; 75: 66-76.

An intraoperative Gram stain also has a very high false-negative rate for the diagnosis of infection.

Intraoperative frozen section is another method of identifying infection. Samples should be obtained from areas of inflammation surrounding the prosthetic joint. More than five polymorphonuclear leucocytes per high-power field indicate infection with a sensitivity of 100% and specificity of 96%. The experience of the pathologist is an important factor.

Finally, culture of intraoperative samples is the gold standard for the diagnosis of joint infections. Multiple samples should be obtained, with different studies advising three to seven samples. Two or more samples should grow the same pathogen for diagnosis of infection.

Management

Superficial infections may be treated with antibiotics, with or without joint washout and retention of components. Deep infections, however, require removal of all metalwork and cement, and reimplantation – either as a single-stage or two-stage procedure.

Single-stage surgery is indicated when the organism is known and the organism is of low virulence and susceptible to antibiotics. The success of surgery may be compromised if the infecting organism is resistant (e.g., MRSA), the patient is immunocompromised or significant bone defects impair the stability of the implant. The advantages of single-stage are a reduced hospital stay, lower morbidity, faster return to mobility and lower cost.

Note

Callaghan JJ, Katz RP, Johnston RC. One-stage revision surgery of the infected hip. A minimum 10-year follow-up study. *Clin Orthop Relat Res* 1999; 369: 139-43. **From 24 one-stage revisions, the authors reported an 8.3% reinfection rate. Criteria for surgery were no draining sinuses, no immunocompromise, good bone stock after debridement and 3-6 months of postoperative oral antibiotic therapy.**

In a two-stage revision, the first stage is removal of all metalwork, cement, infected tissue and infected bone. An antibiotic-loaded spacer is left *in situ* to provide a high local concentration of antibiotics. The second stage is generally performed later at 3 months or longer. During this stage, components are inserted once the inflammatory markers and signs of infection have settled. Two-stage revision allows the use of specific antibiotics. Patients can be monitored for control of infection and the optimum time for reimplantation can be planned.

Note

Hsieh PH, Shih CH, Chang YH, et al. Treatment of deep infection of the hip associated with massive bone loss: two-stage revision with an antibiotic-loaded interim cement prosthesis followed by reconstruction with allograft. *J Bone Joint Surg Br* 2005; 87: 770-5. **In this study, 24 patients underwent a two-stage revision for infection. In a 4.2-year follow-up there was no recurrence of infection.**

Note

English H, Timperley AJ, Dunlop D, Gie G. Impaction grafting of the femur in two-stage revision for infected total hip replacement. *J Bone Joint Surg Br* 2002; 84: 700-5. **This study from Exeter looked at 53 patients and reported a 7.5% reinfection rate at 53 months.**

PROSTALAC (prosthesis with antibiotic-loaded acrylic cement) is a prosthesis used between the first and second stages to allow mobilisation, prevent shortening of the leg and provide a high dose of local antibiotics. Commercial prostheses are available, in addition to the option of using a cemented hip implant inserted without cement pressurisation.

Other options for treatment of infections include excision arthroplasty, antibiotic suppression and surgical debridement without removal of components:

- Excision arthroplasty helps control of infection, but the functional result is often poor.
- Antibiotic suppression can be considered for patients who are not well enough for or who refuse surgery. A well-fixed prosthesis, absence of systemic sepsis and presence of an organism sensitive to a well-tolerated antibiotic are required. Antibiotic therapy may be effective in early infection confined to the soft tissues, but formation of a biofilm on the implants significantly impairs the efficacy of antibiotics.

- The success rate of surgical debridement without revision rapidly declines with an increasing duration between the onset of infection and surgery. If the infection has been present for over 48 hours then the success rate is very low. The problem in predicting success is determining the duration of infection.

Dislocation

Reported dislocation rates vary from less than 1% in reports from specialist centres to up to 5% in data from joint registries. Most dislocations happen in the first year and there is a slow and steady increase in this percentage with time. In a study of more than 6,000 patients over 15 years, Berry et al reported risks of dislocation of 1% at 1 month, 1.9% at 1 year and 7% at 25 years. The risk of dislocation is higher in women and in those with inflammatory arthritis, non-union of the femoral neck or avascular necrosis.

Note

Berry DJ, von Knoch M, Schleck CD, Harmsen WS. The cumulative long-term risk of dislocation after primary Charnley total hip arthroplasty. *J Bone Joint Surg Am* 2004; 86: 9-14. **This study looked at a series of more than 6,000 primary Charnley total hip replacements (all 22mm cemented) performed over 15 years. The risk of dislocation was 1% risk at 1 month and 1.9% at 1 year. The risk rose approximately 1% every 5 years and to reach 7% at 25 years. The risk was higher in women and those with inflammatory arthritis, non-union of the femoral neck or avascular necrosis.**

Note

Fender D, Harper WM, Gregg PJ. Outcome of Charnley total hip replacement across a single health region in England: the results at five years from a regional hip register. *J Bone Joint Surg Br* 1999; 81: 577-81. **From 1,198 hips, the authors reported rates of 2.3% for aseptic loosening, 1.4% for deep infection, 5.0% for dislocation and 3.2% for revision. The failure rate at 5 years was 9%.**

A third of patients who have a dislocation do not have a second episode; another third may have two or three episodes and then stabilise without surgical intervention; and the remaining third may continue to have recurrent dislocations and require intervention.

The presence of an identifiable cause of dislocation improves the success rate of corrective surgery. Exchange of the liner in modular cementless acetabular components (leaving the metal shell *in situ*) is an option, but this has been shown to have a higher dislocation rate.

> ## Note
>
> Blom AW, Astle L, Loveridge J, Learmonth ID. Revision of an acetabular liner has a high risk of dislocation. *J Bone Joint Surg Br* 2005; 87: 1636-8. Of 38 liners revised for wear, 11 (28.9%) of the exchanged liners dislocated within 4.5 years of follow-up.

Venous thromboembolism

The incidence of venous thromboembolism in those undergoing hip replacement has been reported to range from 8% to 70%. The risk of non-fatal pulmonary embolism is 1% and risk of fatal pulmonary embolism is less than 1%.

A diagnosis of pulmonary embolism should be suspected in patients with shortness of breath, chest pain or mental status changes. Oxygen saturation may fall and analysis of blood gas will show respiratory failure. Investigations for diagnosis include chest X-ray and a computed tomography (CT) scan with pulmonary angiography.

Prophylaxis is with warfarin, low-molecular-weight heparin or fondaparinux. The newer oral anticoagulants rivaroxaban and dabigatran have been approved by the National Institute for Health and Clinical Excellence (NICE) for postoperative anticoagulation and can be continued following discharge from hospital. Mechanical prophylaxis is provided in addition to chemical prophylaxis by foot or calf pumps. Chemoprophylaxis should continue for 5 weeks following hip replacement surgery.

Treatment is with warfarin for 3 months (in patients with venous thromboembolism) or 6 months (in patients with proven pulmonary embolism).

Heterotopic ossification

Patients with ankylosing spondylitis, post-traumatic arthritis, extensive soft tissue dissection, hypertrophic arthritis (extensive osteophytes) and hip arthrodesis for conversion to THR are at higher risk for heterotopic ossification (HO). Clinically, HO rarely restricts motion.

HO may be classified by the Brooker classification (Table 1.4).

Table 1.4. Classification of heterotopic ossification: Brooker staging.	
Grade	**Description**
I	Islands of bone within soft tissues
II	Bone spurs on femur or pelvis with >1cm gap between opposing surfaces
III	Bone spurs on femur or pelvis with <1cm gap between opposing surfaces
IV	Apparent bony ankylosis

A limitation of the Brooker classification is that it is a two-dimensional description of a three-dimensional event. The AP view of the pelvis may show spurs close to each other, but those spurs may be in different coronal planes. However, the system is easy to use and gives some idea of the amount of heterotopic bone.

HO can be prevented with radiation or indomethacin. Radiation therapy is with a single dose of 750 rads postoperatively before discharge. Cementless prostheses must be shielded to avoid interference with bone ingrowth. Indomethacin 75mg once daily for 6 weeks is another option. Indomethacin is not advisable for uncemented prostheses, however, as it may interfere with bone ingrowth.

Leg length discrepancy

Leg length discrepancy is minimised by careful preoperative planning. This should take into account the preoperative leg length difference, the planned position of the acetabular component, the planned level of the neck cut, the size and position of the femoral component and the neck length and offset.

The operating surgeon should have a fairly accurate estimate of the implant type and size required before starting surgery.

A very small percentage of patients may require revision for leg length inequality.

Fracture of femur

Fractures are more common with cementless stems, which fit snugly into the femur, and virtually unknown with cemented stems.

Fractures at the proximal end of the femur that impact the prosthesis can be managed with cerclage wiring and restricted postoperative weight bearing.

Unstable fractures near the tip of the femoral component should be managed with a long stem implant that bypasses the fracture site by more than two cortical diameters. Additional cerclage or cable plate may be needed for stability.

Acetabular fractures may occur in cementless components that are press fit.

Trochanteric non-union

Trochanteric non-union is a complication of trochanteric osteotomy. Most primary surgery is performed without trochanteric osteotomy, but revision surgery often necessitates a transtrochanteric approach.

The extended trochanteric osteotomy has a better healing potential and provides excellent access, with a very low risk of non-union.

Failure of components

Earlier stems failed due to poor metallurgy, high offset and a thin cross-section, but breakage of the femoral component is now uncommon. Failure is initiated on the anterolateral aspect, which is the tension side in the stem.

Factors contributing to stem fracture are as follows:

- A higher body weight exerts more stress on the stem and can lead to failure of thin stems.
- Thin stems have lower ultimate strength.
- A long neck or higher offset increases the lever arm on the stem.
- Varus positioning of the stem in effect increases the lever arm due to an increased distance between the centre of the femoral head and the axis of the femur.
- Type IV failure, where the stem is firmly fixed distally but is loose proximally, leads to toggle of the stem and early failure.
- Poor metallurgy means weaker stems.

Currently, most manufacturers advise a maximum patient weight that should not be exceeded for a particular stem size. This is a consideration when using very small stem sizes.

Stem failure can be diagnosed before actual fracture by comparing the most recent radiographic films with the postoperative films. Any evidence of bending of the stem is a sign of impending failure and an indication for revision. Fracture of the stem can be a subtle finding on postoperative radiographs and is sometimes missed.

Limp

A Trendelenburg gait can be due to abductor damage, damage to the superior gluteal nerve resulting in abductor palsy or trochanteric non-union. In addition, a short or a long leg following surgery can result in a limp. An antalgic gait can be due to a painful arthroplasty because of infection or loosening.

Nerve or vessel injury

The nerve at risk is the sciatic nerve in the posterior approach. The risk is higher in patients with developmental dysplasia of the hip or in those undergoing revision surgery.

> **Note**
>
> Schmalzried TP, Noordin S, Amstutz HC. Update on nerve palsy associated with total hip replacement. *Clin Orthop Relat Res* 1997; 344: 188-206. **The authors found the femoral nerve to have more predictable recovery than the sciatic nerve. They reported that 15% of patients with nerve palsy have a poor outcome, while 44% have a complete or near complete recovery.**

Nerve injury may be caused by the following:

- Direct nerve injury.
- Pressure from retractors.
- Tension due to excess lengthening.
- Ischaemia.
- Close proximity to cement.
- Entrapment of the nerve in trochanteric wiring.
- Dislocation of the femoral component.

Screws in the acetabulum can also damage the nerve and vessels and a safe quadrant has been described by Wasielewski and Rubash (see Figure 1.4, page 7).

The maximum lengthening permitted intraoperatively in developmental dysplasia of the hip is approximately 2.5cm. Beyond this limit, the nerve is at risk for stretch injury.

Loosening and wear

A number of factors determine the loosening of an implant over time. In cementless implants, stability is determined by the initial stability achieved at insertion, degree of porous coating, extent of bone ingrowth/ongrowth, response to wear debris and effective joint space. Cemented femoral implants have two potential interfaces for loosening: the metal-cement interface and the cement-bone interface.

Loosening is diagnosed on radiographs by criteria described by Harris. Definite loosening is defined as follows:

- Progressive complete radiolucency at the cement-bone or implant-bone interface.
- Migration of the component.
- Fracture of the component.
- Fracture of the cement mantle.
- Debonding.

Debonding, which is lucency at the metal-cement interface commonly seen in zone 1, is predictive of loosening in cemented stems. Debonding is not a sign of loosening in polished taper stems such as the Exeter as these stems are designed to subside in the cement mantle. A flanged Charnley is not intended to subside and debonding indicates loosening.

Probable loosening is defined as complete radiolucency at the cement-bone interface, while possible loosening is the presence of radiolucency of more than 50% but not complete at the cement-bone interface.

A pedestal may be present just distal to the tip of an unstable subsiding stem. This is a bridge of bone that forms to provide some stability to the stem.

Indicators of a stable implant are as follows:

- Absence of radiolucency at the bone interface.
- Proximal stress shielding, indicating that the stem is well fixed distally.
- Presence of 'spot weld' – areas of dense bone extending from the ingrowth surface of the implant to the endosteal surface of cortex of bone.

The acetabular zones have been described by DeLee and Charnley (Figure 1.8). Gruen's zones of demarcation are used to define the extent of loosening of femoral components (Figure 1.9)

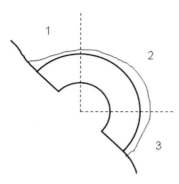

Figure 1.8. Zones of loosening in the acetabulum. The vertical and horizontal lines are drawn through the centre of the acetabulum.

Note

Gruen TA, McNeice GM, Amstutz HC. 'Modes of failure' of cemented stem-type femoral components: a radiographic analysis of loosening. *Clin Orthop Relat Res* 1979; 141: 17-27.

Note

DeLee J, Charnley J. Radiological demarcation of cemented sockets in total hip replacement. *Clin Orthop Relat Res* 1976; 121: 20-32.

Mechanisms of wear
- Adhesive wear – the articulating surfaces bind to each other under load and movement results in material being pulled off the weaker surface.
- Abrasive wear – asperities from the harder surface physically cut through the weaker surface removing material from the weaker surface.
- Fatigue wear – the repeat stresses exceed the failure strength of the material.

Modes of wear
The modes of wear can be divided into four types:

- Type I – wear due to motion between two bearing surfaces that are intended to articulate against each other (e.g., the femoral head against the polyethylene). This is integral to a functioning joint.
- Type II – wear due to motion between a bearing surface and a non-bearing surface (e.g., the femoral head against the acetabular metal shell or the femoral condyle against the tibial base plate). This wear is not intended.
- Type III – wear between primary bearing surfaces with interposed particles. This is also known as third-body wear. The particles may be cement, polyethylene, metal or HA.
- Type IV – wear due to motion between two non-bearing surfaces (e.g., the femoral neck against the acetabular metal shell, motion

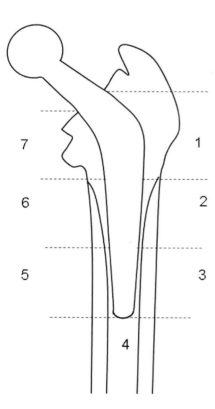

Figure 1.9. Femoral zones, as described by Gruen.

between the cement and metal, motion between the cement mantle and bone). Neither of the surfaces is intended to articulate. Motion between the polyethylene insert and the metal shell in acetabular components (backside wear) is also Type IV wear.

Type I wear will always happen in a functioning joint. The other types may be present to varying extents and may progress with time.

Quantification of wear

Wear can be measured as follows:

- Linear penetration of the femoral head measured on radiographs.
- Volumetric wear.

The AP radiograph only measures wear in the coronal plane (Figure 1.10) and completely ignores wear in planes different from that of the radiograph. Combining the AP and the lateral view of wear analysis improves this assessment as it considers wear in two planes. However, lateral radiographs are not always performed and may not be adequate for wear analysis.

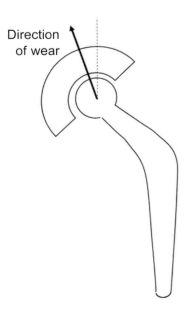

Figure 1.10. Direction of wear in hip replacement in the coronal plane.

Penetration is a better term to describe the measurements, as processes apart from wear may contribute to the distance measured – for instance, creep in the polyethylene and 'bedding in' of the insert in the metal shell.

Volumetric wear is the product of linear penetration and the diameter of the head. For the same distance worn, volumetric wear is greater for larger heads.

Low-friction replacement

When developing the hip replacement procedure, Sir John Charnley used a 22.225mm head to reduce friction torque at the metal-polyethylene interface. A smaller head size was supposed to reduce torque and an added advantage was the use of a thicker polyethylene, which distributed the torque over a large surface area.

Over the years, the wear particles have assumed a greater significance than the torque generated. Charnley's concept still holds good because a smaller head generates a lower volume of wear particles. However, the use of surfaces with low wear characteristics – such as highly cross-linked polyethylene or ceramic – may allow the use of larger-diameter heads.

> **Note**
>
> Wroblewski BM, Siney PD, Fleming PA. Wear of the cup in Charnley LFA in the young patient. *J Bone Joint Surg Br* 2004; 86: 498-503. The authors reported an association of high wear with male sex, osteoarthritis and a valgus stem position. The varus stem position was correlated with low wear.

Osteolysis

Osteolysis is the resorption of bone around a prosthesis. It is initiated as a chemico-immunological reaction to particulate material.

In 1977, Willert and Semlitsch demonstrated the presence of macrophages in response to wear debris. Goldring described the synovial-like character of the interfacial membrane and demonstrated the presence of prostaglandin E_2 (PGE_2) and collagenase secretion from the cells. Observations of osteolysis in cemented implants led to a general belief that osteolysis was related to the acrylic cement and the term 'cement disease' was introduced.

A functioning hip joint generates wear particles. The most biologically active particles are sized between 0.5 and 1.0μm. Polyethylene particles are the predominant type among the various types of particles found in the wear debris and account for 70-90% of the debris volume. Other particles may be of cobalt chrome, polymethylmethacrylate, bone, titanium alloys, ceramics or stainless steel.

Larger particles (>50μm) induce fibrous encapsulation, while smaller particles (<7μm) are phagocytosed and lead to macrophage activation and release of a variety of cytokines such as interleukins, TNF-α, PGE_2 and metalloproteases. Small irregular particles of polymethylmethacrylate have greater reactivity than spherical particles of the same size.

The effective joint space is the entire region within a prosthetic joint that is exposed to the joint fluid and consequently the wear particles. A patch-porous-coated stem allows particles to pass distally in the intramedullary canal leading to osteolytic bone resorption. A prosthesis with a good fit proximally, and which is cemented or circumferentially porous coated, will resist this particle flow.

Clinical presentation

Osteolysis is a silent process and, in itself, does not cause any symptoms. The symptoms may arise from the sequelae of osteolysis – which can be loosening or pathologic fracture through an area of resorbed bone. Osteolysis is diagnosed by serial radiographic follow-up or CT scans.

Radiological assessment

The extent of osteolysis is frequently underestimated on plain radiographs; a CT scan is more accurate. The site of osteolysis around the hip joint depends on the access of particles to the area and is determined, in turn, by the firmness of fixation of the implant.

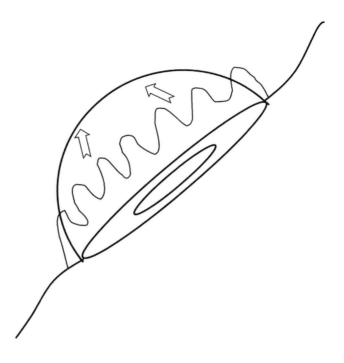

Figure 1.11. Pattern of growth of the histiocytic membrane in cemented cups.

In cemented cups, failure is through formation of a histiocytic membrane from the rim to the dome of the cup (Figure 1.11). This is the cement-bone interface. The subchondral bone reforms and acts as a barrier to ingress of wear particles, resulting in a linear pattern of bone resorption.

In contrast, cementless cups show localised areas of osteolysis that represent areas of particle collection. 'Spot welds' (areas of strong fixation of the cementless component to the bone by dense trabeculae) act as barriers to particle access – hence the localised nature of the osteolysis.

In cemented stems, the patch-porous coating used in earlier implants allowed particle access (Figure 1.3, page 6). All modern implants now have a circumferential coating in the proximal part of the stem to achieve firm fixation.

Causes of bone loss/radiolucency around femoral implants

Osteolysis is only one cause of bone loss or radiolucency around femoral implants. Other causes are as follows:

- Non-filling of cement. This describes gaps between the cement and the bone that did not fill with cement at the time of implantation. These areas will be apparent on the initial postoperative radiographs.
- Adaptive remodelling with formation of a neocortex. A new layer of bone forms adjacent to the cement surface, providing stability. Lucency will be visible on the radiographs between the cement and the bone. This will remain the same on follow-up because the stem is stable.
- Stress shielding. This is commonly seen in distally coated femoral stems. Stress shielding occurs when there is distal stability and the proximal femur is bypassed with regards to weight-bearing forces. This results in diffuse loss of bone in the proximal femur with dense cortical bone distally, which is where the load is being transferred between the prosthesis and bone. A stiff distally fixed stem will lead to greater stress shielding.

Management of osteolysis

Guidelines for management of acetabular osteolysis are shown in Table 1.5.

> **Note**
>
> Maloney WJ, Paprosky W, Engh CA, Rubash H. Surgical treatment of pelvic osteolysis. *Clin Orthop Relat Res* 2001; 393: 78-84.

Failure of hip replacement

In survivorship analysis, different series use different endpoints for defining failure. In order to enable comparability, the endpoint – revision surgery, radiographic loosening or clinically painful replacement – should be clarified.

The modes of femoral stem failure have been described by Gruen and are shown in Figure 1.12.

Table 1.5. Guidelines for management of acetabular osteolysis (based on recommendations from Maloney et al).

Type	Clinical situation	Recommended solution
I	Metal shell is stable, in a good position and has a good track record. The locking mechanism is intact A replacement liner is available	Replace liner, graft lytic lesion
II	The shell is stable, but a liner is not available or the above criteria are not met	1. Revise shell Or: 2. A polyethylene liner can be cemented into the stable metal shell. The outer surface of the liner is scored to improve the cement bond
III	Metal shell is loose	Revise metal shell

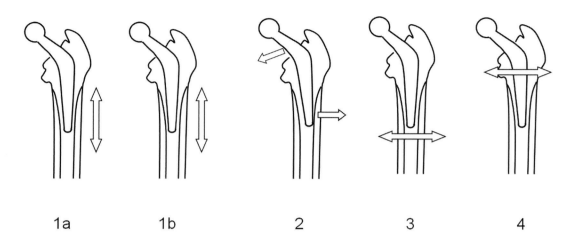

1a   1b   2   3   4

Figure 1.12. Modes of failure of cemented femoral components, as described by Gruen: (1) Pistoning – axial movement of the stem within the cement mantle (1a) or the cement mantle within the bone (1b); (2) medial stem pivot – leads to medial or varus tilt of the stem; (3) calcar pivot; and (4) cantilever bending – the stem is well fixed distally and loose proximally, predisposing to stem fracture.

Antibiotic cover for dental procedures after hip replacement

Prophylaxis is not routinely required for the majority of dental procedures following hip replacement. If there is significant risk of bacteraemia, antibiotics (cephalexin or clindamycin) given 1 hour before and 2 hours after the procedure can be considered. Immunocompromised patients are at higher risk and should be considered for prophylaxis.

The disadvantage of routine prophylaxis is the development of drug resistance.

Resurfacing hip replacement

The use of large-diameter metal-on-metal articulation has been attempted at various stages of the development of total hip replacement. Initial attempts in the 1950s were, however, overshadowed by the development of the successful Charnley hip replacement.

In 1988 there was a resurgence of interest in hip resurfacing with the development of cobalt chrome

alloy bearings. Derek McMinn introduced resurfacing in 1991. The initial design was a smooth press fit, but this had a high incidence of aseptic loosening. Cemented components were introduced and the acetabular component again had a high loosening rate. In 1994, an HA-coated acetabulum and cemented femoral component was developed. From 1994 to 1996, McMinn hip resurfacing used a smooth HA cup and cemented femur. In 1996, the Birmingham hip resurfacing system was introduced, using a porous HA-coated cup and cemented femur.

Most of current resurfacings have a high carbon-content cobalt chrome alloy, with a cemented femoral component and cementless acetabular component. The components of a wrought cobalt chrome alloy are harder and show better wear resistance. Cast cobalt chrome alloy requires postcasting heat treatment.

Double heat treatment of the components leads to a high rate of wear and failure. The heat treatment depletes the carbon, and the reduced percentage of carbide leads to poor wear resistance.

Note

Daniel J, Ziaee H, Kamali A, *et al.* Ten-year results of a double-heat-treated metal-on-metal hip resurfacing. *J Bone Joint Surg Br* 2010; 92: 20-7. **This study reported on 184 hips resurfaced in 1996 in Birmingham. The revision rate was 16% at 7 years, while 24% had signs of failure on X-ray. The double heat treatment resulted in a high rate of wear.**

Advantages

Hip resurfacing has the following advantages:

- Hip resurfacing is a conservative procedure with limited removal of bone, at least on the femoral side. This is debatable for the acetabulum.
- It avoids stress shielding of the proximal femur.
- It allows a greater range of motion (ROM) and a lower risk of dislocation compared to conventional hip replacement.
- It allows a higher level of activity due to hard bearing and low wear.

Note

Vendittoli PA, Lavigne M, Girard J, Roy AG. A randomised study comparing resection of acetabular bone at resurfacing and total hip replacement. *J Bone Joint Surg Br* 2006; 88: 997-1002.

Disadvantages

The disadvantages are as follows:

- Lack of long-term results with current designs.
- Learning curve for surgeons.
- The prevalence of femoral neck fractures ranges from 1% to 2%, and can be higher with inexperienced surgeons.
- Avascular necrosis of the femoral head may lead to loosening of the prosthesis or periprosthetic fracture.
- Resurfacing is associated with a higher rate of early revisions at 1.5% compared to 0.3% for conventional hip replacement within the first year in the National Joint Registry.
- Femoral neck thinning is seen following hip resurfacing. This may be due to altered stress distribution in the femoral neck, possibly related to the presence of the femoral stem.
- The presence of metal ions in the bloodstream, bone marrow and lymphatic tissue is of concern and the long-term effects are unknown.
- Fixation of an acetabular component may not be as secure as the usual titanium cementless THR components, as the cobalt chrome component in hip resurfacing is stiffer and has different mechanical properties. In addition, screws cannot be placed in hip resurfacing acetabular components to augment fixation.

Indications for hip resurfacing

Ideally, hip resurfacing is indicated in young patients with osteoarthritis, and most surgeons would prefer relatively normal bone geometry. Patients with avascular necrosis, secondary arthritis from developmental dysplasia of the hip, Perthes disease and slipped upper femoral epiphysis are also candidates for hip resurfacing. The range of indications is constantly being expanded.

Contraindications for hip resurfacing

Metal hypersensitivity, impaired renal function and proximal femoral osteoporosis in elderly patients are contraindications for hip resurfacing. Large cysts in the proximal femur, severe acetabular bone loss, grossly abnormal proximal femoral geometry and inflammatory arthritis are also relative contraindications for the procedure.

Hip resurfacing is contraindicated in women of childbearing age, and the use of a head size less than 46mm is also not advised.

Note

De Smet K, Campbell PA, Gill HS. Metal-on-metal hip resurfacing: a consensus from the Advanced Hip Resurfacing Course, Ghent, June 2009. *J Bone Joint Surg Br* 2010; 92: 335-6.

Causes of failure of hip resurfacing

Component size

The size of the components of resurfacing may have an influence on the survival of the prosthesis, as suggested by data from the Australian National Joint Register. The report suggested that femoral components of less than 44mm correlated with a five-fold risk of revision. Based on these data, there was no correlation of gender and early failure.

> **Note**
>
> Shimmin AJ, Walter WL, Esposito C. The influence of the size of the component on the outcome of resurfacing arthroplasty of the hip: a review of the literature. *J Bone Joint Surg Br* 2010; 92: 469-76. **This study suggested that the cause of failure may be multifactorial.**

Component design

The arc of the acetabular component is less than a hemisphere in resurfacing arthroplasty and may range from 145° to 170°. A smaller arc increases the risk of edge loading, especially if the component is placed in a more open position.

Component orientation

Steeply placed acetabular components are at risk of edge loading and this correlates with a higher rate of wear and early failure. Similarly, varus positioning of the femoral component can cause high load and fracture of the femoral neck.

> **Note**
>
> De Haan R, Pattyn C, Gill HS. Correlation between inclination of the acetabular component and metal ion levels in metal-on-metal hip resurfacing replacement. *J Bone Joint Surg Br* 2008; 90: 1291-7. **An arc of cover of over 10mm has a lower wear rate than components that cover the femoral head by less than 10mm.**

Stress shielding in the proximal part of the femoral neck

The presence of a stiff cobalt chrome femoral stem causes stress shielding of the proximal neck, which may predispose to late neck fracture. In a smaller sized femoral component, the degree of stress shielding may be greater.

Metal ions

Metal ions released as a result of movement can lead to a local tissue reaction known as ALVAL (aseptic, lymphocytic, vasculitis-associated lesions). This causes local tissue destruction.

Ion levels in blood

Resurfacing hip components are made of cobalt chrome alloy and there is an increase in the ion levels in the body following resurfacing.

> **Note**
>
> Hart AJ, Hester T, Sinclair K, *et al.* The association between metal ions from hip resurfacing and reduced T-cell counts. *J Bone Joint Surg Br* 2006; 88: 449-54. **In this study, blood samples were analysed from 68 patients, 34 with metal-on-metal and 34 with standard metal-on-polyethylene THRs. Cobalt and chromium levels were raised in metal-on-metal group. The level of CD8+ cells was lower in the metal-on-metal group.**

Formation of inflammatory pseudotumours has been reported. Out of 1,419 hip resurfacings, 1.8% had a revision for pseudotumours, with pseudotumours being more common in women. The study authors recommended that resurfacing be carried out with caution in women.

> **Note**
>
> Glyn-Jones S, Pandit H, Kwon YM, *et al.* Risk factors for inflammatory pseudotumour formation following hip resurfacing. *J Bone Joint Surg Br* 2009; 91: 1566-74.

Causes of failure of hip resurfacing

Component size

The size of the components of resurfacing may have an influence on the survival of the prosthesis, as suggested by data from the Australian National Joint Register. The report suggested that femoral components of less than 44mm correlated with a five-fold risk of revision. Based on these data, there was no correlation of gender and early failure.

> **Note**
>
> Shimmin AJ, Walter WL, Esposito C. The influence of the size of the component on the outcome of resurfacing arthroplasty of the hip: a review of the literature. *J Bone Joint Surg Br* 2010; 92: 469-76. **This study suggested that the cause of failure may be multifactorial.**

Component design

The arc of the acetabular component is less than a hemisphere in resurfacing arthroplasty and may range from 145° to 170°. A smaller arc increases the risk of edge loading, especially if the component is placed in a more open position.

Component orientation

Steeply placed acetabular components are at risk of edge loading and this correlates with a higher rate of wear and early failure. Similarly, varus positioning of the femoral component can cause high load and fracture of the femoral neck.

> **Note**
>
> De Haan R, Pattyn C, Gill HS. Correlation between inclination of the acetabular component and metal ion levels in metal-on-metal hip resurfacing replacement. *J Bone Joint Surg Br* 2008; 90: 1291-7. **An arc of cover of over 10mm has a lower wear rate than components that cover the femoral head by less than 10mm.**

Stress shielding in the proximal part of the femoral neck

The presence of a stiff cobalt chrome femoral stem causes stress shielding of the proximal neck, which may predispose to late neck fracture. In a smaller sized femoral component, the degree of stress shielding may be greater.

Metal ions

Metal ions released as a result of movement can lead to a local tissue reaction known as ALVAL (aseptic, lymphocytic, vasculitis-associated lesions). This causes local tissue destruction.

Ion levels in blood

Resurfacing hip components are made of cobalt chrome alloy and there is an increase in the ion levels in the body following resurfacing.

> **Note**
>
> Hart AJ, Hester T, Sinclair K, *et al.* The association between metal ions from hip resurfacing and reduced T-cell counts. *J Bone Joint Surg Br* 2006; 88: 449-54. **In this study, blood samples were analysed from 68 patients, 34 with metal-on-metal and 34 with standard metal-on-polyethylene THRs. Cobalt and chromium levels were raised in metal-on-metal group. The level of CD8+ cells was lower in the metal-on-metal group.**

Formation of inflammatory pseudotumours has been reported. Out of 1,419 hip resurfacings, 1.8% had a revision for pseudotumours, with pseudotumours being more common in women. The study authors recommended that resurfacing be carried out with caution in women.

> **Note**
>
> Glyn-Jones S, Pandit H, Kwon YM, *et al.* Risk factors for inflammatory pseudotumour formation following hip resurfacing. *J Bone Joint Surg Br* 2009; 91: 1566-74.

Note

Daniel J, Ziaee H, Kamali A, *et al.* Ten-year results of a double-heat-treated metal-on-metal hip resurfacing. *J Bone Joint Surg Br* 2010; 92: 20-7. **This study reported on 184 hips resurfaced in 1996 in Birmingham. The revision rate was 16% at 7 years, while 24% had signs of failure on X-ray. The double heat treatment resulted in a high rate of wear.**

Advantages

Hip resurfacing has the following advantages:

- Hip resurfacing is a conservative procedure with limited removal of bone, at least on the femoral side. This is debatable for the acetabulum.
- It avoids stress shielding of the proximal femur.
- It allows a greater range of motion (ROM) and a lower risk of dislocation compared to conventional hip replacement.
- It allows a higher level of activity due to hard bearing and low wear.

Note

Vendittoli PA, Lavigne M, Girard J, Roy AG. A randomised study comparing resection of acetabular bone at resurfacing and total hip replacement. *J Bone Joint Surg Br* 2006; 88: 997-1002.

Disadvantages

The disadvantages are as follows:

- Lack of long-term results with current designs.
- Learning curve for surgeons.
- The prevalence of femoral neck fractures ranges from 1% to 2%, and can be higher with inexperienced surgeons.
- Avascular necrosis of the femoral head may lead to loosening of the prosthesis or periprosthetic fracture.
- Resurfacing is associated with a higher rate of early revisions at 1.5% compared to 0.3% for conventional hip replacement within the first year in the National Joint Registry.
- Femoral neck thinning is seen following hip resurfacing. This may be due to altered stress distribution in the femoral neck, possibly related to the presence of the femoral stem.
- The presence of metal ions in the bloodstream, bone marrow and lymphatic tissue is of concern and the long-term effects are unknown.
- Fixation of an acetabular component may not be as secure as the usual titanium cementless THR components, as the cobalt chrome component in hip resurfacing is stiffer and has different mechanical properties. In addition, screws cannot be placed in hip resurfacing acetabular components to augment fixation.

Indications for hip resurfacing

Ideally, hip resurfacing is indicated in young patients with osteoarthritis, and most surgeons would prefer relatively normal bone geometry. Patients with avascular necrosis, secondary arthritis from developmental dysplasia of the hip, Perthes disease and slipped upper femoral epiphysis are also candidates for hip resurfacing. The range of indications is constantly being expanded.

Contraindications for hip resurfacing

Metal hypersensitivity, impaired renal function and proximal femoral osteoporosis in elderly patients are contraindications for hip resurfacing. Large cysts in the proximal femur, severe acetabular bone loss, grossly abnormal proximal femoral geometry and inflammatory arthritis are also relative contraindications for the procedure.

Hip resurfacing is contraindicated in women of childbearing age, and the use of a head size less than 46mm is also not advised.

Note

De Smet K, Campbell PA, Gill HS. Metal-on-metal hip resurfacing: a consensus from the Advanced Hip Resurfacing Course, Ghent, June 2009. *J Bone Joint Surg Br* 2010; 92: 335-6.

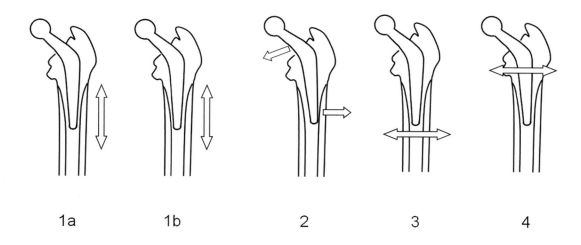

Figure 1.12. Modes of failure of cemented femoral components, as described by Gruen: (1) Pistoning – axial movement of the stem within the cement mantle (1a) or the cement mantle within the bone (1b); (2) medial stem pivot – leads to medial or varus tilt of the stem; (3) calcar pivot; and (4) cantilever bending – the stem is well fixed distally and loose proximally, predisposing to stem fracture.

Antibiotic cover for dental procedures after hip replacement

Prophylaxis is not routinely required for the majority of dental procedures following hip replacement. If there is significant risk of bacteraemia, antibiotics (cephalexin or clindamycin) given 1 hour before and 2 hours after the procedure can be considered. Immunocompromised patients are at higher risk and should be considered for prophylaxis.

The disadvantage of routine prophylaxis is the development of drug resistance.

Resurfacing hip replacement

The use of large-diameter metal-on-metal articulation has been attempted at various stages of the development of total hip replacement. Initial attempts in the 1950s were, however, overshadowed by the development of the successful Charnley hip replacement.

In 1988 there was a resurgence of interest in hip resurfacing with the development of cobalt chrome alloy bearings. Derek McMinn introduced resurfacing in 1991. The initial design was a smooth press fit, but this had a high incidence of aseptic loosening. Cemented components were introduced and the acetabular component again had a high loosening rate. In 1994, an HA-coated acetabulum and cemented femoral component was developed. From 1994 to 1996, McMinn hip resurfacing used a smooth HA cup and cemented femur. In 1996, the Birmingham hip resurfacing system was introduced, using a porous HA-coated cup and cemented femur.

Most of current resurfacings have a high carbon-content cobalt chrome alloy, with a cemented femoral component and cementless acetabular component. The components of a wrought cobalt chrome alloy are harder and show better wear resistance. Cast cobalt chrome alloy requires postcasting heat treatment.

Double heat treatment of the components leads to a high rate of wear and failure. The heat treatment depletes the carbon, and the reduced percentage of carbide leads to poor wear resistance.

Causes of bone loss/radiolucency around femoral implants

Osteolysis is only one cause of bone loss or radiolucency around femoral implants. Other causes are as follows:

- Non-filling of cement. This describes gaps between the cement and the bone that did not fill with cement at the time of implantation. These areas will be apparent on the initial postoperative radiographs.
- Adaptive remodelling with formation of a neocortex. A new layer of bone forms adjacent to the cement surface, providing stability. Lucency will be visible on the radiographs between the cement and the bone. This will remain the same on follow-up because the stem is stable.
- Stress shielding. This is commonly seen in distally coated femoral stems. Stress shielding occurs when there is distal stability and the proximal femur is bypassed with regards to weight-bearing forces. This results in diffuse loss of bone in the proximal femur with dense cortical bone distally, which is where the load is being transferred between the prosthesis and bone. A stiff distally fixed stem will lead to greater stress shielding.

Management of osteolysis

Guidelines for management of acetabular osteolysis are shown in Table 1.5.

> **Note**
>
> Maloney WJ, Paprosky W, Engh CA, Rubash H. Surgical treatment of pelvic osteolysis. *Clin Orthop Relat Res* 2001; 393: 78-84.

Failure of hip replacement

In survivorship analysis, different series use different endpoints for defining failure. In order to enable comparability, the endpoint – revision surgery, radiographic loosening or clinically painful replacement – should be clarified.

The modes of femoral stem failure have been described by Gruen and are shown in Figure 1.12.

Table 1.5. Guidelines for management of acetabular osteolysis (based on recommendations from Maloney et al).

Type	Clinical situation	Recommended solution
I	Metal shell is stable, in a good position and has a good track record. The locking mechanism is intact A replacement liner is available	Replace liner, graft lytic lesion
II	The shell is stable, but a liner is not available or the above criteria are not met	1. Revise shell Or: 2. A polyethylene liner can be cemented into the stable metal shell. The outer surface of the liner is scored to improve the cement bond
III	Metal shell is loose	Revise metal shell

- Blood parameters – an elevated ESR and CRP level are indicative of infection. The white cell count in peripheral blood may be normal despite an infected joint.
- Intraoperative frozen section – the presence of more than 10 white cells per high-power field is indicative of acute inflammation.
- Intraoperative culture and histology – multiple culture specimens should be obtained and a histology specimen sent to check for any rare forms of infection such as fungal infection or tuberculosis.

Preparing for revision surgery

The following steps should guide preparations for revision surgery:

- Establish a diagnosis and cause of failure.
- Obtain all previous operation notes and implant details.
- Consider all possibilities and ensure implants are available to deal with such situations. Special instruments for removing cement, power burrs, a range of osteotomes, implant extractors, cerclage cables and wires, bone graft (cancellous and allograft) and cell saver should be available.
- Template. Choose the implant and determine the size of components, level of neck resection, neck length, head size, additional procedures such as trochanteric osteotomy and impaction grafting. Templating is commonly performed with plain radiographs using implant templates and matching the appropriate size implant to the bone geometry. Software is available to template on CT scans using preoperative standardised CT scan images.

Bone defects

Classification of femoral bone defects

Femoral bone defects can be grouped according to the American Academy of Orthopedic Surgeons (AAOS) classification (Table 1.8).

Table 1.8. The American Academy of Orthopedic Surgeons' classification of femoral bone defects.

Femoral bone defects	
Segmental	Proximal: • Partial or complete • Anterior/medial/posterior Intercalary Greater trochanteric
Cavitary	Cancellous Cortical Ectasia
Combined segmental and cavitary	-
Malalignment	Rotational/angular
Femoral stenosis	-
Femoral discontinuity	-

Table 1.9. The American Academy of Orthopedic Surgeons' classification of acetabular bone defects.

Acetabular bone defects	
Segmental	Peripheral: anterior/superior/posterior Central
Cavitary	Peripheral: anterior/superior/posterior Central
Combined	-
Pelvic discontinuity	-
Arthrodesis	-

Management of femoral bone defects

Femoral bone defects may be managed as follows:

- An intact cortical tube can be used for implant fixation.
- Extensive proximal bone loss proximally requires impaction grafting, calcar replacement stems or a distally fixed cementless stem.
- Bone loss extending beyond the isthmus of the femur makes it difficult to achieve fixation distally due to a divergent femoral canal and may require proximal femoral replacement or an allograft.
- Femoral malalignment may require a femoral osteotomy to achieve a straight canal.

Classification of acetabular bone defects

The AAOS classification of acetabular defects is shown in Table 1.9, with the Paprosky classification of acetabular bone deficiency in Table 1.10.

Table 1.10. The Paprosky classification of acetabular bone deficiency.

Type	Description
1	Minimal lysis or component migration
2a	Superomedial migration <2cm
2b	Superolateral migration <2cm
2c	Teardrop lysis or loss of medial wall
3a	Migration >2cm, ischial lysis
3b	Type 3a plus disruption of Kohler's line, indicating profound medial loss Pelvic discontinuity

Management of acetabular bone defects

For minimal or moderate bone defects, a larger cemented or a hemispheric cementless component can be used. Cementless cups rely on adequate host bone contact. An intact posterior column is necessary, as well as anterosuperior or anteroinferior bone. The survivorship of cementless cups is 96% at 15 years in the revision scenario.

> **Note**
>
> Della Valle CJ, Berger RA, Rosenberg AG, Galante JO. Cementless acetabular reconstruction in revision total hip arthroplasty. *Clin Orthop Relat Res* 2004; 420: 96-100.

For larger defects, the options are impaction grafting, a structural allograft, placement of a larger hemispheric cementless cup or a smaller cup placed at a higher level (the high hip centre). The high hip centre leads to impingement and is largely historical. Trabecular metal augments made of tantalum are being used with good early results.

Defects of the posterior column may require a structural allograft to replace the bone loss.

Antiprotrusio cages or pelvic reconstruction by plates and grafting may be required if there is pelvic discontinuity (Figure 1.13).

> **Note**
>
> Schreurs BW, Bolder SB, Gardeniers JW, *et al*. Acetabular revision with impacted morsellised cancellous bone grafting and a cemented cup. A 15- to 20-year follow-up. *J Bone Joint Surg Br* 2004; 86: 492-7. **This study followed up 62 acetabular revisions for 16.5 years. Survival of the cup was 79% at 15 years, including two cups that were revised for infection and one cup that was revised along with femoral revision. Excluding these, survival was 84% at 15 years.**

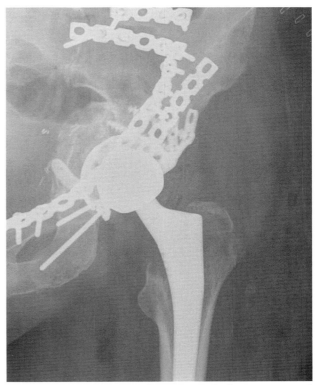

Figure 1.13. The use of an acetabular cage and impaction grafting to reconstruct a post-acetabulum fracture bone defect.

> **Note**
>
> Schreurs BW, Keurentjes JC, Gardeniers JW, *et al*. Acetabular revision with impacted morsellised cancellous bone grafting and a cemented acetabular component: a 20- to 25-year follow-up. *J Bone Joint Surg Br* 2009; 91: 1148-53. **This study reported the 20- to 25-year results from 62 acetabular revisions. Survival was 75% at 20 years, with 87% survival at 20 years for aseptic loosening.**

Trabecular metal is a tantalum augmentation device with a porosity similar to bone and can be used for large defects and pelvic discontinuity. Medium- to long-term results with trabecular metal are not available, but the material is being increasingly used in orthopaedic surgery.

Note

Lingaraj K, Teo YH, Bergman N. The management of severe acetabular bone defects in revision hip arthroplasty using modular porous metal components. *J Bone Joint Surg Br* 2009; 91: 1555-60. **From 23 reconstructions with a 41-month follow-up, the authors found 21 to be well fixed. The short-term results were good.**

Acetabular rings rely on support from the remaining periphery of the acetabulum. These are not used commonly. Acetabular cages gain support from the ilium, ischium and pubis.

Note

Gill TJ, Sledge JB, Müller ME. The Bürch-Schneider anti-protrusio cage in revision total hip arthroplasty: indications, principles and long-term results. *J Bone Joint Surg Br* 1998; 80: 946-53.

A bone graft can be impacted between the cup and the host acetabulum. The cage is secured by screws and a polyethylene cup can be cemented into the stable construct in the desired version and inclination.

Trabecular metal augments can be used instead of allograft for large defects. Different shapes of augments are available to fill defects and these can be used in patients with pelvic discontinuity to restore the posterior column using a posteroinferior and posterosuperior augment. The metal functions as an internal plate and the acetabular component can be cemented into the reconstructed acetabulum.

Note

Herrera A, Martínez AA, Cuenca J, Canales V. Management of type III and IV acetabular deficiencies with the longitudinal oblong revision cup. *J Arthroplasty* 2006; 21: 857-64.

Note

Sporer SM. The use of structural distal femoral allografts for acetabular reconstruction. Average ten-year follow-up. *J Bone Joint Surg Am* 2005; 87: 760-5.

Total knee replacement

Patient assessment

Patient assessment for total knee replacement (TKR) should include taking a full history, performing a physical examination and assessing X-rays.

History
The patient's pain should be evaluated in the following areas:

- Severity.
- Site – anterior, medial, lateral or generalised.
- Pain at rest – suggestive of tumour or infection.
- Night pain – suggestive of tumour or infection.
- Hip/groin pain – indicates hip pathology.
- Radicular pain – indicates spinal pathology.

The patient's level of functional ability should be assessed to determine if he or she can undertake activities of daily living (e.g., shopping, cleaning, personal hygiene). The ability to go up and down stairs and kneel on the ground should be noted, and an activity score can be employed to document preoperative mobility.

The patient must also be assessed in terms of prior treatments (e.g., non-steroidal anti-inflammatory drugs [NSAIDs], activity modifications, walking aids, bracing, hyaluronate/steroid injections) and previous surgeries.

Medical comorbidities such as immune compromise (diabetes, renal dysfunction, AIDS) and infective foci (chest infection, urinary tract infection, dental infections) should be taken into account.

Table 1.11. Examination for total knee replacement.

Area	Description
Gait	Antalgic Trendelenburg – to rule out hip pathology Valgus/varus thrust, indicating ligamentous laxity
Soft tissues	Previous incisions – location and time since previous surgery Psoriasis patch anteriorly on the knee
Knee joint	Tenderness, effusion Range of motion, extensor lag Ligamentous laxity Any deformities – assess if correctable or not
Neurovascular	Rule out radicular pain Check distal pulses
Other areas	Spine, ipsilateral hip, contralateral knee

Examination
Areas for examination are listed in Table 1.11.

X-rays
The standing AP view and lateral view are routine. The skyline view is taken to assess the patellofemoral joint and patellar tracking, and should also be part of the routine assessment. The AP standing view with knees flexed may help to identify any loss of joint space that is not otherwise obvious on standing radiographs.

Long leg films may be required to assess alignment if there are significant deformities at the knee or where there is a suggestion of previous fractures, malunions or deformities in the femur or tibia.

The tunnel view can be helpful in detecting osteochondritis and loose bodies in the notch.

Special situations
The following situations require special consideration:

- Obesity – may impose problems of wound healing, poor functional outcome, superficial infection and medial collateral ligament (MCL) avulsion.

Note

Dowsey MM, Liew D, Stoney JD, Choong PF. The impact of pre-operative obesity on weight change and outcome in total knee replacement: a prospective study of 529 consecutive patients. *J Bone Joint Surg Br* 2010; 92: 513-20. A total of 529 consecutive patients were weighed preoperatively and at 1 year postoperatively. At the preoperative measurement, 60% were obese or morbidly obese. At 1 year 12% of the obese patients had lost weight, but 21% had gained weight. Adverse events occurred in 14% of non-obese and 35% of morbidly obese patients.

- Diabetes – patients may be at higher risk of infection rate due to immune dysfunction. The use of antibiotic-loaded cement reduces the risk of infection.

Note

Chiu FY, Lin CF, Chen CM, Lo WH, Chaung TY. Cefuroxime-impregnated cement at primary total knee arthroplasty in diabetes mellitus. A prospective, randomised study. *J Bone Joint Surg Br* 2001; 83: 691-5. **This single-blind prospective randomised controlled trial enrolled 78 patients. No infections occurred if cefuroxime was added to the cement. There were five infections (13.5%) in the 37 patients without antibiotic cement.**

- Osteonecrosis – can be steroid-induced or idiopathic. The poor-quality bone does not adequately support the components and there is a high rate of loosening and revision. The use of cemented implants and stemmed implants, where necessary, improves outcomes.

Note

Mont MA, Rifai A, Baumgarten KM, *et al*. Total knee arthroplasty for osteonecrosis. *J Bone Joint Surg Am* 2002; 84: 599-603. **In 32 knees, with a mean patient age of 54 years and a mean follow-up of 108 months, 97% of knees had a clinically successful outcome with no progressive radiolucency.**

- Haemophilia – problems are poor bone quality and soft tissue fibrosis. Factor VIII levels should be maintained near 100% perioperatively. The presence of antibodies against Factor VIII is a contraindication to replacement.

Note

Silva M, Luck JV Jr. Long-term results of primary total knee replacement in patients with hemophilia. *J Bone Joint Surg Am* 2005; 87: 85-91. **In 38 knees of patients with haemophilia, the infection rate was 16%. Mechanical survival of the prosthesis was 'quite good'.**

- Paget's disease – medical management before surgery helps to reduce pain and operative blood loss by reducing vascularity. Restoration of alignment is important and long-term results are not adversely affected.
- Post-traumatic arthritis – may be complicated by existing scars, poor soft tissue compliance, ligamentous injury, bone loss, deformities and stiffness. Low-grade underlying infection should be ruled out. Preoperative inflammatory markers should be checked and intraoperative cultures obtained. The use of antibiotic-loaded cement is helpful.

Note

Saleh KJ, Sherman P, Katkin P, *et al*. Total knee arthroplasty after open reduction and internal fixation of fractures of the tibial plateau: a minimum five-year follow-up study. *J Bone Joint Surg Am* 2001; 83: 1144-8. **This study followed up 15 knee replacements after tibial plateau fracture fixation for 38.6 months. Three experienced deep infection, three required manipulation for stiffness and two had patellar tendon rupture.**

- Neurologic dysfunction – poor muscle power can predispose to instability requiring revision. A constrained prosthesis may be considered.
- Ipsilateral hip fusion – should be converted to hip replacement before knee replacement. Conversion to hip replacement in itself may resolve knee pain caused by malalignment. A higher rate of stiffness requiring manipulation is reported if knee replacement is performed with an ipsilateral hip fusion without first converting to hip replacement.

Note

Rittmeister M, Starker M, Zichner L. Hip and knee replacement after longstanding hip arthrodesis. *Clin Orthop Relat Res* 2000; 371: 136-45. **Eighteen patients underwent knee replacement or conversion of hip fusion to hip replacement followed by knee replacement. Patients who were converted had better functional scores and outcomes.**

- Juvenile rheumatoid arthritis – TKR is a reasonable option. Despite the relatively young age of these patients, functional demand on the knee replacement is often low and it is therefore worth considering knee replacement.

Note

Palmer DH, Mulhall KJ, Thompson CA, *et al*. Total knee arthroplasty in juvenile rheumatoid arthritis. *J Bone Joint Surg Am* 2005; 87: 1510-4. **This study followed eight patients with an average age 16.8 years and 15 knee operations for a mean of 15.5 years. Three patients underwent revision surgery and experienced improvements in pain and function. Seven patients were wheelchair-bound before surgery and six were able to walk at last follow-up.**

Contraindications to knee replacement

The following are contraindications to knee replacement:

- Active infection – local or systemic infection is a definite contraindication.
- Incompetent extensor mechanism – this will lead to instability. It is possible to reconstruct the mechanism with an allograft at the time of replacement, but this often results in residual extensor lag.
- Neuropathic joint – due to diabetes, syringomyelia, Charcot-Marie-Tooth disease, spinal dysraphism, amyloidosis or multiple sclerosis. Arthrodesis is an option and hinged replacement can be considered. Problems are malalignment, ligamentous laxity, bone loss and infection.
- Knee fusion – converting a knee fusion to replacement imposes problems of poor muscle power and ligaments, possible underlying infection if fusion is related to a previous infection and poor postoperative ROM.

Note

Bae DK, Yoon KH, Kim HS, Song SJ. Total knee arthroplasty in stiff knees after previous infection. *J Bone Joint Surg Br* 2005; 87: 333-6. **Thirty-two knee replacements in stiff or partially ankylosed hips were followed for 10 years. The postoperative range was 75° in knees with complete ankylosis and 98° in partially ankylosed knees. Complications were one superficial and one deep infection, one nerve palsy and one supracondylar fracture.**

- Peripheral vascular disease – this can lead to wound complications or ischaemia leading to amputation. Indicators are intermittent claudication, prior vascular surgery, absent distal pulses and the presence of vascular calcification on radiographs. If the ankle-brachial index is less than 0.9 then a vascular surgeon should be consulted. If less than 0.5, preoperative bypass may be necessary.

Surgical approach for total knee replacement

The midline anterior approach is the preferred incision. The vascularity of the skin is based medially and, consequently, the lateral flap is less well oxygenated. Existing transverse scars should be intersected at a right angle if possible. If there are multiple longitudinal incisions, the most lateral incision should be used.

Standard approaches are as follows:

- Medial parapatellar – the arthrotomy is along the medial third of the quadriceps tendon and curves around the patella leaving a cuff of tissue on the patella for repair. Alternatively, the arthrotomy can be vertically down over the medial aspect of the patella with subperiosteal elevation of the extensor mechanism from the patella, as described by Insall.
- Lateral parapatellar – indicated for the markedly valgus knee. A potential problem is lack of familiarity of many surgeons with this approach.

- Midvastus – this partly preserves the vastus medialis insertion onto the patella. The proximal extent of the arthrotomy is in line with the fibres of the vastus medialis and the muscle fibres are split rather than cut. This approach can be difficult in obese patients.
- Subvastus – the plane of dissection is distal to the vastus medialis. This is used for minimally invasive surgery. Jigs that make the bone cut from the medial side are used.

The various approaches are illustrated in Figure 1.14.

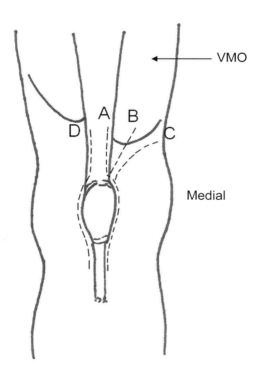

Figure 1.14. Standard knee joint exposure approaches: (A) medial parapatellar; (B) midvastus; (C) subvastus; (D) lateral parapatellar. VMO = vastus medialis obliquus.

Extensile approaches are generally indicated in the revision situation to avoid excess tension on the extensor mechanism and to improve access to the joint:

- Quadriceps snip – reduces the risk of injury to the extensor mechanism from over-stretching. The rectus is divided at the proximal extent of the medial parapatellar arthrotomy. The rectus can be divided in different ways to gain access.
- Tibial tubercle osteotomy – an osteotomy of the tubercle of 8-10cm is performed for exposure and reattached with multiple wires. A step cut at the proximal extent reduces the risk of proximal escape of the fragment. The fragment is 1cm thick proximally and narrows down to a sliver distally. The lateral periosteal hinge is preserved. Originally described by Dolin in 1983, this technique was modified by Whiteside by increasing the length of the osteotomy to 8-10cm (instead of 4-5cm) and using wires instead of screws for reattachment.

Note

Meek RM, Greidanus NV, McGraw RW, Masri BA. The extensile rectus snip exposure in revision of total knee arthroplasty. *J Bone Joint Surg Br* 2003; 85: 1120-2. **This study found that the rectus snip does not affect the function, pain or satisfaction score compared with standard medial parapatellar arthrotomy.**

Femoral components: design and materials

In the sagittal plane, the femoral component has differing radii: a larger radius (more flat) distally that articulates with the tibia in extension and a more curved posterior part that comes into contact with the tibial component in flexion. The large radius distributes the load over a larger area, while the smaller radius helps to improve rollback and gives greater flexion.

Cobalt chrome and titanium femoral components have similar durability. Ceramic femoral components are being trialled. Cementless fixation in the femur is acceptable and has predictable bone ingrowth.

Note

Bassett RW. Results of 1000 performance knees: cementless versus cemented fixation. *J Arthroplasty* 1998; 13: 409-13. **In this study of 1,000 knees with a 5.2-year follow-up, the authors found no difference in clinical results between cemented and cementless fixation. Neither group showed loosening or osteolysis.**

Stems can be used to reduce bending moments at the implant-bone interface in primary knee replacement in the presence of the following:

- Large areas of osteonecrosis of the femoral condyle.
- Notching of the anterior femoral cortex.
- Osteopenia.
- Femoral osteotomies performed along with replacement.

Stems can be cemented to provide more secure fixation or cementless, which makes stems easier to retrieve in case of infection or revision.

Tibial components

Cemented fixation is more commonly used for tibial components. The keel is used to augment fixation and this can be cemented. Alternatively, only the proximal tibial surface can be cemented leaving the keel uncemented.

Note

Bert JM, McShane M. Is it necessary to cement the tibial stem in cemented total knee arthroplasty? *Clin Orthop Relat Res* 1998; 356: 73-8. **The authors concluded that for adequate stability, either the keel should be cemented or the tibial cement mantle on the superior cut surface should be 3mm.**

Cementless tibial components have screws or spikes to augment fixation, but these have limited ingrowth on autopsy retrievals.

Tibial components can be titanium, which is easier to mould, or cobalt chrome, which exhibits less backside wear. Metal-backed trays are associated with backside wear, but allow modularity compared to all-polyethylene trays.

Knee replacement implants can be cruciate-retaining or posterior stabilised. The total condylar (DePuy) provides AP and some degree of varus-valgus stability. The constrained condylar knee (Zimmer) is a similar implant. In the primary replacement setting, it is indicated for large valgus deformities and lack of functioning medial or lateral collateral ligaments.

Lack of both medial and lateral collateral ligaments generally requires a hinged knee prosthesis. Some cases of absent MCL may also be best managed with a hinged prosthesis.

Medial offset stems are useful in patients with a previous high tibial osteotomy, and metal wedges and blocks can be used for congenital or traumatic defects. Blocks provide fewer shear forces, but require more bone resection compared to wedges.

The advantages and disadvantages of metal-backed tibial components are listed in Table 1.12.

Patellar components

Cementless patellar components are associated with problems of fracture of metal pegs, dissociation of polyethylene from the metal backing and wear. Cemented fixation is most commonly used. A mobile bearing cementless component is also an option.

Using an inset porous-coated metal backing, which is countersunk below the cut surface of the patella, allows a thicker polyethylene to be used.

Both multiple- and single-peg fixation designs are available. The shape of the implant may be oval, symmetrical or anatomic.

The advantages and disadvantages of patella resurfacing are listed in Table 1.13.

Table 1.12. Advantages and disadvantages of metal-backed tibial components.

Advantages	Disadvantages
Stress transfer to underlying bone is lower and more evenly distributed	The thin plastic can lead to increased stress and catastrophic failure
Permits modularity	The stiff metal tray can cause stress shielding of the proximal tibia
	The tray can tilt if eccentrically loaded
	Generally more expensive than all-polyethylene tibial components

Table 1.13. Advantages and disadvantages of patella resurfacing.

Advantages	Disadvantages
Reduces risk of patellofemoral pain	Problems of failure of patella fixation
Improves tracking	Unsuitable in young patients with high demand due to high joint forces

Note

Burnett RS, Haydon CM, Rorabeck CH, Bourne RB. Patella resurfacing versus nonresurfacing in total knee arthroplasty: results of a randomized controlled clinical trial at a minimum of 10 years' followup. *Clin Orthop Relat Res* 2004; 428: 12-25. This prospective randomised controlled trial followed 90 patients (100 knees) for 10 years. Patients were randomised to resurfacing or non-resurfacing. There was no difference between the groups in revision rate, knee score, ROM, patient satisfaction or anterior knee pain. The study did not, however, investigate selective resurfacing.

Note

Campbell DG, Duncan WW, Ashworth M, *et al*. Patellar resurfacing in total knee replacement: a ten-year randomised prospective trial. *J Bone Joint Surg Br* 2006; 88: 734-9. In 100 patients, this study found no difference in scores or patellofemoral complications with or without resurfacing.

Causes of patellar maltracking

Patellar maltracking can be caused by the following:

- Valgus alignment of the leg.
- Patella alta.
- Internal rotation of the femoral or tibial component.
- Medialisation of the femoral or tibial component.

- Unequal thickness of the patella cut on the medial and lateral sides.
- Excess patellar thickness.

Patellar fracture

Patellar fracture can be related to central peg patellar components, osteonecrosis of the patella or high stress across the component.

Treatment is non-operative initially, as operative treatment carries a significant complication rate. The vascular supply of the patella is impaired after knee replacement and this contributes to poor healing of patellar fractures.

Patellar clunk

Patellar clunk occurs when scar tissue at the superior pole of the patella catches on the intercondylar box of a cruciate-substituting femoral component. Arthroscopic excision of scar tissue relieves the symptoms. A superolateral portal is employed for easy access and to avoid scratching the femoral component.

Mobile bearing knees

Mobile bearing knees were introduced to reduce backside wear in modular fixed bearing tibial trays. These can be meniscal-bearing or a rotating platform.

Advantages:

- There is less backside wear due to flat-on-flat articulation between the insert and the tibial tray with unidirectional motion, which therefore increases longevity of the polyethylene.
- The prosthesis accommodates minor degrees of malrotation between the femur and tibia.
- The design allows a better contact area in high flexion.

Disadvantages:

- Impingement or dislocation of the bearing – in high flexion, if the posterior cruciate ligament (PCL) is tight, the lateral femoral condyle moves posteriorly and the lateral side of the insert is pushed anteriorly and subluxes.

- Dislocation (spinout) is more likely in cruciate-retaining inserts (as they are curved on the posterior aspect) as compared to posterior stabilised inserts. Spinout can be due to a tight PCL. Tightness is addressed by releasing anterior and lateral fibres from the femoral side of the PCL. The PCL is checked with the patella in the trochlear groove instead of patella everted.
- If there is still a tendency to spinout then a larger bearing of the same thickness can be used. This gives a larger AP dimension, reducing the chances of dislocation. The rotational excursion will be reduced if a larger insert is used and the contact area will also be slightly reduced, but this is not clinically significant. The amount of contact will still be more than with a comparable fixed bearing insert.

Currently, mobile bearing is indicated for young, active patients.

Cemented/cementless technique

Cemented

High-pressure and high-volume lavage before cementation results in the following:

- Reduced radiolucent lines on postoperative radiographs.
- Removal of fat and blood and reduced venous thrombosis.
- Improved penetration of cement in cancellous bone.

Cementless

The optimum pore size is 400-600μ. The distance between bone and implant should be less than 50μ for ingrowth. Micromotion of more than 150μ results in fibrous tissue formation instead of bone ingrowth. Pegs and screws help to provide initial stability. The undersurface of tibial components should be fully coated to prevent migration of wear particles.

Obesity and inflammatory arthritis are not contraindications for cementless fixation. Osteopenic bone may not be able to support cementless fixation and cemented implants should be considered.

Cementless fixation technique involves the following:

- Precise cutting instruments.
- Irrigation while making bone cuts to prevent thermal necrosis.
- Maintenance of the posterior slope – the trabeculae are perpendicular to the anatomic surface and this allows bone to be loaded in compression.
- Patellar countersinking and medialisation.

Alignment in knee replacement

The mechanical axis is the line joining the centre of the femoral head and the centre of the ankle joint, passing through the centre of the knee. The anatomical axis is the line along the tibial shaft and femoral shaft, making an angle of 5-7° valgus with the mechanical axis (Figure 1.15).

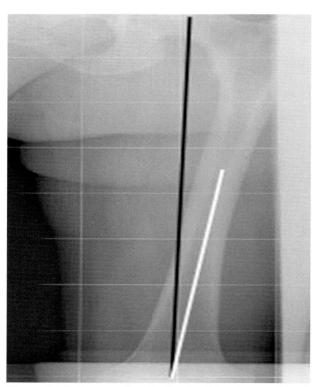

Figure 1.15. The mechanical axis of the femur (black line) makes an angle of 5-7° with the anatomical axis of the femoral shaft (white line).

The aim of distal femoral resection is to make the cut perpendicular to the mechanical axis. A component that is not perpendicular to the mechanical axis will be subject to shear stress on loading. The femoral prosthesis is aligned by intramedullary jigs along the anatomical axis. The distal cut is made 5-7° valgus to the anatomical axis, resulting in a cut perpendicular to the mechanical axis.

Anatomically, the femoral condyle is in 7° of valgus and the tibial plateau is in 3° of varus. In flexion, the medial femoral condyle extends 3° more posteriorly in relation to the lateral condyle. In the normal knee, 70% weight transmission takes place through the medial compartment.

Flexion and extension gaps

The flexion gap is the distance between the cut surface of the distal femur and the cut surface of the proximal tibia, measured with the knee in flexion; the extension gap is the distance between the cut surface of the distal femur and the cut surface of the proximal tibia, measured with the knee in extension (Figure 1.16). Both of these gaps should be rectangular – implying equal tension on the medial and lateral side – and should be equal to each other.

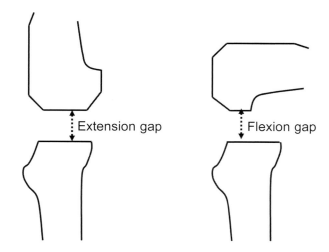

Figure 1.16. The concept of flexion and extension gaps.

Femur alignment should be restored to 5° ± 1-2° of valgus.

The femur is cut in 5° valgus, and intramedullary jigs are more accurate than extramedullary jigs. The entry point should be in line with the medullary canal of the femur and slightly medial to the centre of the intercondylar notch.

The size of the femoral component can be determined by anterior or posterior referencing. Anterior referencing avoids notching the anterior femoral cortex and overstuffing the patellofemoral joint. The disadvantage is that measurements that fall in between femur sizes must be downsized (i.e., smaller component used), which involves removing more posterior condyle.

The measured resection technique involves removing enough bone from the femur and tibia to allow similar thickness components. The tension technique involves making the proximal tibial cut first and then equalising the flexion and extension gaps by femoral resection.

Femoral component rotation (internal/external rotation) is assessed by the following:

- Interepicondylar axis – the anterior and posterior flanges of the component should be parallel to the interepicondylar axis (the epicondylar axis is the line connecting the lateral epicondylar prominence and the median sulcus of the medial epicondyle).
- Whiteside's line (a line from the deepest part of the trochlear groove to the centre of the intercondylar notch posteriorly) – a line perpendicular to Whiteside's line is the external rotation needed in femoral components.

- Posterior condylar axis – between the posterior surfaces of the femoral condyles. This is unreliable in the presence of bone loss or dysplasia of the condyles.
- Rectangular flexion gap – in the flexed knee, the cut surface of the femur (posterior) should be parallel to the superior cut surface of the tibia.
- The anterior femoral cut surface should resemble a double curve, with the medial peak lower than the lateral peak.
- More bone is removed from the back of the medial femoral condyle than from the lateral, as the medial femoral condyle extends further posteriorly.

Note

Whiteside LA, Arima J. The anteroposterior axis for femoral rotational alignment in valgus knee arthroplasty. *Clin Orthop Relat Res* 1995; 321: 168-72.

Note

Miller MC, Berger RA, Petrella AJ, *et al.* Optimising femoral component rotation in total knee arthroplasty. *Clin Orthop Relat Res* 2001; 392: 38-45.

If posterior referencing is used, the presence of a hypoplastic lateral femoral condyle in a valgus knee can lead to excess internal rotation of the femoral component. Excess internal rotation or medialisation of the femoral or tibial component leads to a relative lateral displacement of the extensor mechanism and problems with patellar tracking (Table 1.14 and Figure 1.17).

Table 1.14. Effects of inappropriate external rotation of the femoral component.

Excess external rotation	Excess internal rotation
Loose medial flexion gap	Tight medial flexion gap
Tight lateral flexion gap	Loose lateral flexion gap
Lateral displacement of patellofemoral groove of the implant	Medial displacement of patellofemoral groove of the implant

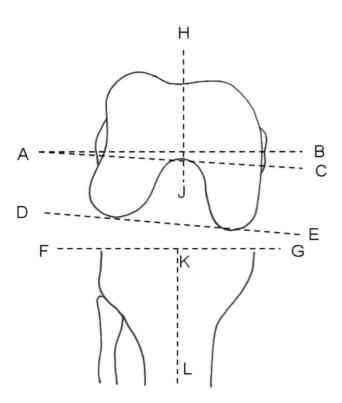

Figure 1.17. Illustration to demonstrate the importance of externally rotating the femoral component. The tibial cut (F-G) is perpendicular to the mechanical axis of the tibia (K-L), which commonly coincides with the long axis of the tibia. In the flexed knee, the medial femoral condyle extends more distally than the lateral (D-E). If the cut is parallel to this line (A-C), this will produce a flexion gap that is tight medially; hence, the femoral component is externally rotated. This gives the alignment (A-B), which is parallel to the tibial cut (F-G), parallel to the interepicondylar axis and perpendicular to the long axis of the trochlea (H-J).

The tibial cut is perpendicular to the mechanical axis, which usually coincides with the long axis in the AP view. The tibial cut can be made with the help of extramedullary or intramedullary alignment jigs.

Extramedullary alignment is not affected by tibial deformities or obstruction in the tibial canal. Intramedullary alignment is useful in obese patients, where it may be difficult to palpate bony prominences

(required for extramedullary alignment). For intramedullary alignment the initial hole is at the junction of attachments of the anterior cruciate ligament (ACL) and the anterior horn of the lateral meniscus. Fluted rods reduce the incidence of fat embolism.

The tibial cut is perpendicular to the mechanical axis of the tibia in the AP view, such that the tibial tray is parallel to the ground on weight bearing. A varus cut increases load on the medial side and leads to early failure.

> **Note**
>
> Berend ME, Ritter MA, Meding JB, *et al*. Tibial component failure mechanism in total knee arthroplasty. *Clin Orthop Relat Res* 2004; 428: 26-34. **The authors found that a tibial cut in more than 3° of varus increases the failure rate. In addition, varus limb alignment postoperatively increases the failure rate.**

The extramedullary jig is positioned slightly medial to the midpoint of the ankle along the intermalleolar line so as to avoid a varus cut of the proximal tibia. The upper platform is lined up with the medial third of the tibial tubercle. The normal posterior slope should be reproduced. The thickness removed should match the thickness of components to be inserted and is generally 10mm from the surface of a less arthritic plateau.

Medialisation or internal rotation of the tibial component results in relative lateral positioning of the tibial tubercle. This malaligns the pull of the quadriceps to a more lateral force and leads to patellar maltracking.

If there is a bowing deformity of the tibia, the resection should be perpendicular to the mechanical axis. This may involve removing an asymmetric amount of bone from the medial and lateral tibial plateaus. In severe cases, deformity correction may be required as a separate procedure prior to replacement.

The varus knee

In the varus knee the deformity is generally in the tibia. This contrasts to the valgus knee, in which the deformity is often in the femur. Neutral alignment is considered to be between 4° and 9°. Less than 4° is considered varus and more than 9° is valgus.

Varus is a more common deformity than valgus. Rheumatoid patients have a relatively higher incidence of valgus, but the majority still have varus deformity.

A varus deformity can be correctable if medial structures are not contracted. In longstanding deformity, however, contractures may develop.

Balancing

Using the medial parapatellar approach, osteophytes should be removed and up to the level of the semimembranosus bursa released in the plane between the medial tibial plateau and the deep MCL. The superficial MCL is preserved. The knee should be balanced in extension first.

The tibial bony cut is based 10mm below the intact lateral side perpendicular to the long axis of the tibia. A tibial component one size smaller may have to be selected along with excision of bone from the medial tibial margin to slacken the MCL. If the perpendicular distance (difference in height) between the medial and the lateral joint line is more than 15mm then medial augmentation may be needed. This can be in the form of cement, a bone graft or metal augments.

A standard distal femoral valgus resection of 5-7° is adequate. The rotation of the femoral component is checked after the knee has been balanced in extension. The usual 3° of external rotation may have to be increased because a hyperplastic medial femoral condyle may distort the posterior referencing.

If the preoperative fixed flexion deformity is more than 15° then a greater distal femoral resection will be required.

Table 1.15 describes the problems and solutions found with soft tissue balancing.

Table 1.15. Problems and solutions in soft tissue balancing.

Problem	Solution
Both flexion and extension gaps tight	Increase tibial resection
Flexion and extension gaps loose	Use thicker polyethylene insert
Extension gap tight, flexion gap satisfactory	Release posterior capsule from femur
	Clear the osteophytes at back of femoral condyle
	Increase distal femoral resection
Flexion gap tight, extension gap satisfactory	Downsize femur (will increase posterior condyle resection)
	Release posterior cruciate ligament from femoral side
	Increase posterior tibial slope
	Increase tibial resection, use thicker insert and treat loose extension gap

The valgus knee

Problems in the valgus knee are as follows:

- The lateral femoral condyle may be hypoplastic both distally and posteriorly, affecting femoral component alignment.
- The lateral structures may be tight and the MCL attenuated.

The jig for the distal femoral cut is aligned to 5°, although the cut can be 3° if there is significant diaphyseal valgus remodelling.

Making a 5° cut is the best compromise; a cut of 2° or 3° requires a greater lateral release to balance the knee. A smaller cut (≤5°) helps to take the strain off the attenuated MCL during weight bearing.

Distal metaphyseal valgus bowing can lead to higher valgus resection because the axis of the femoral canal exits more medially to the normal entry point. Choosing a valgus angle of 2° or 3° can avoid excess valgus resection. Alternatively, the entry point for the femoral intramedullary jig should be shifted medially if the angle chosen is 5°.

The hypoplastic lateral femoral condyle should be augmented instead of resecting down to the level of the condyle. A distal femoral resection performed at the level of the hypoplastic lateral femoral condyle elevates the joint line, which in turn interferes with the kinematics of the collateral ligaments. Additionally, it creates an excessive extension gap.

Once the femoral and tibial cuts have been made, a rectangular shape of the flexion and extension gaps is achieved by soft tissue balancing. The rotation of the femoral component is adjusted on the basis of flexion gap symmetry.

The lateral release progressively includes the following:

- Osteophytes.
- Posterolateral capsule – at the level of the tibial cut, extending from the posterior margin of the iliotibial band to the posterior capsule.
- Iliotibial band – 'pie-crusting' technique – using multiple transverse stab incisions from the deep surface. This is useful if the knee is tight in extension.
- If still tight in flexion, release the popliteus tendon (this is rarely needed).
- Release of the lateral collateral ligament from the femoral attachment is rarely needed.

If lateral release results in loss of lateral support, a constrained implant is required.

The patella should track within the trochlear groove on knee flexion and remain in contact with both the condyles of the femoral trial component. If it is still tight laterally, a lateral retinacular release should be considered after releasing the tourniquet. The lateral release is through multiple transverse stab incisions on the lateral retinaculum.

The lateral popliteal nerve is at risk of stretch injury when valgus deformity is corrected. If a nerve palsy is detected postoperatively, flexing the knee will relieve the stretch on the nerve.

A cruciform release of the lateral retinaculum for balancing the valgus knee has been described by RD Scott (Brigham and Women's Hospital, Boston, USA).

Posterior cruciate ligament: to retain or replace?

The PCL extends from the lateral surface of medial femoral condyle to the posterior part of the intercondylar area of the tibia. It comprises an anterolateral band that is tight in flexion and posteromedial band that is tight in extension. The distal insertion extends below the level of the articular surface and the ligament is extrasynovial.

As the knee flexes from the fully extended position, the first 30° of flexion involves rolling of femoral condyles over the tibial plateau. Beyond 30° the PCL produces a rollback of the femur on the tibia, preventing impingement of the posterior surface of the distal femur against the posterior part of the tibial plateau. As a result of rollback, higher flexion can be achieved.

With femoral rollback the extensor mechanism moves anteriorly, improving the power. The lateral femoral condyle rolls back further than the medial. Normal femoral rollback is not reproduced in the prosthetic knee with or without the PCL.

The forerunner to the cruciate-substituting (posterior stabilised) knee was the cruciate sacrificing prosthesis. The stability of the cruciate sacrificing prosthesis depended on equal flexion and extension gaps and intact collaterals with a well-conforming tibial component. An example of this was the total condylar knee. This evolved into the first successful posterior stabilised knee: the Insall-Burstein posterior stabilised knee.

The advantages of retaining the PCL are as follows:

- Allows the use of a less constrained prosthesis, resulting in less stress transfer to the interface.
- Easier to balance the flexion and extension gaps. The PCL acts as an additional tether to prevent an excessively wide flexion gap.
- Less femur has to be resected to insert cruciate-retaining components because the flexion space does not open up as much.
- No elevation of the joint line, preserving collateral ligament kinematics. Mid-flexion instability is avoided.
- No patellar clunk or dislocation of the post.
- No peg fracture or wear.
- More options to treat supracondylar fractures above the femoral component.

- PCL-substituting designs do not tolerate hyperextension as it leads to impingement of the post.
- PCL-substituting implants can have dislocation of the femoral cam anterior to the tibial polyethylene post on hyperflexion. Reduction of this requires general anaesthetic and manipulation.
- Better proprioception.

On the other hand, there are several advantages to substituting the PCL:

- PCL function is compromised in the arthritic knee and in the absence of the ACL.
- Reproducible femoral rollback and reduced patellofemoral joint forces. Some PCL-retaining knees actually allow the femur to move forwards in flexion instead of backwards.
- Less effect of the level of the joint line on the function of the prosthesis.
- Allows more conforming articular surfaces, reducing contact stress.

There are several indications for PCL substitution:

- Severe flexion deformity.
- Ankylosed knee.
- Post-patellectomy knee.
- Chronic patellar dislocation.

Checking for PCL tension

With the trial components in place, it should not be possible to pull out the tibial component from under the femoral component with the knee flexed to 90°. If

Table 1.16. Knee flexion requirements.	
Action	**Degree of flexion required**
For walking on level ground	70
Ascending stairs	90
Descending stairs	100
Rising from a chair without using arm support	105

the tibial component can be pulled out or pushed in with the femoral component *in situ*, the knee is too loose and a thicker insert must be used.

If flexion of the knee with the trial components causes the front of the tibia trial component to lift off, or the femoral trial to be pushed off distally, the PCL is too tight. A tight PCL pulls the femur backwards and the impingement of the femoral condyle on the back of the tibial tray causes lift off in the front. In this situation, the PCL should be released. This test should be performed with the patella restored to the trochlear groove and not everted, otherwise the tight quadriceps can cause a false lift off. Posterior femoral osteophytes are also a rare cause of lift off and should be removed.

Knee flexion requirements are shown in Table 1.16.

Stiffness after total knee replacement

Again, causes of stiffness after TKR can be pre-, intra- or postoperative.

Preoperative factors:

- ROM – patients with preoperative flexion of less than 90° tend to gain flexion, while those with preoperative flexion of more than 105° tend to lose flexion. In general, however, greater preoperative flexion is likely to result in greater postoperative flexion.
- Previous surgery, obesity, multiple joint involvement, age, sex and bilateral surgery have not shown a consistent relationship with postoperative ROM.

Intraoperative factors:

- Tight flexion gap due to:
  - oversized femoral component;
  - posteriorly shifted femoral component;
  - tight PCL.
- Tight extension gap due to:
  - inadequate distal femoral resection;
  - inadequate tibial resection;
  - tight posterior capsule or osteophytes.

- Tight patellofemoral joint due to:
  - inadequate patellar resection;
  - anterior translation of femoral component.
- Anterior tibial slope.
- Elevation of joint line – causes relative patella baja and increased joint forces and stiffness.
- Malrotation (internal rotation) of the femoral component – can cause an asymmetric flexion gap.

Postoperative factors:

- Poorly motivated patient.
- Arthrofibrosis.
- Infection.
- HO.
- Patellar complications (fracture, maltracking, pain).
- Complex regional pain syndrome.

Total knee replacement in the stiff knee (flexion contracture)

For preoperative flexion contracture:

- Remove the osteophytes from the intercondylar area and from the posterior part of the femoral condyle.
- Release the posterior capsule.
- Increase the distal femoral resection by 2mm if the preoperative flexion contracture is more than 15°. Take a further 2mm off for every further 10° of fixed flexion.

Severe preoperative flexion contractures may require serial casting prior to surgery.

Total knee replacement after failed high tibial osteotomy

High tibial osteotomy (HTO) provides good short-term results in 80-90% of patients. The results deteriorate with time, however, and on long-term follow-up only 60% of patients retain good function. Risk factors for early failure include male sex, increased weight, young age at the time of TKR, coronal laxity and preoperative limb malalignment.

Note

Parvizi J, Hanssen AD, Spangehl MJ. Total knee arthroplasty following proximal tibial osteotomy: risk factors for failure. *J Bone Joint Surg Am* 2004; 86: 474-9. In 118 patients with an average clinical follow-up of 15.1 years, a high rate of radiographic loosening was observed. Male sex, increased weight, young age at the time of TKR, coronal laxity and preoperative limb malalignment were identified as risk factors for early failure.

TKR after failed HTO may present several problems (Table 1.17).

Management of bone defects

Contained defects (<15-20% of the cut surface of the distal femur or proximal tibia) can be managed with an autogenous bone graft from the cut tibial plateau.

Uncontained defects of the tibia that are less than 3mm can be managed with an undercut and use of a thicker polyethylene. For those greater than 3mm, metal augmentation blocks or wedges may be used.

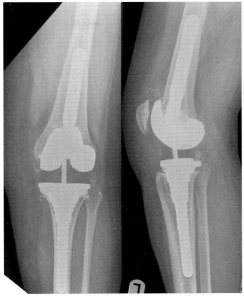

Figure 1.18. The use of metaphyseal tibial sleeves to restore the level of the tibial tray in a patient with circumferential proximal tibial bone loss from previous revision knee replacement. The sleeve fits over the stem and is coated with hydroxyapatite ceramic. Note the level of the proximal tibial bone in relation to the head of the fibula.

The development of metaphyseal sleeves (Figure 1.18) has improved the management of bone defects.

Table 1.17. Potential problems and solutions with TKR after failed high tibial osteotomy.

Problems	Solutions
Existing scars	Conduct preoperative planning to avoid compromising the blood supply
	Use the most lateral scar if there are multiple longitudinal scars
Existing metalwork	Remove at time of replacement or as a separate procedure prior to replacement
Patella baja	May increase tibial resection and shift the femoral component distally
Non-union of osteotomy	Stemmed tibial component and bone grafting of non-union
Tibial deformity	Alter bone cuts to correct deformity or correct deformity in a separate procedure
Offset tibial shaft from tibial plateau	Use a smaller component shifted to one side or use offset stems
Excess valgus after overcorrected osteotomy	Internally rotate the femoral component and avoid excess release of the lateral collateral ligament

Uncontained defects of the femur require augmentation or cemented revision implants. In patients with a deficient distal femoral condyle, instead of resecting the normal condyle, the hypoplastic condyle can be built up distally with a screw and cement, and the prosthesis placed in the anatomic position. Increasing distal resection of the normal femoral condyle will result in an elevated joint line.

Causes of failure of total knee replacement

TKR can fail due to any of the following:

- Polyethylene wear.
- Loosening.
- Instability.
- Infection.
- Stiffness.
- Malalignment.
- Extensor mechanism rupture.

Complications in knee replacement

Infection

Infection may be prevented with perioperative antibiotics and antibiotic-impregnated cement in high-risk individuals. Tobramycin (600mg) and gentamicin (1g) are commonly used as additives.

Factors that predispose a patient to infection include the following:

- Poor soft tissue envelop.
- Hinged and highly constrained implants.
- Impaired circulation.
- Immunocompromise, diabetes, rheumatoid disease, malnourishment.
- Obesity.
- Steroid use.
- Concurrent infection elsewhere.
- Prolonged hospital stay.

Deep infection is defined as infection in the subfascial plane and/or intra-articular infection. The presence of a discharging sinus tract indicates chronic deep infection. The risk of deep infection in knee replacement is less than 1%, but is higher in revision surgery (approximately 6%).

Note

Blom AW, Brown J, Taylor AH, et al. Infection after total knee arthroplasty. *J Bone Joint Surg Br* 2004; 86: 688-91. The authors used vertical laminar flow, occlusive clothing and chlorhexidine lavage as infection-prevention measures during 931 primary TKRs and 69 revisions. Patients were followed-up for 6.5 years. Deep infections were seen in 1% of primary and 5.8% of revision surgeries.

Acute infections are those in which symptoms have been present for less than 2 weeks. If the symptoms of infection present for longer than 2 weeks, the infection is chronic.

Clinical features

The clinical features of infection are pain (constant or night pain); a warm, red and swollen knee; pain on movement; and a discharging wound, cellulitis or sinus.

Diagnosis

Several tests can be used in diagnosis:

- ESR – non-specific for infection.
- CRP – normally returns to normal 2-3 weeks after surgery. A persistently raised CRP or rising levels following an operation should raise suspicion of postoperative infection.
- X-rays to see loosening and resorption. Radiologic changes occur late in the course of infection.
- Tc-99mm bone scan – may show increased uptake. Bone scans are of limited use within the first year because of bone remodelling changes. Increased uptake in all three phases is suggestive of infection.
- Aspiration is the most accurate test, with almost 100% sensitivity and specificity. Antibiotics should be stopped 1 week prior to aspiration to improve diagnostic yield and reduce false negatives.
- Intraoperative frozen section – greater than 10 polymorphonuclear cells per high-power field is suggestive of infection. This has 84% sensitivity and is 99% specific.

Note

Greidanus NV, Masri BA, Garbuz DS, *et al.* Use of erythrocyte sedimentation rate and C-reactive protein level to diagnose infection before revision total knee arthroplasty. A prospective evaluation. *J Bone Joint Surg Am* 2007; 89: 1409-16. **In 151 knees that underwent revision TKR, 45 were infected. The sensitivity of ESR was 0.93 and specificity 0.83. For CRP, sensitivity was 0.91 and specificity 0.86.**

Management

There may be a role for intravenous antibiotics for infections with a sensitive organism that are diagnosed within 48 hours. Cure rates are low (10-15%). Intravenous antibiotics are conventionally given for 6 weeks, but penetration into the knee joint is low after 3 weeks due to scar tissue formation.

Arthroscopic debridement is of questionable efficacy, although some reports have shown good results using multiple portal arthroscopy and debriding the interface.

Open debridement, synovectomy and polyethylene liner exchange can salvage about 25% joints if performed within 30 days of the onset of infection. The prosthesis should be well fixed and the organism should be sensitive.

Either single or two-stage revision surgery may be performed. Two-stage revision surgery is the preferred option, although single surgery may be performed in the case of a sensitive organism.

Note

Haleem AA, Berry DJ, Hanssen AD. Mid-term to long-term follow-up of two-stage reimplantation for infected total knee arthroplasty. *Clin Orthop Relat Res* 2004; 428: 35-9. **This study looked at 94 patients and 96 knees, with a 7.2 year follow-up. All had an antibiotic spacer and antibiotic-loaded cement. Overall, 16% required reoperation: 9% for recurrent infection and 6% for aseptic loosening. The average time for reoperation for reinfection after revision surgery was 1 year.**

Note

Hart WJ, Jones RS. Two-stage revision of infected total knee replacements using articulating cement spacers and short-term antibiotic therapy. *J Bone Joint Surg Br* 2006; 88: 1011-5. **In this study, 48 patients were managed with an articulating spacer and short-term parenteral antibiotics after first-stage revision surgery. Infection was eradicated in 42 out of 48 patients. The authors concluded that protracted intravenous antibiotics may not be necessary.**

Articulated spacers maintain soft tissue quality and movement and improve outcome. PROSTALAC stands for prosthesis of antibiotic-loaded acrylic cement. It is loosely cemented as an articulating spacer and allows preservation of the soft tissue envelope and joint mobility in the interval between the first and second stage. The antibiotic provides a high local concentration, which is unachievable through intravenous administration.

Arthrodesis is an option in patients with failed reconstruction, poor soft tissue cover or infection with resistant organisms. Arthrodesis helps to control infection and provides a stable knee.

Resection replacement can be considered for non-ambulatory patients. Poor functional results should be expected.

Transfemoral amputation is the last resort.

Wound problems

In the presence of existing scars, the most lateral longitudinal incision should be used as long as it does not compromise access. A gap of 7cm between longitudinal scars is advisable. Greater vascular supply comes from the medial side and hence the lateral flap has lesser vascularity.

The use of tissue expanders has been successful prior to knee surgery if there is a concern about the adequacy of skin for achieving closure.

Patellofemoral problems

Patellar clunk

Patellar clunk can occur due to a fibrous nodule on the deep surface of the quadriceps tendon causing a clunk in flexion-extension of the knee. Treatment is with flexion-extension exercises or arthroscopic debridement.

Loosening of the patellar component

In metal-backed patellar components, loosening of the patellar component may be caused by avascular necrosis of the patella, deficient bone, patellar fracture, subluxation of the patella, a malpositioned component or failure of ingrowth. Failed metal-backed components may be associated with dissociation of the metal plate or the polyethylene, leading to metal-metal contact and accelerated failure of the joint.

Extensor mechanism rupture

Acute open repair is advised for extensor mechanism rupture (quadriceps tendon or patellar tendon rupture), but the results may be unsatisfactory with residual extensor lag.

Patellar fractures

Patellar fractures are predisposed by the following:

- Avascular necrosis due to medial parapatellar arthrotomy, with lateral release leading to damage to the superior lateral and medial genicular arteries.
- Inaccurate resection of the patella.
- A too thick or too thin patella after resurfacing.
- An oversized femoral component.
- Maltracking of the patella.
- Use of patellae with a single central peg.

The classification of patellar fractures is shown in Table 1.18.

Treatment can be non-operative if the component is not loose and the extensor mechanism is competent. Open reduction and internal fixation is associated with a high failure rate. Partial patellectomy and extensor mechanism repair is an option.

Patellar instability

Problems of patellar maltracking may result from several causes:

- Femoral component internal rotation – increases the Q angle.
- Tibial component internal rotation – increases the Q angle.
- Excess valgus distal femoral cut.
- Medialisation of the femoral component in the coronal plane.
- Medialisation of the tibial component in the coronal plane.
- Lateralisation of the patellar component.

CT scans can help to accurately assess any internal rotation of the femoral or tibial component.

Table 1.18. Classification of patellar fractures.

Type	Description
I	Fractures do not involve the implant-cement interface
II	Fractures involve the implant-cement interface or extensor mechanism
III	Inferior pole fractures
IIIa	Associated patellar tendon rupture
IIIb	No rupture of the patellar tendon
IV	Fracture dislocation of the patella

At the time of surgery, patellar tracking should be checked in a full range of flexion-extension with the 'no-thumb' technique: it should not be necessary to apply external pressure on the patella to maintain the patella in the trochlear groove.

If the patellar tracking is not satisfactory, alignment and rotation of the femoral and tibial components should be checked. A tight lateral retinaculum can be released, but the release will not compensate for a malaligned femoral or tibial component.

Venous thromboembolism

Venous thromboembolism can occur up to 1 month after knee replacement. The current NICE guidelines recommend chemical thromboprophylaxis for 2 weeks following knee replacement surgery, in addition to mechanical prophylaxis.

Note

Bjørnarå BT, Gudmundsen TE, Dahl OE. Frequency and timing of clinical venous thromboembolism after major joint surgery. *J Bone Joint Surg Br* 2006; 88: 386-91. Over a 13-year period, 5,607 patients undergoing hip or knee replacement were given low-molecular-weight heparin as prophylaxis. Overall, 2.7% of patients experienced symptomatic venous thromboembolism, 1.1% had a pulmonary embolism and 1.5% had deep vein thrombosis. The risk for thromboembolism lasted for 3 months after hip surgery and for 1 month after knee surgery.

Periprosthetic fracture

Distal femoral supracondylar fractures

Distal femoral supracondylar fractures related to knee replacements are predisposed by osteoporosis, rheumatoid disease, steroid use, a stiff knee preoperatively and anterior femoral notching.

They are classified into type I (with a stable prosthesis) and type II (with a loose implant).

Treatment options are as follows:

- Non-operative (cast bracing or cast) – for minimally displaced fractures with a stable prosthesis in good alignment.
- Surgical stabilisation:
  - condylar plate;
  - intramedullary nail – not for cruciate-substituting femoral components that have a box to house the cam and post mechanism. Some 'open box' designs may be amenable to nailing;
  - LISS (less invasive stabilisation system);
  - external fixation;
  - antegrade nailing.
- Revision knee replacement.

Proximal tibial fractures

Proximal tibial fractures generally occur in association with stemmed tibial components. Their classification is shown in Table 1.19.

Table 1.19. Classification of proximal tibial fractures.	
Type	**Description**
Type I	Fractures extending into the tibial cut surface
Type II	Fractures at the tip of the tibial stem component
Type III	Fractures distal to the tip of the tibial component
Type IV	Fractures involving the tibial tubercle
Subtype* Description	
A	With stable components
B	With loose tibial component
C	Intraoperative fractures
* Each type is further divided into the three subtypes described.	

Vascular injury

Intraoperative vascular injury necessitates immediate vascular repair. In an extremity with a compromised vascular supply or previous bypass graft, the use of a tourniquet should be avoided.

Nerve injury

Correction of severe valgus can cause a stretch injury to the peroneal nerve. If detected postoperatively, any compressive bandages should be removed and the knee flexed to relax the nerve. Generally, recovery is good.

Stiffness

Open arthrolysis may improve stiffness following TKR.

> **Note**
>
> Hutchinson JR, Parish EN, Cross MJ. Results of open arthrolysis for the treatment of stiffness after total knee replacement. *J Bone Joint Surg Br* 2005; 87: 1357-60. Thirteen patients underwent open arthrolysis for stiffness following TKR. Mean ROM improved from 55° to 91°. The mean time between TKR and arthrolysis was 14 months.

Instability after total knee replacement

Instability can be patellofemoral or tibiofemoral.

Patellofemoral instability is due to medialisation of the femoral sulcus (resulting in effective lateralisation of the patella). The medialisation can result from several factors:

- Internal rotation of the femoral component.
- Medial placement of the femoral component.
- Internal rotation of the tibial component.
- A tight lateral retinaculum, loose medial retinaculum or oblique patellar resection.
- Overstuffing of the patellofemoral joint.

Instability presents clinically as 'giving way', anterior knee pain or crepitus.

Evaluation is with plain X-rays including a sunrise (skyline) view and CT scan. CT scanning is accurate in assessing femoral or tibial component malrotation.

Treatment is based on the underlying cause of instability, but may include vastus medialis obliquus exercises, lateral release with vastus medialis obliquus advancement, tibial tubercle transfer or revision of components.

Tibiofemoral instability can be flexion instability, varus valgus instability or global instability.

Flexion instability

Sacrifice of the ACL leads to some degree of anterior instability in all prosthetic knees. Posterior instability is due to a poorly functioning PCL in posterior cruciate-retaining implants.

Clinical symptoms include anterior knee pain, 'giving way', effusion and difficulty with climbing stairs. On examination, the posterior drawer and quadriceps active tests are positive.

Flexion instability can be caused by a loose flexion gap at the time of surgery, damage to the PCL at time of surgery or late attrition rupture of the PCL.

Reduction and bracing is the initial treatment for cam dislocation. Recurrent cam dislocation may require revision surgery.

Symptomatic posterior instability in cruciate-retaining knees can be managed by revising to a thicker insert, or revision of the femoral component to cruciate-substituting and using a posterior stabilised insert.

Varus valgus instability

Varus valgus instability is due to incompetence of the medial or lateral collateral ligament. Patients present with pain, effusion and 'giving way'. Clinically, collateral laxity is evident and stress radiographs are helpful.

Treatment is by revising to a more constrained implant or to a hinged knee. In primary knees, ligament repair or advancement may be an option. Hinged knees have poor long-term survival and hence limited application.

Global instability

Global instability is a combination of varus valgus and AP instability. It is usually seen in patients with marked polyethylene wear, component migration, poor quadriceps function, rheumatoid arthritis or collagen vascular disease. It requires revision to a hinged knee implant.

Loosening and wear

Loosening and wear are long-term problems. Loosening is more common in constrained prostheses due to a higher load transfer to the cement-bone interface.

Results of total knee replacement

Knee replacement has demonstrated excellent long-term survival.

> **Note**
>
> Rodricks DJ, Patil S, Pulido P, Colwell CW Jr. Press-fit condylar design total knee arthroplasty. Fourteen to 17-year follow-up. *J Bone Joint Surg Am* 2007; 89: 89-95. **This study looked at 160 knees with a 15.8-year follow-up and mean patient age of 70.5 years. The survival rate with revision as the endpoint was 97.2%. Radiolucent lines did not correlate with loosening.**

> **Note**
>
> Ritter MA. The Anatomical Graduated Component total knee replacement: a long-term evaluation with 20-year survival analysis. *J Bone Joint Surg Br* 2009; 91: 745-9. **Using a non-modular metal-backed tibia with compression-moulded polyethylene, 20-year survival was 97.8%.**

Other types of knee replacement

Unicompartmental knee replacement

Unicompartmental knee replacement (UKR) is an alternative to TKR when the arthritis primarily involves either the medial or the lateral tibiofemoral compartment. It is usually performed on the medial side due to the more common pattern of medial arthritis and with more predictable long-term results.

UKR has several advantages over TKR:

- Preserved cruciate ligaments give a more normal kinematic pattern.
- UKR can be performed through a limited incision and gives faster recovery and shorter hospital stay.
- A better flexion range is achievable.

There are some prerequisites for medial UKR (as applied to mobile bearing Oxford UKR):

- Correctable varus.
- Flexion to 110° or more.
- Fixed flexion deformity of less than 15°.
- Intact ACL.
- Intact lateral compartment.
- Non-inflammatory arthritis.

On radiography, the standing AP view will show the loss of medial joint space and a varus alignment of the knee. Stress radiographs will show the varus is correctable. On the lateral radiograph, the erosion on the medial tibial plateau should be predominantly anterior, implying an intact ACL. An indistinct lip of the posterior articular surface indicates a dysfunctional ACL.

Results

> **Note**
>
> Pandit H, Jenkins C, Barker K, *et al.* The Oxford medial unicompartmental knee replacement using a minimally-invasive approach. *J Bone Joint Surg Br* 2006; 88: 54-60. **This study describes 688 Phase 3 medial UKRs. Follow-up was 100%. Nine out of 688 knees were revised, while 1% required another procedure (manipulation under anaesthesia, arthroscopy or debridement). Survival at 7 years was 97.3%. Mean flexion was 133°.**

Note

Steele RG, Hutabarat S, Evans RL, *et al.* Survivorship of the St Georg Sled medial unicompartmental knee replacement beyond ten years. *J Bone Joint Surg Br* 2006; 88: 1164-8. **This study looked at 203 implants at a mean of 14.8 years after surgery. Overall, 7.9% had been revised at 13 years. Survivorship was 85.9% at 20 years and 80% at 25 years.**

Note

Price AJ, Dodd CA, Svard UG, Murray DW. Oxford medial unicompartmental knee arthroplasty in patients younger and older than 60 years of age. *J Bone Joint Surg Br* 2005; 87: 1488-92. **The 10-year survival was 91% in patients younger than 60 years.**

Combined ACL reconstruction and unicompartmental knee replacement

In patients with an ACL-deficient knee and medial compartmental arthritis, a combination of ACL reconstruction and UKR is an option.

Note

Pandit H, Beard DJ, Jenkins C, *et al.* Combined anterior cruciate reconstruction and Oxford unicompartmental knee arthroplasty. *J Bone Joint Surg Br* 2006; 88: 887-92. **Fifteen patients with combined UKR and ACL reconstruction were matched with 15 patients with UKR and an intact ACL. A 2.5-year follow-up found no difference in Oxford score or functional knee score between the two groups.**

Survival of unicompartmental replacements

Conversion of UKR to TKR should be considered in patients with ongoing pain in the medial compartment or progression of arthritis in the remaining compartments in the knee.

Data from the New Zealand Joint Registry have shown that TKR after UKR has a four times higher revision rate compared to primary TKR.

Note

Pearse AJ, Hooper GJ, Rothwell A, Frampton C. Survival and functional outcome after revision of a unicompartmental to a total knee replacement: the New Zealand National Joint Registry. *J Bone Joint Surg Br* 2010; 92: 508-12. **From a total of 4,284 UKRs, 236 required revision: 205 were revised to a TKR and 31 had a further UKR. The patients who underwent TKR after UKR had a revision rate of 1.97 per 100 component years. The UKR to UKR revisions had the worst results, with 6.67 revisions per 100 component years. This was 13 times the revision rate for primary TKR.**

Patellofemoral replacement

TKR is an effective treatment for patellofemoral arthritis with satisfactory results in up to 90% patients. However, it is a more extensive operation than patellofemoral joint replacement. Replacement of the patellofemoral joint comprises a patellar button and trochlear component. The indications and contraindications are listed in Table 1.20.

A high Q angle should be treated with a realignment procedure prior to replacement.

ACL deficiency is not a contraindication

AP and lateral radiographs should be taken prior to the procedure. The skyline view is more useful for diagnosing patellofemoral arthritis and to assess the position of the patella in the trochlea.

Table 1.20. Indications and contraindications for patellofemoral joint replacement.

Indications	Contraindications
Selected patients with arthritis localised to the patellofemoral compartment	Tibiofemoral arthritis
	Inflammatory arthritis
Treatment of trochlear dysplasia	Significant maltracking of the patella or an excess Q angle (relative contraindication)

The following factors should be considered when choosing a patellofemoral implant:

- Sagittal radius of the curvature.
- Proximal extent of the trochlear flange.
- Mediolateral width of the implant.
- Degree of constraint.

Results

The early results following patellofemoral replacement in the carefully selected patient are encouraging. Long-term problems relate to loosening and progression of arthritis in the remaining knee, requiring conversion to TKR.

> **Note**
>
> Ackroyd CE, Chir B. Development and early results of a new patellofemoral arthroplasty. *Clin Orthop Relat Res* 2005; 436: 7-13. This study looked at 306 arthroplasties in 240 patients, with a 2-year follow-up for 124 knees and a 5-year follow-up for 33 knees. There was no deterioration in pain or function. Disease progressed in the tibiofemoral joint in 5% of knees, requiring revision in 3.6%. Persistent anterior pain was experienced in 4% of knees.

> **Note**
>
> Ackroyd CE, Newman JH, Evans R, *et al.* The Avon patellofemoral arthroplasty: five-year survivorship and functional results. *J Bone Joint Surg Br* 2007; 89: 310-15. A total of 109 knees in 85 patients were followed. No loosening was seen. The knees had 95.8% survival with revision as the endpoint. The success rate at 5 years was 80%, based on pain score. Radiological progression of arthritis was seen in 28%.

Bilateral knee replacement

Bilateral knee replacement is advocated if there is advanced arthritis in both knees. More importantly, a significant bilateral flexion deformity should be addressed by a bilateral simultaneous knee replacement to prevent recurrence of deformity after UKR. The safe time is considered to be either within the same anaesthetic or after a gap of 4-6 weeks, even though there is evidence to the contrary.

Note

Forster MC, Bauze AJ, Bailie AG, *et al*. A retrospective comparative study of bilateral total knee replacement staged at a one-week interval. *J Bone Joint Surg Br* 2006; 88: 1006-10. **Participants undergoing bilateral knee replacement were divided into three groups: replacement under the same anaesthetic; replacement after a 1-week interval in the same admission; and replacement under a separate admission. There was no difference between the three groups.**

Computer-aided knee replacement

The use of computer-aided surgery is becoming increasingly common in knee replacements to achieve better alignment compared with conventional jigs. Malalignment is a known factor leading to early failure.

Note

Bäthis H, Perlick L, Tingart M, *et al*. Alignment in total knee arthroplasty. A comparison of computer-assisted surgery with the conventional technique. *J Bone Joint Surg Br* 2004; 86: 682-7. **In this prospective study of 80 patients, the mechanical axis was better in the computer-assisted group (96% versus 78% within 3° varus/valgus).**

Revision knee replacement

Indications for revision TKR are as follows:

- Loosening (can be caused by wear-debris-induced osteolysis).
- Infection.
- Instability.
- Stiffness.
- Malaligned femoral or tibial components (can lead to accelerated wear, patellar instability, tibiofemoral instability or restricted ROM).

- Periprosthetic fractures around TKR in association with bone loss.

A painful knee replacement is commonly due to loosening or infection. The success rate of revision surgery is low if the cause of the pain is not evident.

Preoperative assessment

The history and examination focuses on identifying the specific problem. The hip and spine are potential sites of referred pain. Assessment should consider medical comorbidities, functional status, skin condition, extensor mechanism, ROM, instability, alignment and neurologic and vascular status.

Radiographs can help to determine the underlying problem. Full-length leg films are useful to check the limb alignment. The extent of bone loss is frequently underestimated on plain radiographs; oblique views help in visualising the bone loss in relation to the femoral condyles. Rotational malalignment and osteolysis is demonstrated well on CT scanning. Gallium and Tc-99m bone scans are sometimes used to detect septic or aseptic loosening.

Laboratory tests are primarily aimed at detecting infection and include CRP levels and ESR. Knee aspiration should be under strict asepsis and is useful for preoperative determination of any infecting organism.

Bone defects in revision total knee replacement

The final and most accurate assessment of bone loss can be made once the existing components have been removed. Table 1.21 outlines the Anderson Orthopaedic Research Institute classification of bone loss.

Reconstruction options in revision knee surgery

A useful strategy in reconstruction is to follow a stepwise approach:

- Restore the tibial articular surface.
- Restore the flexion gap. Correct sizing of the femoral implant, adjusting the rotation of the femoral component and soft tissue releases are performed at this stage.
- Match the extension gap to the flexion gap. This may require distal translation of the femoral

Table 1.21. The Anderson Orthopaedic Research Institute classification of bone loss.

Defect	Description
Type 1 (F1 and T1)	Healthy cancellous bone present to support the components
	Preserved metaphyseal bone distal to the femoral epicondyles (F1) and proximal to the fibular head (T1)
	Preserved level of joint line
	No osteolysis or component migration
Type 2 (F2 and T2)	Subsidence and migration of component
	Osteolysis at margins of component
	If only one femoral condyle or one side of the tibial plateau is involved, the defect is classified as F2A or T2A
	When both femoral condyles or both sides of the tibial plateau are involved, the defect is classified F2B or T2B
Type 3 (F3 and T3)	Large areas of osteolysis and gross migration of components
	Femoral epicondyles flare away from the femur
	Bone loss extends proximally to the femoral epicondyles or distally to the fibular head

component and the use of augments and stems to support the femoral component.

Managing bone loss

Small contained defects can be managed with a bone graft or cement. Small uncontained defects can be managed with a metal augment or structural bone graft. Large defects require allografts.

Stemmed implants

Both cemented and cementless stems are used. The stems achieve fixation in the metaphysis and diaphysis in situations where adequate support for the implant is lacking at the cancellous surface.

Very wide canals are better managed by cemented stems to avoid inserting a large-diameter cementless stem. Metaphyseal fixation is also easier with

cemented stems. Larger defects require longer stems and if fixation in the diaphysis is considered, cementless stems may be advantageous.

Non-replacement treatment for the osteoarthritic knee

Medication

NSAIDs and opioids are extensively used to alleviate pain from knee arthritis.

Oral glucosamine

Oral glucosamine has some benefit, although the degree of improvement is debatable. A recent report in the *British Medical Journal* showed no difference compared with placebo in terms of pain relief.

Note

Wandel S, Jüni P, Tendal B, *et al*. Effects of glucosamine, chondroitin, or placebo in patients with osteoarthritis of hip or knee: network meta-analysis. *BMJ* 2010; 341: c4675.

Intra-articular steroids

Steroids act by reducing neutrophil migration; reducing phagocytosis, lysosomal enzyme release and inflammatory mediator release; and increasing the hyaluronic acid concentration and viscosity of synovial fluid.

Triamcinolone is longest-acting and the least soluble steroid.

Side effects are suppression of the hypothalamic-pituitary axis, a reduced stress response to hypoglycaemia, steroid arthropathy (fibrillation, fissure and thinning of cartilage), patellar tendon rupture and osteonecrosis.

Intra-articular hyaluronic acid

Exogenous hyaluronic acid is incorporated into articular cartilage and may have a direct effect on chondrocytes through CD44 receptors.

Intra-articular hyaluronate is usually prescribed once a week for 3-5 weeks, although newer preparations allow a single injection. It is thought to improve chondrocyte density and reduce inflammation. It may have a role in active patients older than 60 years and with moderate arthritis.

Note

Akmal M, Singh A, Anand A, *et al*. The effects of hyaluronic acid on articular chondrocytes. *J Bone Joint Surg Br* 2005; 87: 1143-9. **This was an experimental study on bovine articular chondrocytes. Increased matrix deposition of chondroitin-6-sulphate and type II collagen was found in response to exposure to hyaluronic acid *in vitro*.**

Synovectomy

Synovectomy may be recommended for patients with rheumatoid arthritis, and is indicated if there is no loss of joint space and no deformity. It leads to joint swelling and recovery is slow. The good short-term results of synovectomy deteriorate with time, but this treatment does help to remove mechanical blocks to motion and debris.

Arthroscopic synovectomy is associated with 83% improved outcome at 3 years, while 46% of patients report improvement at 8 years. Recovery is faster with the arthroscopic procedure.

Valgus bracing

Valgus bracing may be used to reduce the load on the medial compartment. It is indicated for active patients with unicompartmental disease who are considered too young for replacement.

Arthroscopic lavage

A study has shown some benefit for arthroscopic debridement. From 110 patients who were followed up for 34 months after the procedure, 90% of patients with mild arthritis, normal alignment and more than 3mm joint space were improved after arthroscopy. However, only 25% of knees with severe arthritis and less than 2mm joint space showed improvement.

Note

Aaron RK, Skolnick AH, Reinert SE, Ciombor DM. Arthroscopic debridement for arthritis of the knee. *J Bone Joint Surg Am* 2006; 88: 936-43. **This study followed 110 patients for 34 months after arthroscopic debridement. Overall, 90% of patients with mild arthritis, normal alignment and more than 3mm joint space experienced improvements after arthroscopy, while only 25% of knees with severe arthritis and less than 2mm joint space showed improvement.**

Osteotomy

A normal mechanical axis drawn from the centre of the hip to the centre of the ankle passes the medial to tibial spines. In HTO, the mechanical axis is shifted

Table 1.22. Indications and contraindication for high tibial osteotomy.

Indications	Contraindications
Age <60 years	Loss of joint space on the lateral side
Single-compartment arthritis	Lateral tibial subluxation >1cm
10-15° varus	Medial compartment loss >2-3mm
90° ROM	Ligamentous instability
Flexion contracture <15°	Inflammatory arthritis

laterally such that it passes through the lateral compartment, hence offloading the medial compartment.

Indications and contraindications for HTO are shown in Table 1.22.

Varus knees undergo a varus thrust during weight bearing and this will not correct with HTO. Overcorrection by 3-5° helps to offload the medial compartment. A medial opening wedge or lateral closing wedge can be performed. The maximum thickness of the wedge can be calculated with the following equation:

$$\text{Maximum wedge thickness} = 0.02 \times (\text{diameter of plateau}) \times (\text{angle of correction})$$

By this method, assuming the diameter of the tibia at the level of the osteotomy is 56mm, a 1mm wedge corresponds to a 1° correction.

The following problems may occur with TKR after HTO:

- Patella infera (in 80% of cases).
- Patellar maltracking.
- Offset of the tibial plateau from the shaft.
- Skin incisions.

Patella infera can be avoided with a biplanar osteotomy, which exits below the level of the tibial tubercle.

Supracondylar osteotomy
Supracondylar osteotomy has the following indications:

- Isolated lateral compartment arthritis.
- A tibiofemoral angle of more than 12°.
- A valgus joint-line tilt of more than 10°.
- 90° ROM.
- Less than 10° flexion contracture.

The aim is to correct to a tibiofemoral angle of 4-6°.

A medial closing wedge or lateral opening wedge is performed. A 90° fixed-angle blade plate or locking plate on the lateral side is used to stabilise the osteotomy.

Subchondral drilling
In subchondral drilling, 2.5mm drill holes are made. This leads to a clot with stem cells that can undergo metaplasia to fibrocartilage.

Microfracture
In microfracture an awl is used to penetrate the subchondral bone, making three to four holes per square centimetre. Microfracture is indicated for full-thickness lesions in weight-bearing areas. The cartilage fragments are debrided. Patients undergo postoperative continuous passive motion and touch weight bearing.

Mosaicplasty
In mosaicplasty, osteochondral plugs are taken from non-articular areas such as the lateral portion of

the distal femur and the intercondylar notch. These areas, however, may not be totally free of pressure.

Plugs are 2.5mm long and 2.7-8.5mm wide. This technique leads to hyaline cartilage in the plugs with interspersed fibrous repair tissue.

Autologous chondrocyte implantation

In autologous chondrocyte implantation, a 12×5mm specimen of the articular cartilage, containing about 250,000 cells, is taken from the superior aspect of the medial femoral condyle. It is then cultured for 3 weeks to make 12 million cells. These are replanted and covered with a periosteal flap harvested from the medial tibia. Fibrin glue can be used to suture surfaces.

Continuous passive motion 6-8 hours/day for 6 weeks and toe-touch weight bearing for 6 weeks are recommended. Full weight bearing is allowed by 12 weeks. Patients can take part in non-impact activities after 6-9 months and impact activities after 9-12 months. This is further discussed in Chapter 3 (Sports medicine).

Total shoulder replacement

Charles Neer is credited with the development of modern techniques for shoulder replacement. Initially, humeral head replacement was designed for proximal humeral fractures; as good results were obtained, the scope was extended to arthritis of the shoulder.

The first replacement of the humeral head was performed by Neer using a Vitallium prosthesis in 1951. Glenoid components were developed in the early 1970s to improve shoulder biomechanics and function. Stability, restoration of version, balance of soft tissues and tension in the soft tissues are critical to good function.

Anatomical relationships

Humeral head
The average curvature of the humeral head is 24mm and the average thickness is 19mm. The absolute values vary in different patients, but the inter-relationship of these two variables is relatively constant at a ratio of 0.7-0.9.

The humeral head is retroverted by 10-55°; the average is approximately 30°.

The superior extent of the humeral head lies 8-10mm superior to the highest point of the greater tuberosity. The centre of rotation of the humeral head is medial and posterior to the axis of the humeral shaft.

The neck shaft angle is described as the angle between the axis of the humeral shaft and the base of the articular fragment. The angle is 40-45°.

Glenoid
The glenoid is pear-shaped (wider inferiorly). The articular cartilage is thin at the centre and thicker at the periphery. This makes the glenoid articular surface more concave to match the convexity of the humeral head. The bony glenoid is relatively flat. The radius of curvature of the humeral head is 2-3mm less than the radius of curvature of the glenoid.

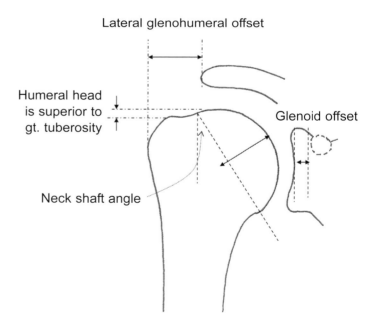

Figure 1.19. Anatomical relationships of bony landmarks around the shoulder.

Glenoid offset is the perpendicular distance between the deepest part of the glenoid and the lateral aspect of the base of the coracoid. Lateral glenohumeral offset is the perpendicular distance between the lateral border of the greater tuberosity and the lateral aspect of the base of the coracoid process. If this distance is reduced then the lever arm of the deltoid is also reduced, impairing abduction power. If the distance is increased following replacement then the joint is overstuffed, resulting in loss of movement.

Glenoid depth is the percentage of humeral head that is covered by the glenoid and labrum. It is approximately 28% on average.

Figure 1.19 displays the anatomical relationships of bony landmarks around the shoulder.

Table 1.23. The result of humeral component malpositioning.

Humeral component malpositioning	Effect on function
Anterior overhang of humeral head	Excess tension on the subscapularis
	Posterior impingement of uncovered metaphysis on the glenoid
Oversizing the humeral head	Increase in the lateral glenohumeral offset
	Tightening of the soft tissue envelope
	Reduction in the range of motion
	Rupture of the subscapularis
Undersizing the humeral head	Reduction of the lever arm of the deltoid
	Internal impingement of the humerus and cuff on the glenoid
	Instability
Inferior positioning of the humeral head	Prominence of the greater tuberosity
	Impingement of the greater tuberosity against the acromion
Varus stem alignment	Head will be medial and inferior
	Overstuffed joint
	Increased lateral glenohumeral offset
	Greater tuberosity may be prominent and impinge on the acromion
Valgus stem positioning	Head will be superior and laterally placed
Retroversion of the head	Posterior instability
	Rotator cuff rupture
Anteversion of the head	Loss of external rotation

Component design in total shoulder replacement

Humeral component design

The humeral head should be reconstructed close to its anatomical shape and size. The perpendicular distance between the lateral margin of the acromion and the lateral aspect of the greater tuberosity is an indicator of restoration of offset.

Modular heads enable different head sizes to be matched to different stems to achieve the best fit. Any overhang of the humeral head either anteriorly or posteriorly should be avoided (Table 1.23).

An offset humeral head matches the normal anatomy better than components where the centre of the humeral head is in line with the humeral shaft axis. This is because the anatomical humeral head centre is medial and posterior to the axis of the humeral shaft. Proximal cementation of the stem seems to work as well as full cementation.

Glenoid component design

The bony glenoid is pear-shaped and hence a prosthetic pear-shaped glenoid will achieve maximum bone cover and bone support. An oval glenoid will overhang anterosuperiorly and anteroinferiorly, and pressure from the humeral head in these areas may lead to loosening. In addition, a pear-shaped glenoid allows greater ROM before internal impingement occurs compared with an oval glenoid.

Adequate bone support of the glenoid component is important for better survival. Concentric reaming is used to improve contact.

Non-contained defects in the glenoid rim require augmentation by bone graft or metal augments. Cement does not function well in non-contained defects.

Metal-backed glenoid components tend to increase the thickness of the component, which can lateralise the joint line and weaken the abductor lever arm. If a metal-backed component is chosen, more reaming of the glenoid may be required. There is a risk of dissociation of polyethylene from the metal backing.

Cemented all-poly glenoid components are the most commonly used. Multiple small pegs are preferred to counter the shear stress. Keeled components are an option in rheumatoid arthritis and these tend to compensate, to some extent, increased shear forces due to the absence of the rotator cuff.

Erosion of the posterior margin of the glenoid may occur in osteoarthritis. Hemiarthroplasty performed in patients with posterior glenoid erosion has a less satisfactory outcome.

Types of shoulder replacement prostheses

There are several types of prostheses:

- Unconstrained – no constraint between the humeral head and the glenoid. This group includes Neer-type shoulder replacements and cup arthroplasty.
- Semiconstrained – this group includes hooded glenoid components, which provide some constraint to humeral head movement. Examples are the Neer hooded replacement and DANA (Designed after Natural Anatomy).
- Constrained ball and socket – the glenoid is specially designed to capture the humeral head and improve stability. Disadvantages include breakage and loosening.
- Constrained reverse ball and socket – the ball is mounted on the glenoid and the socket is placed on the humeral head.

Indications

The following are indications for shoulder replacement:

- Osteoarthritis.
- Rheumatoid arthritis.
- Traumatic arthritis.
- Osteonecrosis (Table 1.24).
- Rotator cuff arthropathy.

Table 1.24. Stages of osteonecrosis of the humeral head.	
Stage	**Description**
1	No changes on plain radiographs
2	Sclerosis and remodelling of the humeral head; shape of head maintained
3	Subchondral collapse resulting in loss of sphericity
4	Collapse of the articular surface
5	Arthritic changes in the glenoid

Contraindications

The following are contraindications for shoulder replacement:

- Active infection.
- Loss of both deltoid and rotator cuff function.
- Gross instability.
- Massive rotator cuff tear is a contraindication for glenoid replacement.

Surgical aspects

Several surgical aspects should be considered prior to shoulder replacement:

- Soft tissue balance – the soft tissues must be balanced to provide optimum function. Rotator cuff tear repair, release of capsular contractures and plication of capsular laxity may be required.
- Patients with osteoarthritis may have osteophytes on the humeral head. These can lead to capsular distension, which will require capsular reefing.
- Release of the subscapularis or Z lengthening may be needed for contractures.

- Patients with rheumatoid arthritis generally require cemented components due to osteopenia.
- The outcome in patients with post-traumatic arthritis is less satisfactory due to soft tissue scarring and malunited proximal humeral fractures.

Glenoid replacement in shoulder osteoarthritis

Advantages:

- More reliable pain relief, especially if glenoid erosion is noted at the time of shoulder surgery. If the glenoid articular surface does not exhibit significant erosion at the time of surgery, the results of hemiarthroplasty are comparable to total shoulder replacement (TSR).

Disadvantages:

- Technically difficult – the glenoid is often retroverted with posterior erosion and it requires reaming of the anterior rim to provide circumferential bone support.
- Excess retroversion of the replaced component may predispose to posterior instability.
- In relatively young, high-demand patients, there is a high risk of loosening and glenoid replacement should be avoided.
- Osteolysis from polyethylene debris can lead to loosening of the glenoid component with consequent risk of failure.
- Limitations on the activities allowed.
- Increases operative time and blood loss.

Indications for hemiarthroplasty

Hemiarthroplasty is indicated in young patients with preserved glenoid anatomy; in patients with massive rotator cuff tears; and where there is inadequate bone for achieving glenoid component fixation.

Note

Radnay CS, Setter KJ, Chambers L, *et al.* Total shoulder replacement compared with humeral head replacement for the treatment of primary glenohumeral arthritis: a systematic review. *J Shoulder Elbow Surg* 2007; 16: 396-402. **This review of 23 studies looked at 1,952 patients with a mean follow-up of 43 months. TSR provided better pain relief, forward elevation, external rotation and patient satisfaction. The revision rate of TSR was 6.5%, compared to 10.2% for humeral head replacement.**

Shoulder replacement in rotator cuff tears

The absence of a functioning rotator cuff causes the humeral head to migrate superiorly and put pressure on the superior rim of the glenoid. This edge loading, known as the 'rocking horse phenomenon' is a factor in early loosening of the glenoid component.

TSR should be avoided in individuals with rotator cuff tears unless the cuff tear is reparable. A shoulder hemiarthroplasty obviates the possibility of glenoid loosening.

Hemiarthroplasty is possibly the most viable option. The prosthetic humeral head depends on the intact coracoacromial arch to prevent unrestricted upward migration and a functioning deltoid is essential.

The reverse shoulder prosthesis (described next) is an option for patients with massive cuff tears.

The reverse shoulder prosthesis

Developed in France in the 1980s based on a concept by Professor Grammont, the reverse shoulder prosthesis (also known as the Delta shoulder) is a semiconstrained implant.

In the reverse shoulder prosthesis, the centre of rotation is in the scapula. The humeral head is a socket instead of a ball. The convex articular surface (ball) is mounted on the scapula. Hence, the centre of rotation is more medial.

These prostheses have been used in patients with large rotator cuff tears in an effort to reduce the shear forces on the glenoid and improve the lever arm for muscle forces.

Note

Matsen FA 3rd, Boileau P, Walch G, *et al.* The reverse total shoulder arthroplasty. *J Bone Joint Surg Am* 2007; 89: 660-7.

Replacement of both shoulder and elbow in rheumatoid arthritis

In a study with a long follow-up, TSR in patients with rheumatoid disease resulted in preserved ROM and no pain in most patients after a mean of 20 years.

Note

Betts HM, Abu-Rajab R, Nunn T, Brooksbank AJ. Total shoulder replacement in rheumatoid disease: a 16- to 23-year follow-up. *J Bone Joint Surg Br* 2009; 91: 1197-200. **Fifty-eight shoulders were followed for 19.8 years. Most patients had preserved movement range and no pain.**

The humeral components of the shoulder and elbow replacement should either both have short stems, or the cement mantle of the shoulder humeral stem should be in continuity with the cement column of the humeral component of the elbow replacement. With short stems, a gap of 6cm is desirable between the two cement columns to prevent a stress riser.

Complications of total shoulder replacement

Early complications

Instability
Instability can be due to poor component alignment, poor soft tissue repair or deficient bone stock.

Infection
The routine use of perioperative prophylaxis is recommended.

Gram-negative organisms causing acute infection may be managed by debridement and washout with retention of components.

Late infection is haematogenous and the presence of Gram-negative organisms necessitates removal of the prosthetic joint. A two-stage revision with use of antibiotic-loaded cement is considered to be the most reliable method of managing infection.

Impingement
Impingement can occur with improper sizing or positioning of components. An inferiorly placed humeral component will lead to impingement of the greater tuberosity against the acromion.

Humeral fracture
Patients have a less than 1% risk of humeral fracture. Fractures of the humeral shaft are more often intraoperative as opposed to postoperative. Excess force of external rotation on the arm to gain exposure or excess force while reaming or pressurising cement are common causes of humerus shaft fractures.

The removal of well-cemented humeral stems can be difficult and may lead to iatrogenic fracture.

If detected intraoperatively, fractures around the stem should be stabilised with struts and cerclage wires or by using a long stem implant. Fractures distal to the tip of the stem can be managed by plate fixation.

Glenoid fractures are rare and are caused by retraction or over-reaming in osteoporotic bone. Bone grafting is an option.

Nerve injury
Most nerve injuries are neurapraxias (usually neurapraxia of the brachial plexus due to stretching) and should be followed up with electromyography to monitor recovery. Direct injuries to the axillary nerve, radial nerve (in patients with humeral shaft fracture) and musculocutaneous nerve are also reported, albeit rarely.

Late complications

Loosening of humeral component
There is generally a low risk of loosening causing clinical symptoms (1-2%), and cemented and cementless components have similar survival.

Radiolucent lines around stems are more common around cementless stems than cemented stems, but do not necessarily indicate loosening. The subsidence rate of cementless stems is higher than that of cemented stems.

Causes of glenoid loosening include humeral head translation leading to glenoid edge loading. This may be evident radiographically as progressive lucency, migration of the component, fracture of cement and lucency at the prosthesis-cement interface. Asymptomatic radiolucent lines are not an indication in themselves for revision.

Radiolucent lines
Radiolucent lines are seen in two-thirds of glenoid components in the early postoperative period. Despite this high incidence, clinical failure of the glenoid component is relatively rare.

Instability
Instability may be early or late. Table 1.25 outlines the directions and causes of instability.

Table 1.25. Directions and causes of instability.

Direction of instability	Cause
Anterior	Subscapularis rupture (most common cause) Anteverted humeral component Rupture of anterior fibres of deltoid Oversized humeral head
Posterior	Rupture of rotator cuff Retroverted humerus or glenoid Laxity of posterior capsule
Superior	Rupture of rotator cuff Unopposed pull of deltoid against weak rotator cuff Deficient coracoacromial arch
Inferior	Deltoid dysfunction Inferior placement of the humeral head Excess removal of proximal humerus

Rotator cuff tears

Rotator cuff tears occur in approximately 2% of patients after TSR. Small tears are managed by standard techniques. Large tears should be repaired if possible to avoid loosening of the glenoid component. Irreparable large tears may require removal of the glenoid component and bone grafting of the glenoid.

Wear

Glenoid polyethylene components are subject to surface wear as well as to fatigue failure.

Heterotopic ossification

HO is seen in up to 40% of patients after TSR. Generally the ossification is not severe enough to restrict movements or require removal of the prosthesis.

Stiffness

Stiffness can be due to oversized components or poor soft tissue balance. Lengthening the subscapularis improves the range of external rotation.

Periprosthetic humeral fractures

There are three types of periprosthetic humeral fracture:

- Type A – extends proximally from the tip of the prosthesis.
- Type B – fractures around the tip of the humeral stem.
- Type C – fractures distal to the tip of the humeral stem.

Type A fractures are likely to require revision of the humeral component. Type B and C fractures can be managed non-operatively if adequate alignment is achieved, or by open reduction and internal fixation.

Revision total shoulder replacement

Loosening of the glenoid component is managed by removal of the glenoid component. In patients with an intact rotator cuff and good bone stock, it may be possible to implant another glenoid component.

Revision of the humeral component may be needed in patients with infection or loosening. Removal of a well-fixed humeral component carries the risk of loss of bone stock of the proximal humerus; accepting a malpositioned component and taking advantage of modularity is an option.

Resection replacement of the shoulder

Resection replacement is indicated in patients with persistent infection or inadequate bone stock for revision.

Loss of the fulcrum of the shoulder leads to loss of abduction and results are generally unsatisfactory.

Total elbow replacement

Anatomy

The centre of rotation of the elbow lies along a line connecting the centre of the capitellum and the trochlea. The axes of the humeroulnar and radiohumeral joints coincide.

The centre of rotation for the elbow joint lies in line with the anterior border of the humeral shaft. The carrying angle is higher in extension and reduced as the elbow flexes.

Types of elbow joint replacement

Implants for elbow replacements can be grouped into three types:

- Constrained.
- Semiconstrained.
- Unconstrained.

Constrained prostheses transfer high stress to the implant cement and cement-bone interface, leading to early loosening and failure. These are metal-to-metal articulations with a hinge for movement. There is no varus-valgus allowance at the hinge, and these prostheses are also known as 'fixed hinge'.

Semiconstrained prostheses have a metal-to-polyethylene articulation. Due to dissipation of forces at the articulation the stress transfer to the fixation interface is limited, enabling longer survival. These prostheses allow some degree of varus and valgus movement and hence are called 'sloppy hinge'. An example is the Coonrad-Morrey replacement. The Coonrad-Morrey prosthesis has titanium stems for the humerus and elbow, and the articulation allows 7° of varus-valgus and rotary motion.

Unconstrained implants are usually metal and polyethylene articulations with no actual mechanism to connect the two parts together. These implants rely on intact ligaments and an anterior capsule for stability and generally need adequate bone stock to achieve fixation. They are prone to dislocation, subluxation and transient nerve palsies.

Interposition replacement of the elbow has been attempted in the past, but results were generally poor. Complications included instability, bone resorption, heterotopic bone formation and rupture of the triceps. Currently, interposition replacement of the elbow can be considered for young patients with post-traumatic arthritis of the elbow.

Resection replacement of the elbow is a further option, but problems of instability limit its use. The exception is in patients with infection of an elbow replacement where reconstructive surgery is not considered feasible.

Indications for total elbow replacement

Total elbow replacement is indicated in patients with pain, instability or ankylosis. It can be considered in several clinical conditions:

- Osteoarthritis.
- Rheumatoid arthritis.
- Juvenile rheumatoid arthritis.
- Traumatic arthritis.
- Tumours or trauma leading to loss of bone stock.
- Comminuted distal humeral fractures in the elderly.

Note

Garcia JA, Mykula R, Stanley D. Complex fractures of the distal humerus in the elderly. The role of total elbow replacement as primary treatment. *J Bone Joint Surg Br* 2002; 84: 812-6. In this study, 19 patients were treated with a Coonrad-Morrey prosthesis. The mean age was 73 years and the mean follow-up was 3 years. Of these patients, 68% had no pain and the mean flexion arc was 24-125°. Fifteen patients were satisfied.

Contraindications

Contraindications to elbow replacement include the following:

- Ongoing sepsis (the main contraindication).
- Neurotrophic joint.
- Ankylosis of the ipsilateral shoulder.
- Excess bone loss.
- Lack of functioning musculature.

Complications

Complications include infection, loosening, instability, dislocation or uncoupling of components and fracture of the components.

Loosening of components is a greater problem with constrained than with the semiconstrained implants. Migration of components or a complete radiolucent line at the cement-bone interface indicates loosening.

Other complications include nerve paraesthesias, iatrogenic fracture (commonly humeral condyles), stiffness and wound problems.

Management of failed elbow replacement

Options for managing a failed elbow replacement include resection arthroplasty, elbow arthrodesis or revision elbow arthroplasty.

Early postoperative infection may be treated with debridement with preservation of the implant. Chronic infection indicates resection arthroplasty or arthrodesis.

Note

Gille J, Ince A, González O, *et al.* Single-stage revision of peri-prosthetic infection following total elbow replacement. *J Bone Joint Surg Br* 2006; 88: 1341-6. Of 305 primary total elbow replacements, deep infection occurred in six. In all six cases, the patients had rheumatoid arthritis and had been on steroids. Five had no recurrence of infection following revision. The sixth patient had resection arthroplasty. Function was good in three elbows.

Results of elbow replacement

Elbow replacements function well and have reliable results in most patients. Loosening is the long-term issue that limits survival of the prosthesis.

Note

Talwalkar SC, Givissis PK, Trail IA, *et al.* Survivorship of the Souter-Strathclyde elbow replacement in the young inflammatory arthritis elbow. *J Bone Joint Surg Br* 2005; 87: 946-9. A total of 309 patients were divided into two groups by age. At 16 years, patients younger than 50 years had 74% survival compared with 85% for those older than 50 years.

Note

Shi LL, Zurakowski D, Jones DG, *et al.* Semiconstrained primary and revision total elbow arthroplasty with use of the Coonrad-Morrey prosthesis. *J Bone Joint Surg Am* 2007; 89: 1467-75. Sixty-seven implants in 56 patients were studied. Patients had excellent pain relief and a good functional return. The 5-year survival was 64%.

Chapter 2 Shoulder disorders

Shoulder problems can broadly be grouped into three clinical presentations:

- The unstable shoulder.
- The painful shoulder.
- The painful stiff shoulder.

The diagnostic and treatment issues are discussed on the basis of these presentations.

The unstable shoulder

The shoulder joint is inherently unstable, with a head that is significantly larger than the glenoid. Shoulder stability is maintained by a complex interplay of static and dynamic factors.

Static stabilisers

There are three static shoulder stabilisers:

- Bony anatomy.
- Labrum and articular cartilage.
- Ligaments.

Bony anatomy

The glenoid is shallow and slightly concave and, on its own, cannot afford stability to the spherical humeral head. The glenoid is pear-shaped, being wider inferiorly. It is about 25mm at its widest, compared to the humeral head size of 45-48mm. The glenoid is retroverted by about 3-7° in 75% of people and anteverted mildly in others, with a superior tilt of 3° in most people. The humeral head is usually retroverted at 20-30° (Figure 2.1).

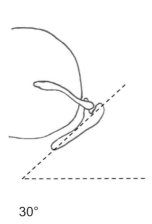
30°

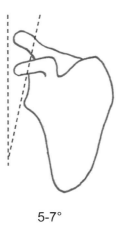
5-7°

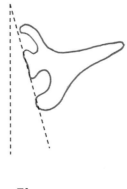
7°

Figure 2.1. The anatomical orientation of the glenoid.

Labrum and articular cartilage

The articular cartilage is thicker at the edge, which helps to increase the concavity of the bony glenoid; the glenoid labrum increases this concavity further by 5-9mm. This improves the congruence of the joint. The superior labrum and biceps attachment also contributes to the stability and conformity of the joint. Lesions of the superior labrum increase the anteroposterior (AP) translation of the humeral head.

Ligaments

The ligaments include the superior, middle and inferior glenohumeral ligaments. These ligaments are in tension in different ranges of motion and act to centre the humeral head in extremes of motion. They do not, however, contribute significantly to stability in the normal arc of motion (Figure 2.2).

The superior glenohumeral ligament (SGHL) is a thin structure running anterosuperiorly from the

The rotator interval is a capsular interval between the superior edge of the subscapularis and the anterior edge of the supraspinatus tendon. It can be stretched and enlarged in a lax shoulder or as part of multidirectional instability. The SGHL and coracohumeral ligament lie in the rotator interval.

The rotator interval is tight in external rotation. Therefore, external rotation should abolish the sulcus sign. A positive sulcus sign in external rotation implies a lax rotator interval.

> **Note**
>
> Harryman DT, Sidles JA, Harris SL, Matsen FA. The role of the rotator interval capsule in passive motion and stability of the shoulder. *J Bone Joint Surg Am* 1992; 74: 53-66.

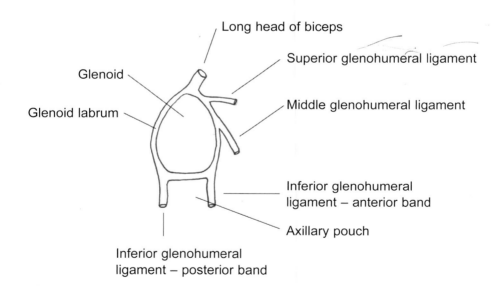

Figure 2.2. The arrangement of the ligaments around the glenoid.

glenoid to the lesser tuberosity. It is augmented by the coracohumeral ligament, which runs from the lateral aspect of the coracoid to the lesser and greater tuberosity. The SGHL helps to prevent inferior translation of the adducted arm.

The middle glenohumeral ligament is a much stronger thickening in the capsule. It runs from the anterosuperior glenoid and labrum to the humerus at the lesser tuberosity. It is a prime stabiliser against anterior dislocation in abduction and external rotation.

The inferior glenohumeral ligament has an anterior and posterior band. The anterior band runs from the anteroinferior aspect of the labrum to the humeral neck, just below the middle glenohumeral ligament attachment. It prevents inferior translation of the arm both in adduction and abduction and, being a hammock under the head in abduction, moves reciprocally and prevents anterior or posterior translation of the humeral head.

> ### Note
>
> O'Brien SJ, Neves MC, Arnoczky SP, *et al.* The anatomy and histology of the inferior glenohumeral ligament complex of the shoulder. *Am J Sports Med* 1990; 18: 449-56.

Physical properties

Additionally, physical properties of the shoulder joint help to stabilise it. These include the following:

- The negative suction effect.
- Surface tension effect of the fluid film on smooth surfaces.
- A vacuum effect to a distracting force.

Dynamic stabilisers

Dynamic stabilisers are as follows:

- Rotator cuff.
- Scapular stabilisers.
- Biceps long head.

Rotator cuff and scapular stabilisers

Dynamic stabilisers include both the rotator cuff muscles and the scapular stabilisers. The prime amongst these are the deltoid, trapezius, pectoralis major, serratus anterior and latissimus dorsi. These act differentially to centre the humeral head and give rise to concavity compression (i.e., the ball is compressed and thus centred into the concavity by the muscle action). Proprioceptive feedback from capsular stretching is vital for this muscle action and

control of stability. Neural pathway integrity is essential for this action.

Biceps long head

The long head of the biceps tendon attaches adjacent to the superior lip of the glenoid and courses superior to the humeral head. This provides superior stability to the glenohumeral joint.

Classification of shoulder instability

Instability by definition is symptomatic glenohumeral translation and the clinical tests may be sometimes difficult to reproduce and elicit. In occult instability tests may yield no definite answers, and there may be no obvious cause for pain in the young patient. Equally, diagnosis of a superior labral anterior and posterior (SLAP) lesion may be difficult and there is the dilemma of whether laxity contributes to it. Laxity is a normal characteristic of the shoulder joint and its contribution to instability, if any, is often difficult to determine.

There are two broad groups of shoulder instability:

- Traumatic:
  - anterior (acute or recurrent);
  - posterior (acute or chronic);
  - inferior (luxatio erecta).
- Atraumatic multidirectional instability:
  - voluntary (asymptomatic);
  - acquired (structural – anteroinferior capsular stretch).

Matsen proposed a widely used classification that describes two types of instability: TUBS and AMBRI. These are useful reminders as to the pathogenesis and management:

- TUBS is instability that is **T**raumatic, **U**nidirectional and with a **B**ankart lesion that is treated by **S**urgery.
- AMBRI is instability that is **A**traumatic, **M**ultidirectional and often **B**ilateral. The mainstay of treatment is physiotherapy and **R**ehabilitation. Surgery is rarely required in the form of **I**nferior capsular shift.

This classification is no longer used, however, because the problem is more complex than the acronyms suggest.

The Stanmore group has emphasised that instability at presentation is a spectrum of disorders. Specific polar groups are organised at the apices of a triangle, with many patients falling on the slope between polar groups (Figure 2.3). The polar groups are as follows:

- Traumatic structural – for example, anterior dislocation with a Perthes-Bankart lesion.
- Atraumatic structural – such as in patients who stretch their capsule in overhead sport, with a wide rotator interval.
- Muscle patterning – patients with an overactive scapular stabiliser, which destabilises the shoulder articulation due to asynchronous contraction.

A summary of the classification of shoulder instability is shown in Table 2.1.

Scapular dyskinesias

The glenoid can be positioned in space depending on the arm position. This contributes to large

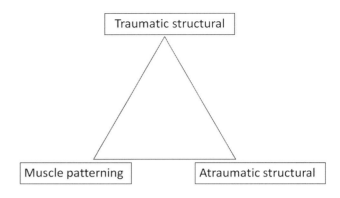

Figure 2.3. The Stanmore concept of shoulder instability.

excursions of the arm in space, as compared with any other body part. Scapular dyskinesia is the abnormal position or movement of the scapula in movement of the shoulder, and occurs in nearly all patients with instability or impingement. The effects include loss of protraction and retraction; loss of elevation; and loss of the kinetic chain:

- Loss of protraction and retraction – protraction is necessary for decelerating in throwing, and

Table 2.1. Summary of the classification of shoulder instability.

Degree	Frequency	Aetiology	Direction
Dislocation	Acute (primary)	Traumatic (macrotrauma)	Unidirectional: • Anterior
Subluxation	Chronic: • Recurrent	Atraumatic: • Voluntary (muscular) • Involuntary (positional)	• Posterior • Inferior
Subtle	• Fixed		Bidirectional: • Anteroinferior • Posteroinferior
		Acquired (microtrauma)	
		Congenital	Multidirectional
		Neuromuscular (Erb's palsy, cerebral palsy, seizures)	

retraction is required for cocking in abduction and external rotation.

- Loss of elevation – elevation of the scapula is by the action of serratus anterior muscle through the inferior angle of the scapula and with the lower fibres of the trapezius. Loss of elevation of the scapula causes the acromion to impinge on the rotator cuff.
- Loss of the kinetic chain – here, dyskinesia prevents the transmission of forces from the trunk and lower extremities, leading to abnormal glenohumeral stresses.

Treatment of dyskinesias should include correcting abnormalities of the lower extremities and trunk. Correcting posture and strengthening the trunk are the first elements to be addressed in the kinetic chain, followed by the scapular and the shoulder musculature.

Treatment of correctable pathologies in the shoulder (e.g., labral tears) should precede addressing scapular stabilisers.

Anterior dislocation

Pathology
Anterior dislocation is the most common presentation of shoulder instability. There is often a history of trauma, with the shoulder requiring relocation. The mechanism of injury usually involves excess external rotation and abduction. Anterior dislocation is often the result of a sporting injury in the young adult, or may be caused by a fall.

In the young adult, shoulder dislocation is associated with a risk of recurrence. Patients younger than 20 years have nearly a 100% recurrence rate, reflecting their level of activity as well as the severity of structural lesions such as large bony Bankart lesions, capsular tears and rotator cuff tears.

> **Note**
>
> Wheeler JH, Ryan JB, Arciero RA, Molinari RN. Arthroscopic versus non-operative treatment of acute shoulder dislocations in young athletes. *Arthroscopy* 1989; 5: 213-7.

Recurrent dislocations carry a risk of ongoing damage to the shoulder. The most important of these is the Bankart lesion (also known as Perthes-Bankart lesion), which is an anteroinferior labral tear that is found in 95% of patients with first-time traumatic anterior dislocation. In 40% of patients the Bankart lesion is associated with a bony avulsion of a fragment of the glenoid, which in more severe cases can lead to glenoid deficiency. Some Bankart lesions (anterior labral periosteal sleeve avulsion [ALPSA]) take a periosteal sleeve with them from the anterior glenoid margin. ALPSA predisposes to recurrent dislocation.

> **Note**
>
> Bankart AS. Recurrent or habitual dislocation of the shoulder joint. *BMJ* 1923; 2: 1132-3.

> **Note**
>
> Taylor DC, Arciero RA. Pathologic changes associated with shoulder dislocations. Arthroscopic and physical examination findings in first-time, traumatic anterior dislocations. *Am J Sports Med* 1997; 25: 306-11. **In this prospective observational study, 97% of patients younger than 24 years with traumatic anterior shoulder dislocation had a Bankart lesion, 22% had an osseous glenoid rim fracture, 10% had a SLAP lesion and none had a rotator cuff tear.**

Another consistent pathology is the Hill-Sachs lesion on the posterosuperior humeral head due to indentation of the humeral head on the anteroinferior glenoid. Large Hill-Sachs lesions, above 30% of the humeral head, will cause recurrence despite anterior repair (engaging Hill-Sachs) and will need intervention to prevent recurrence.

More severe and recurrent injuries leave an anteroinferior capsular redundancy, humeral avulsion of the glenohumeral ligament (HAGL) and SLAP lesions. Capsular deficiency is usually demonstrable in recurrent dislocations. The 'drive-through sign' on arthroscopy indicates laxity and may also be present in SLAP lesions due to anterior pseudolaxity.

In chronic situations, an inverted pear glenoid may be seen.

A subset of athletes, especially climbers and those who require overhead use of the arm, develop subtle or occult instability. It is believed that repetitive microtrauma produces inferior glenohumeral ligament stretching, which leads to instability. These patients have secondary impingement at presentation.

Note

Tibone J, Jobe F, Kerlan R, *et al.* Shoulder impingement syndrome in athletes treated by anterior acromioplasty. *Clin Orthop Relat Res* 1985; 198: 134-40.

Older people (>40 years) who dislocate have a propensity to damage the rotator cuff and experience neurologic sequelae. This is usually axillary nerve damage, but can also be a brachial plexus injury.

Note

Neviaser RJ, Neviaser TJ, Neviaser JS. Anterior dislocation of the shoulder and rotator cuff rupture. *Clin Orthop Relat Res* 1993; 291: 103-6.

Chronic anterior dislocation is sometimes seen in elderly patients, patients with multiple trauma and patients with impaired cognition.

Natural history

The risk of recurrence is 95% in patients younger than 20 years and 60% in those aged between 20 and 25 years. In the general population, exercise reduces recurrence risk in only 16% of patients.

Note

te Slaa RL, Wijffels MP, Brand R, Marti RK. The prognosis following acute primary glenohumeral dislocation. *J Bone Joint Surg Br* 2004; 86: 58-64. **This study included 105 patients with 107 acute, first-time shoulder dislocations. The overall probability of recurrence was 26%. Age was a factor, with a 64% risk of recurrence in those younger than 20 years and a 6% risk in those older than 40 years. Associated fractures occurred in 19% of patients and nerve injuries in 21%.**

Clinical examination

An accurate history to determine the force required to dislocate the shoulder in the first instance helps differentiate traumatic and atraumatic dislocations. The frequency of recurrent episodes and the ease of reduction should be documented.

Clinical examination in the acute setting is limited due to pain. The arm will be adducted and internally rotated and the patient will be unable to externally rotate or fully abduct the extremity. The humeral head can often be palpated on the anterior aspect of the shoulder. Acute reduction is performed in the emergency department unless there is a fracture dislocation. A simple tuberosity fracture may still be amenable to careful manipulation under sedation.

In patients who present late, the examination will reveal a classic apprehension sign, where the patient feels discomfort and apprehension of dislocation when the shoulder is taken into a position of abduction and external rotation. This is relieved when a posteriorly directed force is applied to the head of the humerus (Jobe's relocation test).

Investigation

In acute dislocation, an AP view is usually adequate for diagnosis and to assess associated fractures. Detailed imaging is obtained after reduction.

Plain radiographs and computed tomography (CT) scans may help to define the bony disruption and the

Hill-Sachs lesion. The Stryker notch, West point axillary and apical axillary views used to be used for detection of humeral head impaction, but are rarely performed now because of the extensive use and easy availability of cross-sectional imaging.

Magnetic resonance (MR) scanning has 60% sensitivity and 85% sensitivity for labral pathology. MR arthrography has 90% sensitivity and specificity, and the ABER (abduction, external rotation) position improves accuracy. An MR arthrogram will show a Bankart lesion, ALPSA and capsular laxity.

Management

Midazolam is used when reducing shoulder dislocations in the emergency department. Intra-articular 1% lidocaine (15-20mL) can be injected through the posterior approach.

The initial treatment is immobilisation in a sling for 3-6 weeks, with a period of physical therapy and rehabilitation before normal function. Immobilisation in external rotation was proposed by Miller on the basis of a cadaveric study, which showed maximum contact between the labrum and glenoid in 45° external rotation.

Note

Miller BS, Sonnabend DH, Hatrick C, et al. Should acute anterior dislocations of the shoulder be immobilized in external rotation? A cadaveric study. J Shoulder Elbow Surg 2004; 13: 589-92.

Itoi conducted a prospective randomised controlled trial in which six patients out of 20 in an internal rotation sling experienced dislocation within 16 months, while none of 20 patients in an external rotation orthosis had a dislocation. An external rotation orthosis was advised, but further long-term follow-up has not shown any benefit of external rotation immobilisation and hence this is no longer the practice.

An assessment is conducted at 3 weeks to look for increased external rotation, which indicates subscapularis rupture. Patients should start gentle self-forward elevation and external rotation of less than 40°. Passive stretching is allowed at 6 weeks, along with rotator cuff exercises, and plyometrics is advised from 12 weeks.

Patients younger than 25 years have a substantial risk of redislocation, and this group will benefit from early surgical intervention. Surgical treatment is the mainstay of treatment and can be performed with either open or arthroscopic procedures.

Surgery can be offered after imaging in high-demand patients and athletes after the first dislocation. Most surgeons will stabilise after a second dislocation in a young patient.

Indications for surgery are as follows:

- Dislocation in a young person (<25 years).
- Greater tuberosity displaced more than 5mm.
- Subscapularis rupture.
- A rotator cuff tear in a person aged less than 45 years or an athlete, or if the joint is under high demand.

Open surgery

The open procedure involves a Bankart repair and, in most instances, some form of imbricating and reducing anteroinferior capsular volume. Latarjet or the modified Bristow-Helfet procedure involves bony transfer of the coracoid with the attached conjoint tendon to the face of the anteroinferior glenoid. This is useful when there is a bony deficiency in the glenoid.

Capsular plication can be performed to restrict external rotation in an engaging Hill-Sachs lesion, which will prevent the lesion from engaging. Allografts or humeral head replacement are needed for large Hill-Sachs lesions (>40%).

Arthroscopic surgery

The vast majority of shoulder stabilisation procedures are now done arthroscopically. Arthroscopy has the advantage of less soft tissue damage and earlier rehabilitation, and in the long term the results are comparable with open Bankart repair. Its advantage lies in the ability to treat concomitant lesions such as cuff tears and especially SLAP and HAGL lesions.

Acute posterior dislocation

Posterior dislocations account for fewer than 5% of all shoulder dislocations. Almost 50% of these may be missed on initial presentation.

Predisposing conditions for posterior dislocation include seizures, alcoholism, electroshock therapy or a direct blow on the anterior aspect of the shoulder.

Evaluation
Lack of active external rotation should raise the suspicion of a posterior dislocation. A McLaughlin lesion is an anteromedial humeral head defect seen in patients with a posterior dislocation of the humeral head.

Imaging
AP radiographs of the shoulder show the classic 'light-bulb sign', which means the humeral head appears symmetrical. This is because the greater tuberosity is not visible on the AP view due to internal rotation of the arm. The axillary lateral (or scapular Y) view is helpful in diagnosis.

Management
Reduction is achieved by in-line traction and a sling is advised for 3-4 weeks. If unstable, an abduction brace can be used for 6 weeks.

Indications for surgery
A McLaughlin lesion is an anteromedial humeral head defect. Surgery is indicated for symptomatic instability. In the McLaughlin procedure, the subscapularis is transferred into the humeral head defect through a deltopectoral approach. In the Neer procedure, the lesser tuberosity is transferred into the defect.

Recurrent posterior instability

The incidence of recurrent posterior instability is 2-5% of all dislocations. Trauma may be subtle in almost 90% of patients and there is usually no relocation history. Recurrent posterior instability usually occurs in people aged 20-30 years. The presentation is one of recurrent subluxation, usually with the individual perceiving pain at relocation. Patients, particularly those with epilepsy, may rarely present with recurrent dislocations.

The history should exclude the following:

- Voluntary dislocation in people who may have secondary psychological gain.
- Presentation as part of multidirectional instability.

The lesions encountered during arthroscopic surgery include a posterior labral tear, Kim lesion (an incomplete and concealed avulsion of the posteroinferior aspect of the labrum), posterior humeral kissing lesions, posteroinferior capsular redundancy, large rotator intervals and bony pathologies, including glenoid defects posteriorly and anterior reverse Hill-Sachs defects. Patients with multidirectional instability have global capsular insufficiency.

> **Note**
>
> Kim SH, Ha KI, Yoo JC, Noh KC. Kim's lesion: an incomplete and concealed avulsion of the posteroinferior labrum in posterior or multidirectional posteroinferior instability of the shoulder. *Arthroscopy* 2004; 20: 712-20.

Clinical examination
Examination may reveal some generalised joint laxity. Posterior instability is tested with the arm in flexion and internal rotation with posterior directed force through the arm (posterior stress test). The palpating hand at the shoulder perceives the posterior translation, but more commonly the clunk of relocation is felt when the shoulder is moved into extension from the flexed position. Scapulothoracic dyskinesia is apparent at subluxation, probably as a compensatory mechanism to the instability. A sulcus sign on pulling the arm down when it is at the side is indicative of an insufficient cuff or inferior capsule.

The drawer test is performed with the shoulder abducted at 30°, applying a posterior or anterior directed force to the head of the humerus. It is worth bearing in mind that some young athletes have posterior laxity as part of the spectrum of normal; they may also have asymmetrical laxity from the opposite shoulder.

Imaging

Plain radiographs may reveal anterior reverse Hill-Sachs defects or, rarely, posterior glenoid defects. An MR arthrogram is best used to delineate the soft tissue pathology.

Management

Initial treatment should involve physical therapy, posture and proprioceptive feedback exercises and exclusion of those who habitually dislocate. Activity modification, seizure control, pain relief, and cuff and scapulothoracic muscle rehabilitation should be the mainstays of therapy.

Surgery is increasingly being recognised as a way by which to address structural defects early in order to better rehabilitate the patient. This is especially true with an antecedent history of trauma. The most commonly performed procedure involves treatment of the posterior capsulolabral lesion through either open or arthroscopic surgery.

In locked posterior dislocations, open surgery is a McLaughlin procedure in which the anterior humeral head defect is filled by moving the subscapularis attachment to the defect.

> **Note**
>
> McLaughlin HL. Posterior dislocation of the shoulder. *J Bone Joint Surg Am* 1952; 24: 584-90.

If seen early (within 2 weeks), humeroplasty to elevate the defect and bone graft of the resultant hole in the head yields better results. A bone graft to the chronic defect or grafting and resurfacing are more recent treatment options.

The best results are achieved when all pathological lesions are addressed and in the unidirectional posterior instability. Arthroscopic repair will involve the following:

- Repairing the posterior Bankart lesion.
- Addressing capsular redundancy, including the rotator interval.
- Completing a Kim's lesion and repair.
- Bony procedures (rarely), especially for reverse Hill-Sachs in the form of bone grafting.

Multidirectional instability

Multidirectional instability can be symptomatic (true instability) or asymptomatic (laxity). In symptomatic patients, multidirectional instability is experienced in the midrange of glenohumeral motion, such as during activities of daily living. Most patients tend to avoid the extremes of movement due to discomfort.

Clinically, the humeral head can be translated in three directions – anterior, posterior and inferior – with the reproduction of discomfort or pain.

The symptoms are subtle and there is usually no history of significant trauma. The underlying pathology is capsular laxity.

Congenital instability is seen in Ehlers-Danlos and Marfan syndromes. Acquired instability can be seen as a result of repetitive microtrauma in athletes, swimmers and gymnasts.

> **Note**
>
> McFarland EG, Kim TK, Park HB, *et al.* The effect of variation in definition on the diagnosis of multidirectional instability of the shoulder. *J Bone Joint Surg Am* 2003; 85: 2138-44.

The painful shoulder

Shoulder pain is a diagnostic conundrum full of pitfalls. The pain of impingement, for example, may be a symptom of instability. Clicks in the shoulder have a variety of causes, including an inflamed bursa abrading on the acromion, SLAP lesions, subtle subluxations or frank instability.

Problems of the rotator cuff are the most common cause of shoulder pain. Other causes of pain depend on the age at presentation:

- In the young patient, the cause is usually instability.
- In the middle-aged patient, it is rotator cuff pathology, subacromial bursitis or acromioclavicular wear.
- In the elderly, it is degenerative cuff disease, glenohumeral arthritis or cervical spondylosis.

Pain in the shoulder can also be referred from the neck as part of a radiculitis.

Anterior shoulder pain is often difficult to attribute to a single cause. Subacromial bursitis with rotator cuff tendinitis is the most common cause, but other entities include bicipital tendinitis, internal impingement, coracoid impingement, acromioclavicular arthritis, anterosuperior articular lesions on the humeral head and SLAP lesions.

All of the above pathologies can cause anterosuperior pain with impingement-like presentation. A careful history and diligent examination are essential.

Causes of a painful shoulder

The causes of a painful shoulder are listed in Table 2.2.

Table 2.2. The causes of a painful shoulder.

Younger adults (≤30 years)	Older adults (>30 years)

Traumatic aetiology:
• Instability
• Acromioclavicular joint strain
• SLAP lesion
• Traumatic impingement
• Internal impingement, thrower's shoulder
• Rotator cuff tears
 	
Non-traumatic aetiology:
• Avascular necrosis of humeral head
• Juvenile rheumatoid arthritis
• Atraumatic instability
• Os acromiale
• Scapulothoracic bursitis
• Neurologic causes:
  - Parsonage-Turner syndrome
  - Entrapment of the suprascapular nerve
  - Cervical radiculitis
	• Rotator cuff degeneration and subacromial bursitis
	• Rotator cuff tears
	• Calcific tendinitis
	• Early stages of adhesive capsulitis
	• Osteoarthritis of the glenohumeral and acromioclavicular joints
	• Rheumatoid arthritis
	• Secondary tumours

Primary bone tumours
Chronic regional pain syndrome

Rotator cuff disease

The rotator cuff is an important tendon complex that helps in the movement and stability of the shoulder joint. It is prone to degeneration and tendinosis, and thus can undergo attrition rupture. The muscle action is complex and the articular surface of the tendon is in close proximity to the bone and cartilage or the proximal humerus. On its bursal surface it is separated from acromion and the coracoacromial ligament by the subacromial bursa. The acromioclavicular joint is also closely applied to the supraspinatus and any osteophytes can impinge on the tendon. The bursa itself can be painful and has a rich nerve supply.

Rotator cuff tendinitis

The basic pathology of tendinosis is degeneration within the tendon with age. Some studies have implicated genetic and mechanical factors. The coracoacromial arch, especially the undersurface of the acromion, is known to perpetuate the pain.

> **Note**
>
> Zuckerman JD, Kummer FJ, Cuomo F, *et al.* The influence of coracoacromial arch anatomy on rotator cuff tears. *J Shoulder Elbow Surg* 1992; 1: 4-14.

Intrinsic factors:

- Muscle fatigue and overload in tension, especially in overhead activities.
- Tendinosis.
- Overuse of the shoulder.

Extrinsic factors:

- Malunion of greater tuberosity fractures.
- Shoulder instability.
- Osteophytes from the acromioclavicular joint.
- Hooked acromial spur. (The acromion is classified into three types on outlet radiographs: type I, flat; type II, curved; and type III, hooked; Figure 2.4. The hooked

acromion is considered to be most commonly associated with tears.)

> **Note**
>
> Morrison DS, Bigliani LU. The clinical significance of variations in acromial morphology. *Orthop Trans* 1987; 11: 234.

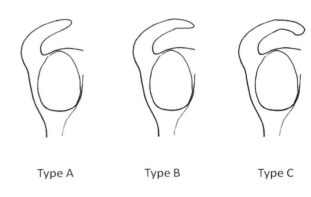

| Type A | Type B | Type C |

Figure 2.4. Morphological types of acromion.

The painful rotator cuff due to inflammation is the most common presentation in the clinic.

Charles Neer described three stages of impingement:

- Stage 1 – reversible oedema and haemorrhage.
- Stage 2 – fibrosis and tendinitis.
- Stage 3 – tears and bone spurs on acromion.

He also divided impingement into outlet impingement (due to the coracoacromial arch) and non-outlet impingement (due to an inflamed bursa and/or tendon), and advocated excising the anteroinferior acromion.

> **Note**
>
> Neer CS, 2nd. Anterior acromioplasty for chronic impingement syndrome: a preliminary report. *J Bone Joint Surg Am* 1972; 54: 41-50.

Clinical presentation

The pain is felt usually in the upper lateral aspect of the arm and quite often radiates to the elbow. It is a dull ache associated with activity and can be sharp in certain positions of the arm (e.g., abduction, internal rotation). Patients complain of being unable to reach their back pocket, fasten their bra strap, comb their hair and, in severe cases, do any overhead activities. Lying on the affected side is painful and can lead to severe stiffness in chronic cases. The stiffness usually starts in the posterior capsule and manifests as reduced internal rotation.

There is a painful arc of abduction (pain at mid levels of elevation and disappearing in full elevation). The Neer sign is pain on elevation in the scapular plane at 70-90°.

Patients have a positive Neer impingement test (in which injection of local anaesthetic in the subacromial space reduces the pain and eliminates the weakness) and Hawkins sign (pain felt on internal rotation of the flexed shoulder).

Patients often have tenderness at Codman's point. This is best examined with the hand behind the back and the shoulder extended and internally rotated.

Imaging

Radiographic signs include reciprocal sclerosis and subchondral cysts of the greater tuberosity and acromion. Radiographs may also show calcific tendinitis and acromioclavicular joint arthritis. The axillary lateral view is useful in looking for os acromiale. Ultrasound or MR imaging is helpful in delineating the status of the rotator cuff.

Management

Many studies confirm that 60% of patients resolve with non-operative management. Management includes avoidance of activity, physiotherapy, non-steroidal inflammatory drugs (NSAIDs) and subacromial injection of steroids. All patients should have a non-operative trial for a minimum of 6 months, but preferably longer.

Morbidity with arthroscopic acromioplasty is decreasing, and this procedure is now frequently performed.

Operative treatment involves either open or arthroscopic subacromial decompression. The acromioclavicular joint is usually excised only if symptomatic or grossly arthritic.

> **Note**
>
> Ellman H. Arthroscopic subacromial decompression: analysis of one- to three-year results. *Arthroscopy* 1987; 3: 173-81.

> **Note**
>
> Ketola S, Lehtinen J, Arnala I, *et al*. Does arthroscopic acromioplasty provide any additional value in the treatment of shoulder impingement syndrome? A two-year randomised controlled trial. *J Bone Joint Surg Br* 2009; 91: 1326-34. **This study compared arthroscopic acromioplasty with a supervised exercise program. At 2 years, there was no difference between the two groups.**

Rotator cuff tears

The rotator cuff maintains a balanced force couple that helps the shoulder move in space, as well as keeping the fulcrum centred within the joint. The aim of repair surgery is to balance this force couple in all planes when it is disrupted, and to relieve pain.

Rotator cuff tears can be symptomatic or asymptomatic. The most common location is the supraspinatus tendon. Tears are commonly posterosuperior (supraspinatus, infraspinatus and rarely teres minor) or less commonly anterosuperior (supraspinatus and subscapularis).

Tears are classified by the size of the tear:

- Small, less than 1cm.
- Medium, 2-3cm.
- Large, 3-5cm.
- Massive, more than 5cm.

Pathology

Tears usually occur following degeneration of the tendon. Eccentric load is an important factor in the tear propagation. These histological changes of degeneration include decreased cellularity, some of which is genetically determined.

Note

Kannus P, Józsa L. Histopathological changes preceding spontaneous rupture of a tendon. A controlled study of 891 patients. *J Bone Joint Surg Am* 1991; 73: 1507-25.

Traumatic tears occur in patients younger than 50 years. In the elderly, minimal trauma can cause a tear in a degenerative cuff.

Blood supply changes have been demonstrated with degenerate cuffs and in cuff tears. The avascular Codman's zone has been demonstrated 1cm from insertion, but its role in pathogenesis is not entirely clear.

Reduced cellularity and metabolism have been shown at the edges of tears, especially with large tears, which may influence the capacity to heal. The role of compression from impingement in the pathogenesis is questionable.

Note

Matthews TJ, Smith SR, Peach C, *et al. In vivo* measurement of tissue metabolism in rotator cuff tendons: implications for surgical management. *J Bone Joint Surg Br* 2007; 89: 633-8.

Clinical presentation

A rotator cuff tear is not symptomatic in all patients. Asymptomatic patients older than 60 years have a 30% incidence of rotator cuff tears, and this increases with age. It is not known why the presentation varies so widely in different patients.

Note

Yamaguchi K, Tetro AM, Blam O, *et al.* Natural history of asymptomatic rotator cuff tears: a longitudinal analysis of asymptomatic tears detected sonographically. *J Shoulder Elbow Surg* 2001; 10: 199-203.

In symptomatic patients, the symptoms are those of impingement. Weakness is readily apparent in large and massive tears, but can be subtle in small and medium tears. In acute-on-chronic tears, patients are unable to lift their arms and there may be ecchymosis evident over the arm anteriorly. The pain levels are not severe in the later stages, but functional limitation is marked. Stiffness is not part of the initial presentation. Internal rotation is more restricted than other movements. Arm elevation is usually good because of compensatory deltoid activity.

Weakness can lead to a drop sign. This is the inability to sustain a contraction and the arm drops limply. It is usually demonstrated as an internal or external rotation lag sign. An external rotation lag sign is elicited by passively positioning the arm in maximal external rotation. When there is marked weakness, the patient is unable to hold the arm in this position and the arm drops.

Hornblower's sign, an inability to externally rotate the elevated arm, also demonstrates severe infraspinatus weakness. The prognosis for repair is guarded in these patients. External rotation weakness is more consistently demonstrable than abduction (deltoid compensation).

Subscapularis tear is rare (around 5%) and presents with internal rotation weakness, excessive passive external rotation and a positive lift-off test. This test is difficult to elicit due to the pain of internal rotation and a belly press test may be more appropriate.

Investigation

In addition to size, it is important to determine the following characteristics of the tear:

- Acute or chronic.
- Traumatic or atraumatic.
- Retracted (mild, moderate – uncovering the head, severe retracted – to and beyond the glenoid).
- Quality and delamination.
- Wasting and, if wasted, is there fatty infiltration (MR imaging).
- Associated stiffness (examination with or without anaesthesia).

In order to assess these issues a detailed history and examination are needed, coupled with appropriate investigations. The investigation starts with radiographs: an AP and an axillary lateral view. The gold standard investigation is MR imaging, which has good specificity for cuff tears. It helps to assess:

- Fatty infiltration.
- Other soft tissues, including biceps, cartilage, SLAP lesions and the acromioclavicular joint.
- In the young it can help assess the labrum, but an MR arthrogram is more useful for this.

The office ultrasound is cheaper and much faster. It is operator-dependent and is best performed in the clinic setting either by an accompanying radiologist or the surgeon. The sensitivity and specificity for medium to large tears is very good. Partial-thickness tears can be difficult to diagnose.

Rarely, a nerve conduction study to look for suprascapular nerve damage is helpful when the wasting is disproportionate to the size of the tear. Examination of the patient under anaesthesia and arthroscopic visualisation complete the assessment of the tear.

Muscle changes in cuff tears

The chronicity of a tear can affect management decisions. Chronic tears are detectable from a longstanding history, with accompanying wasting, stiffness, and X-ray changes.

Wasting of the supraspinous and infraspinous fossa in a patient presenting after an acute injury indicates a longstanding tear:

- No wasting – acute-on-chronic, acute.
- Wasting – chronic, acute-on-chronic:

X-ray changes include some superior migration of the humeral head, reciprocal changes in the greater tuberosity and acromion, and an acromion humeral distance of less than 7mm (normal being about 10mm). In advanced massive cuff tears the humeral head starts subluxing upwards and the patient will develop secondary arthritis, given the abnormal joint mechanics. It is important to rule out significant arthritis as this will affect the management.

Management

Non-operative management

Non-operative measures are variously reported as being effective in 33-90% of patients. Good prognostic indicators include small tears, duration of less than a year and a well-motivated patient. In most reported series, 30-40% of patients deteriorate or do not get better with non-operative management. The decision not to operate has to be balanced against the acuteness of the tear, the potential for tear propagation and the need for a long non-operative treatment protocol.

The options for symptom relief include activity modification, NSAIDs and steroid injection. Steroids should be repeated only twice with a minimum 3-month interval.

Pain relief helps the patient to adhere to physical therapy regimes. Rotator cuff strengthening is started with the arm by the side at waist level. For massive tears, deltoid strengthening exercises are helpful in restoring some function. Scapular stabiliser exercises are also of use.

The need for and timing of operative treatment is still under debate. Most studies on the subject have been single-centre, non-randomised cohort studies, mostly retrospective. Most surgeons allow a 6-month trial of non-operative treatment, depending on symptom severity and the age of the patient.

Note

Oh LS, Wolf BR, Hall MP, *et al.* Indications for rotator cuff repair: a systematic review. *Clin Orthop Relat Res* 2007; 455: 52-63.

Note

Wirth MA, Basamania C, Rockwood CA Jr. Non-operative management of full-thickness tears of the rotator cuff. *Orthop Clin North Am* 1997: 28: 59-67.

Patients aged 50 years and younger may benefit from early intervention in the symptomatic shoulder. Tendon quality tends to be poor in patients aged 65 years and above, and they are best treated with non-operative management in the first instance. Surgery is reserved for the refractory patient. Large and massive tears are prone to re-tear (40-50%).

Both open and arthroscopic treatments have good results. The advantages of arthroscopic treatment are that it is minimally invasive and that procedures such as suprascapular nerve release and repair of labral tears can be performed simultaneously.

Surgical repair is considered in the following situations:

- After at least a 3-month (and often up to 6-month) trial of non-operative treatment.
- In the acute tear in the active adult.
- In severe disabling pain that does not respond to non-operative measures within 6-8 weeks.

Note

Bassett RW, Cofield RH. Acute tears of the rotator cuff. The timing of surgical repair. *Clin Orthop Relat Res* 1983; 175: 18-24.

Open repair

Open repairs are easier to perform and have good results. Open surgery involves a lateral deltoid splitting approach. Visualisation is through the narrow window with the humeral head rotated to bring the cuff tissue into view. This limits the surgeon in the dissection. When performed through the anterosuperior approach, extensions along the deltoid insertion either anteriorly or posteriorly can help visualise the cuff.

The approach anteriorly is through the deltopectoral plane for subscapularis tears. A mini open anterosuperior approach has been successfully used in small- and medium-sized tears.

Open repair was the gold standard, but arthroscopic repairs now provide as good results – and, in experienced hands, better results.

Arthroscopic repair

The basic aim of arthroscopic repair is to recreate the footprint of the cuff insertion at the greater and lesser tuberosity. Better biomechanical fixation yields a better biologic result. Important considerations include the skill of the surgeon, quality of the tissues, motivation of the patient and, finally, rehabilitation protocols.

The size and location of the tear and the quality of the tendon can be all macroscopically assessed at arthroscopy and serve as predictors of the final result. Tears are assessed for mobilisation and classified as follows:

- C-shaped, when the central tendon mass at insertion gives way.
- U-shaped, which is an extension of the C-shaped with retraction.
- L-shaped, when a linear limb retracts from its attachment.
- Reverse L-shaped, when the retraction is posterior to anterior.
- Combination and complex.

Repairs can be either 'side-to-side', when the anterior and posterior limbs are simply brought together, or 'end-to-bone', when the tendon is brought to the humeral head, up to its insertion at the tuberosity. Side-to-side repair is also known as 'margin convergence' (in U-shaped tears). Rarely the repair is medialised, especially in massive tears when the cuff cannot reach the tuberosity. Bone anchors are used to secure the tendon to bone. The anchors can be used as a single row in simple tears, but a double row (one medial and other lateral) secures a biomechanically stronger fixation.

In massive tears the measure of irreparability is constantly changing as advanced mobilisation techniques develop. The potential damage to the suprascapular nerve at the spinoglenoid notch has to be borne in mind.

Subscapularis tears are much less common than posterior cuff tears and are technically more demanding due to constraints of the subcoracoid space. The axillary nerve must be protected from iatrogenic injury.

The results of cuff repair are better with small to moderate tears with good tendon quality. The overall re-tear rate is 15-20%, but this rises to 40-50% with massive tears. The overall satisfaction rate in various series is 80-95%. Re-tear adversely affects the outcome, but surgery may nonetheless significantly improve pain relief. Tear recurrence reduces the improvement in functional rehabilitation and patient satisfaction. Cuff repair (re-tear or not) gives superior results to acromioplasty and debridement alone.

Note

Moosmayer S, Lund G, Seljom U, *et al*. Comparison between surgery and physiotherapy in the treatment of small and medium-sized tears of the rotator cuff. A randomised controlled study of 103 patients with one-year follow-up. *J Bone Joint Surg Br* 2010; 92: 83-91. **In this prospective randomised controlled trial in 103 patients, the group with surgery had a better shoulder score, improvement in pain and pain-free abduction.**

Poor prognostic factors

Several factors indicate a poor prognosis:

- Massive tears.
- Increasing age.
- Reduced tendon quality.
- Fatty infiltration of muscle.
- Patient comorbidities (e.g., diabetes).
- Smoking.

Note

Burkhart SS, Danaceau SM, Pearce CE, Jr. Arthroscopic rotator cuff repair: analysis of results by tear size and by repair technique – margin convergence versus direct tendon-to-bone repair. *Arthroscopy* 2001; 17: 905-12.

Note

Levy O, Venkateswaran B, Even T, Ravenscroft M, Copeland S. Mid-term clinical and sonographic outcome of arthroscopic repair of the rotator cuff. *J Bone Joint Surg Br* 2008; 90: 1341-7.

Specific issues

- The role of concomitant acromioplasty is being questioned. Gartsman published that there were no differences in the type 2 acromion with and without acromioplasty. Most surgeons include acromioplasty as part of the repair, but caution should be exercised in the cuff-deficient shoulder.

Note

Gartsman GM, O'Connor DP. Arthroscopic rotator cuff repair with and without arthroscopic subacromial decompression: a prospective, randomized study of one-year outcomes. *J Shoulder Elbow Surg* 2004; 13: 424-6.

- Partial-thickness rotator cuff tears can lead to persistent pain. If rehabilitation fails then treatment ranges from debridement in the young patient to debridement and acromioplasty. Excision or repair of the tear may be considered in severe partial tears.

> **Note**
>
> Weber SC. Arthroscopic debridement and acromioplasty versus mini-open repair in the management of significant partial-thickness tears of the rotator cuff. *Orthop Clin North Am* 1997; 28: 79-82.

- Internal impingement is a process of damage to the rotator cuff insertion at the greater tuberosity in extremes of abduction and external rotation with fraying of the undersurface. Reciprocal changes on the posterosuperior glenoid labrum may be visible at times. Treatment is usually with rehabilitation. Since this is an arthroscopic diagnosis, treatment involves arthroscopic debridement. A capsular plication may be recommended with demonstrable instability.

> **Note**
>
> Walch G, Boileau P, Noel E, Donell ST. Impingement of the deep surface of the supraspinatus tendon on the postero-superior glenoid rim: an arthroscopic study. *J Shoulder Elbow Surg* 1992; 1: 238-45.

- Rehabilitation after a cuff tear varies depending on the anatomy and biomechanics of the repair. An abduction pillow is useful for massive tears and a simple shoulder immobiliser in other sound repairs for at least 6 weeks. Early passive motion is advised.
- The use of an extracellular matrix for biologic repair of the cuff has been attempted. The extracellular matrix is naturally occurring and is processed to remove cells to reduce antigenicity (e.g., GraftJacket). It does not provide structural support to the repair.

- In massive tears, the fatty infiltration can be staged as per Goutallier. Various treatments are advocated, including debridement and partial repair, mobilisation and repair, synthetic materials, tendon transfers, biologic augmentation and arthroplasty. In most instances a tear is considered irreparable after an attempted repair. In the healthy active individual it is easier to perform an early repair, as even 6 weeks can lead to severe retraction and scarring. Tendon transfers include the upper part of the subscapularis and, more frequently, the latissimus dorsi.

> **Note**
>
> Goutallier D, Postel JM, Bernageau J, *et al.* Fatty muscle degeneration in cuff ruptures. Pre- and postoperative evaluation by CT scan. *Clin Orthop Relat Res* 1994; 304: 78-83.

> **Note**
>
> Gerber C, Fuchs B, Hodler J. The results of repair of massive tears of the rotator cuff. *J Bone Joint Surg Am* 2000; 82: 505-15.

The painful stiff shoulder

There are several causes of a painful stiff shoulder:

- Frozen shoulder (adhesive capsulitis).
- Arthritis of the shoulder.
- Avascular necrosis of the shoulder.
- Rotator cuff arthropathy.

Adhesive capsulitis

Adhesive capsulitis was first described as 'frozen shoulder' by Codman in the 1930s. It is characterised by pain and limited movement at the glenohumeral joint. Most cases are idiopathic in an otherwise healthy individual, and this is known as primary frozen shoulder. Secondary frozen shoulder is associated with conditions such as diabetes (carries a poorer prognosis), thyroid disorders, hyperlipidaemia, Dupuytren's disease, trauma and cardiac disease. Capsulitis is a third category for the stiff shoulder. This develops after surgery or fracture of the joint and is often more resistant to management.

Pathology

The cause of frozen shoulder is unknown, although many theories have been proposed. Bunker and Anthony found histological changes, with the capsule thickened and with increased vascularity, together with proliferation of fibroblasts, transformation to myofibroblasts and increased collagen deposition, similar to Dupuytren's disease. They found the synovium to be normal with no inflammatory changes. The contracture acts as a check against external rotation, resulting in a loss of active and passive movement.

> **Note**
>
> Bunker TD, Anthony PP. The pathology of frozen shoulder. A Dupuytren-like disease. *J Bone Joint Surg Br* 1995; 77: 677-83.

Clinical presentation

Frozen shoulder is most common in middle to old age, with a slight female preponderance. Clinical evaluation reveals globally restricted movements, especially external rotation.

Hannafin and Chiaia have described four stages of adhesive capsulitis:

- Stage 1 occurs during the first 3 months and is characterised by pain with little loss of motion.
- Stage 2 (the freezing stage) occurs between 3 and 9 months and is characterised by pain with a loss of active and passive motion.
- Stage 3 (frozen stage) occurs at 9-15 months and is characterised by little pain, but with loss of motion.
- Stage 4 (thawing phase) occurs after 15-24 months, with little pain and a progressive improvement in the range of motion.

These stages have not been borne out in other studies, however, where the course has been found to be more protracted without intervention.

> **Note**
>
> Hannafin JA, Chiaia TA. Adhesive capsulitis. A treatment approach. *Clin Orthop Relat Res* 2000; 372: 95-109.

Investigation

Plain radiographs are useful in excluding other conditions such as glenohumeral arthritis and posterior dislocation.

Management

Management options include the following:

- Analgesia.
- Physiotherapy.
- Steroid injection.
- Manipulation under anaesthesia.
- Arthroscopic release.
- Open release.

Analgesia and physiotherapy are useful if the symptoms have been present for less than 6 months. The aim is to regain and maintain motion. The physiotherapist plays a useful role in supporting the patient through the natural course of the condition. Griggs *et al* described 90% satisfaction with non-operative treatment, although the shoulder remained significantly different from the unaffected shoulder.

> **Note**
>
> Griggs SM, Ahn A, Green A. Idiopathic adhesive capsulitis. A prospective functional outcome study of non-operative treatment. *J Bone Joint Surg Am* 2000; 82: 1398-407.

There is little evidence for long-term benefit with steroid injection, but it may be effective in providing pain relief and is often combined with other treatment modalities. In the painful stiff shoulder, a steroid injection followed by physiotherapy is helpful.

Manipulation under anaesthesia is a mainstay of treatment and is often carried out in patients with symptoms persisting for longer than 6 months. Humeral fracture is a major complication, as are glenoid rim fractures, dislocations, rotator cuff tears, labral detachments and brachial plexus injuries.

Arthroscopic release is performed when closed manipulation fails or in recalcitrant cases, such as patients with diabetes. Release of the anterior capsule is often sufficient, although the posterior capsule can be released if required. Complications include damage to the axillary nerve, which is best avoided by not releasing the inferior capsule with the arthroscopic wand.

Open release tends to be reserved for patients where manipulation or arthroscopic release fails to restore range of motion, or where the adhesions are extra-articular. A frozen shoulder in the presence of a shoulder arthroplasty is best treated by open release, although malposition of the prosthesis should be ruled out.

Osteoarthritis

Osteoarthritis of the shoulder can be primary or secondary (related to fractures or dislocations). The prevalence is far lower than arthritis of the knee or hip.

Maximal wear in the primary group tends to occur in the area of the head, which articulates with the glenoid between 60° and 90° of abduction. This is the region of maximal joint reaction force. As the disease progresses, the glenoid is eroded posteriorly with resultant posterior head subluxation. The rotator cuff tends to be intact in primary osteoarthritis; this differs from rheumatoid patients radiologically by having osteophytes and being generally sclerotic rather than osteopenic in appearance.

Management is with non-operative measures or arthroplasty.

Rheumatoid arthritis

Rheumatoid arthritis of the shoulder usually affects the glenohumeral joint, but involvement of the acromioclavicular joint and cervical spine can cause symptoms around the shoulder.

There are three patterns of involvement, as described by Neer:

1. The dry type is characterised by loss of joint space, formation of subchondral cysts, sclerosis and osteophytes, together with stiffness.
2. The wet type is characterised by synovial involvement and marginal erosions of the glenoid.
3. The resorptive type is the most destructive, resulting in extensive resorption of the humeral head and glenoid with medial migration.

Note

Neer CS, 2nd. *Shoulder Reconstruction.* Philadelphia, PA, USA: WB Saunders, 1990: 273-362.

Non-operative management is similar to other joints. Surgical procedures include synovectomy and debridement, capsular releases, subacromial decompression and distal clavicle resection. Joint replacement surgery is usually in the form of hemiarthroplasty as the degree of glenoid erosion can make glenoid replacement difficult. However, total shoulder replacement gives early and good pain relief. Problems with total shoulder replacement usually relate to glenoid wear and loosening.

Avascular necrosis

The shoulder is the second most common site for avascular necrosis (after the hip). Idiopathic osteonecrosis is rare, and up to 70% of cases are associated with steroid use.

Rotator cuff arthropathy

Rotator cuff arthropathy is characterised by the following:

- Recurrent effusions containing biochemically active enzymes.
- Absence of the rotator cuff.
- Degenerative glenohumeral joint changes with collapse of the humeral head.
- Erosion of the undersurface of the acromion, acromioclavicular joint and distal end of the clavicle.
- In advanced cases, radiographs also show proximal migration of the humeral head together with anterior escape in a joint deficient of a coracoacromial ligament.

Contributing factors that have been proposed include a crystal arthropathy, loss of the cuff resulting in direct wear of the humeral head on the acromion and leakage of synovial fluid in a cuff-deficient joint, resulting in impaired cartilage nutrition. Multiple factors may be present within the same shoulder.

Rotator cuff arthropathy characteristically affects older women. The symptoms can be bilateral and may have been present for many years, with intermittent exacerbations of more intense discomfort. Examination usually shows atrophy, weakness and joint effusion.

A classification for rotator cuff arthropathy was proposed by Seebauer (Table 2.3).

Management

It is rarely possible to repair a severely damaged cuff in advanced cuff arthropathy. Surgical management is for salvage rather than reconstruction, with the aim of pain relief. There is frequently little improvement in movement and strength.

Table 2.3. The Seebauer classification for rotator cuff arthropathy.

IA (centred, stable)	Type IB (centred, medialised)	Type IIA (decentred limited stable)	Type IIB (decentred unstable)
Intact anterior restraints	Intact anterior restraints	Compromised anterior restraints	Incompetent anterior structures
	Force couple intact or compensated	Force couple compromised	
Minimal superior joint migration	Minimal superior joint migration	Superior translation	Anteriosuperior escape
Dynamic joint stabilisation	Compromised dynamic joint stabilisation	Insufficient dynamic joint stabilisation	Absent dynamic joint stabilisation
Acetabularisation of CA arch	Medial erosion of glenoid	Minimal stabilisation by CA arch	No stabilisation by CA arch
Femoralisation of humeral head	Acetabularisation of CA arch	Superomedial erosion and extensive acetabularisation of CA arch	Deficient anterior structures
	Femoralisation of humeral head	Femoralisation of humeral head	

CA = coracoacromial

There are several surgical options:

- Hemiarthroplasty.
- Total shoulder replacement.
- Reverse shoulder replacement.
- Shoulder arthrodesis.
- Resurfacing the humeral head.

Hemiarthroplasty involves replacing the humeral head with a stemmed head (Figure 2.5). It may be performed using a standard or large-headed prosthesis. An intact coracoacromial arch is required to prevent anterior superior escape. Fixation in the humerus is achieved with either a press fit or porous coating, or with the use of cement.

Total shoulder replacement involves replacing the humeral head and the glenoid, usually with a cemented all-polyethylene component (Figure 2.6). These implants are normally minimally constrained. Because of the high forces generated across the joint and the small area of bone available for fixation of the glenoid component, loosening remains a real problem and glenoid replacement is generally avoided in cuff-deficient shoulders or inflammatory joint disease. However, it may provide superior pain relief, better range of motion and patient satisfaction than hemiarthroplasty.

Note

Radnay CS, Setter KJ, Chambers L, *et al.* Total shoulder replacement compared with humeral head replacement for the treatment of primary glenohumeral osteoarthritis: a systematic review. *J Shoulder Elbow Surg* 2007; 16: 396-402.

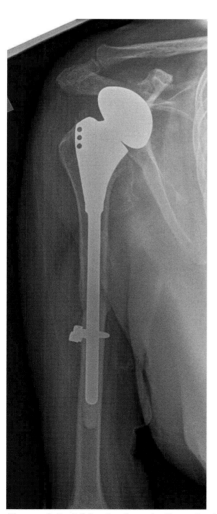

Figure 2.5. A bipolar hemiarthroplasty of the shoulder performed for a proximal humeral fracture with coexisting arthritis of the glenohumeral joint. *(Image courtesy of Mr R. Williams, Cardiff, UK.)*

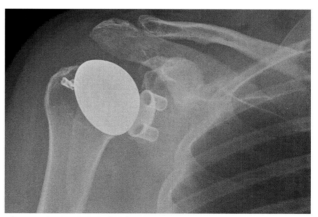

Figure 2.6. A resurfacing total shoulder replacement. *(Image courtesy of Mr R. Williams, Cardiff, UK.)*

In cuff tear arthropathy there is a high rate of loosening of the glenoid component due to abnormal joint mechanics and poor glenoid bone stock. Absence of the rotator cuff is considered to be a contraindication to replacing the glenoid.

The reverse shoulder replacement has been used in rotator cuff arthropathy and is a potential option (Figures 2.7 and 2.8). A reverse ball-and-socket prosthesis is typically used in a cuff-deficient joint where the proximal migration of the humeral head through the relatively unopposed contraction of deltoid can produce abnormal forces across the joint and subsequent failure of the glenoid component with a standard total shoulder prosthesis. The centre of rotation is medialised, which decreases the forces across the glenoid component. Lowering of the humerus increases the deltoid tension and optimises the action of the muscle.

> **Note**
>
> Boileau P, Watkinson D, Hatzidakis AM, Hovorka I. Neer Award 2005: the Grammont reverse shoulder prosthesis: results in cuff tear arthritis, fracture sequelae, and revision arthroplasty. *J Shoulder Elbow Surg* 2006; 15: 527-40.

> **Note**
>
> Frankle M, Siegal S, Pupello D, *et al*. The reverse shoulder prosthesis for glenohumeral arthritis associated with severe rotator cuff deficiency: a minimum two-year follow-up study of sixty patients. *J Bone Joint Surg Am* 2005; 87: 1697-705.

A reconstruction socket achieving fixation in the glenoid, coracoid and the acromion is a salvage procedure for failed reverse shoulder replacements.

Resurfacing the humeral head has become popular, especially with the success of the Copeland prosthesis. It consists of a hemispherical cup, which is fixed to a reamed humeral head via a hydroxyapatite coating, and a press-fit peg. It preserves bone stock and is relatively easy to maintain correct version.

> **Note**
>
> Levy O, Copeland SA. Cementless surface replacement arthroplasty (Copeland CSRA) for osteoarthritis of the shoulder. *J Shoulder Elbow Surg* 2004; 13: 266-71.

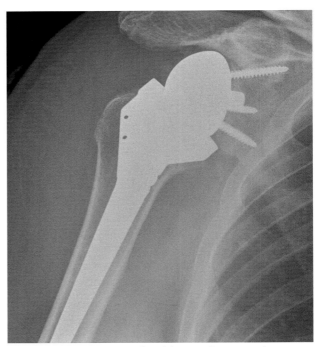

Figure 2.7. A reverse shoulder replacement. *(Image courtesy of Mr R. Williams, Cardiff, UK.)*

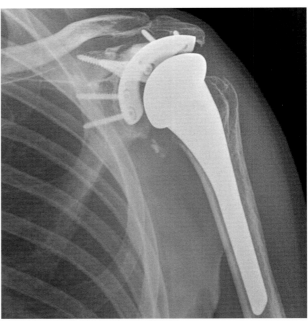

Figure 2.8. Epoca Reco shoulder replacement. *(Image courtesy of Mr R. Williams, Cardiff, UK.)*

Complications of shoulder arthroplasty are similar to those of other joint replacements, and include infection, aseptic loosening (especially of the glenoid component), dislocation and periprosthetic fracture.

Chapter 3 Sports medicine

Meniscal injuries

The medial and lateral menisci are fibrocartilaginous structures that function to transmit the load of weight bearing and act as shock absorbers. They may also have a proprioceptive role.

The menisci are composed of type I collagen and proteoglycans. The medial meniscus is a semicircular structure, while the lateral meniscus is nearly circular with a smaller diameter. The coronary ligaments attach the meniscus to the margin of the tibial plateau. The deep fibres of the medial collateral ligament (MCL) attach to the medial meniscus and this limits the anteroposterior mobility of the medial meniscus.

The genicular vessels provide the vascular supply to the menisci. Blood vessels are present in the outer 20-30% of the medial meniscus and the peripheral 10-25% of the lateral meniscus. The rest of the meniscus derives its nutrition from the synovial fluid.

Removal of the meniscus leads to a reduced contact area and increased pressure on the articular surfaces. In the long term, it predisposes to degenerative arthritis.

Clinical features

Meniscal tears can be traumatic or degenerative. Traumatic tears present with pain and swelling of the knee, typically following a twisting injury. Tears of the vascular zone result in immediate swelling due to haemarthrosis, while tears of the avascular zone will cause an effusion that is evident after a few hours.

A displaced bucket-handle tear may present as a locked knee (the inability to fully extend the knee). Some flap tears cause locking if displaced in between the femoral condyle and the tibia. Longstanding tears may cause mechanical symptoms such as clicking or catching of the knee.

Joint-line tenderness is present on examination. In lateral meniscal tears, McMurray's test elicits pain on the lateral side of the knee while extending the knee with valgus stress and external rotation force. Medial pain on extension along with varus and internal rotation force indicates a tear of the medial meniscus.

Tears of the medial meniscus are more common in patients with chronic anterior cruciate ligament (ACL) injuries, while acute ACL injuries are more often associated with lateral meniscal injuries.

Degenerative meniscal tears are quite common and can be present in two-thirds of individuals over the age of 65 years. The posterior one-third of the medial meniscus is the most common site for degenerative meniscal tears, and these can be associated with generalised degenerative changes in the knee joint.

Degenerative tears present with insidious pain, swelling and localised joint-line tenderness. Mechanical symptoms are often seen, but locking is not. Parameniscal cysts may be palpable.

Imaging

Plain radiographs help to rule out other knee pathology. Magnetic resonance (MR) scans have high accuracy but can overdiagnose meniscal tears. A small number of tears may be missed on MR scanning.

Types of tears

Tears can be classified as partial or full thickness, stable or unstable and symptomatic or asymptomatic. Based on the orientation of the meniscal injury, tears can be radial, vertical, parrot beak, flap or bucket handle (Figure 3.1).

Management of meniscal tears

Meniscal tears that are partial thickness, less than 1cm in size and stable can be managed non-operatively. Persistently symptomatic tears and the acute locked knee require arthroscopy and excision or repair of the meniscal tear.

Excision of the meniscus should be minimal, with the aim of preserving as much tissue as possible. Parameniscal cysts can be decompressed into the knee joint.

Meniscal repair can be attempted for acutely detected unstable tears in the periphery of the meniscus. A better prognosis following meniscal repair is indicated by a stable knee, young age and the presence of vascularity at the margins of the tear (red-red tears). Complex tears are unsuitable for repair. Red-white tears, where only the peripheral margin has detectable vascularity while the inner margin is avascular, have a lower potential to heal (Figure 3.2).

The techniques for repair include outside-in, inside-out and all-inside, based on the suture used and the method of repair. The use of a fibrin clot has been proposed to encourage healing after repair in tears with a limited blood supply.

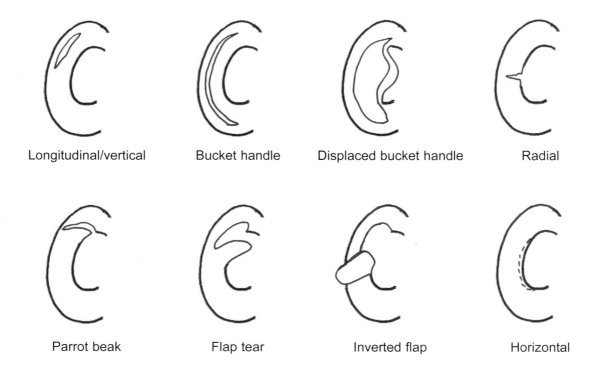

Longitudinal/vertical   Bucket handle   Displaced bucket handle   Radial

Parrot beak   Flap tear   Inverted flap   Horizontal

Figure 3.1. Types of meniscal tears.

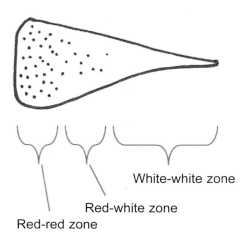

White-white zone

Red-white zone

Red-red zone

Figure 3.2. Vascular zones in the meniscus.

Meniscal replacement

Meniscal replacement is possible through synthetic collagen scaffolds, or with the use of allografts. Collagen scaffolds replace the meniscus and are sutured to the remaining anterior and posterior horn, and along the meniscal rim. Allografts can be used when the anterior and posterior horns are absent. Early results are encouraging, and long-term results are awaited.

Meniscal injuries in children

Meniscal injuries in children are relatively rare, with children accounting for just 5% of all meniscal injuries. A discoid lateral meniscus may, however, predispose to meniscal tears.

The clinical presentation and signs of meniscal tears in children may not be typical and an MR scan is useful for diagnosis.

Treatment is based on the symptoms, and preservation of the meniscus is the goal. Repair in the vascular area of the meniscus can be accomplished with suturing techniques. Every attempt should be made to preserve the rim of the meniscus.

Discoid lateral meniscus

A discoid lateral meniscus presents as a snapping knee in children around the age of 10 years. It occurs in 1-3% of the population.

Discoid meniscus is grouped according to the Watanabe classification:

- Type I – incomplete discoid meniscus.
- Type II – complete discoid meniscus.
- Type III – Wrisberg ligament type – absent Wrisberg ligament; associated with instability of the posterior horn of the meniscus.

Clinically, the symptoms are a clicking and snapping of the joint. The age of symptom onset is around 10 years. Pain is a late feature and represents a meniscal tear. Patients with type III lesions can have symptoms of instability.

On plain radiographs, discoid lateral meniscus appears as widening of the lateral joint space, squaring of the femoral condyle and concavity of the lateral tibial plateau. An MR scan is diagnostic.

Management

Treatment is aimed at trimming the meniscus to a relatively normal shape and repairing or excising the meniscal tears. Patients with instability symptoms in type III lesions are managed with a capsular stitch to stabilise the meniscus. Meniscus preservation is preferable to total meniscectomy.

Meniscal allograft is currently under trial and some synthetic meniscal replacements are also available. The experience with these surgeries is steadily increasing.

Anterior cruciate ligament injuries

The ACL is the primary restraint to anterior translation of the tibia in relation to the femur. It has two bands: anteromedial and posterolateral. The anteromedial band is tight in flexion, while the ~~posteromedial~~ *Posterolateral* band is tight in extension. The posterolateral band provides rotatory stability in addition to anteroposterior translation stability. The anteromedial band is purely engaged in translational restraint. The middle genicular artery is the main blood supply.

A narrow intercondylar notch may predispose to the development of ACL injuries. On computed tomography (CT) films, the notch width is compared to the width of the femur at the level of the femoral condyles. A notch width index of less than 0.2 indicates notch stenosis and predisposes to non-contact ACL injury. This may be due to the course of the ACL in the narrow notch and pressure against the femoral condyle.

Natural history

Lack of a functioning ACL leads to instability, which can in turn lead to further injury within the knee joint. The increased laxity and consequent cartilage damage lead to early joint degenerative disease.

Clinical features

A history of twisting injury on the weight-bearing knee with consequent pain and swelling should raise the suspicion of an acute ACL injury. The Lachman test will show increased anterior translation of the tibia compared with the other side. The pivot shift is helpful in diagnosis but sometimes difficult to elicit in the painful knee. An intact MCL and iliotibial band and full extension of the knee are prerequisites for eliciting the pivot shift.

A variety of instruments are available to measure the anterior subluxation of the tibia on the anterior drawer test and are useful in research studies, but are rarely used in clinical practice. An example of one such instrument is the KT1000.

Plain radiographs should be obtained to rule out other injuries and look for any bony avulsions. The presence of the Segond fracture on X-ray indicates ACL injuries. The Segond fracture is an avulsion from the lateral tibial margin visible in the anteroposterior (AP) radiograph.

An MR scan of the knee has a high sensitivity and specificity (Figure 3.3). It is also helpful to diagnose associated injuries, such as meniscal tears, injuries to other ligaments and chondral lesions.

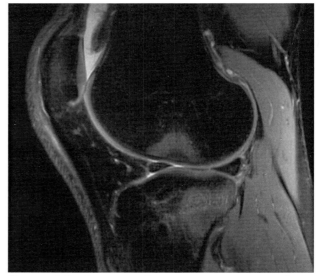

Figure 3.3. A magnetic resonance scan of an anterior cruciate ligament (ACL) injury. Bone bruising – associated with ACL ruptures – is visible on the femoral condyle and tibial plateau.

Management

ACL injuries can be managed non-operatively or by surgical reconstruction. Non-operative treatment is appropriate in the low-demand patient who does not have recurrent instability symptoms. These patients should be referred to a rehabilitation program and are able to participate in mild to moderate sporting activities.

Instability symptoms indicate a predisposition to further injury to the knee and are an indication for reconstruction. Other candidates for reconstruction are high-demand athletes and those with a pivot shift on examination. Overall, about 80% of patients with an ACL injury require reconstruction.

Chronic ACL insufficiency with instability can lead to degenerative changes in the knee, but there is little evidence to suggest that ACL reconstruction delays or avoids these changes.

The timing of surgery is debatable. Most surgeons operate once the acute pain has settled and the knee has regained full extension. Surgery in the acute phase has a higher risk of stiffness (arthrofibrosis). The incidence of arthrofibrosis has been reduced by better pre- and postoperative exercise programs and more accurate placement of grafts. The presence of a locked knee due to a coexisting bucket-handle tear of the meniscus is an indication for early repair. Delayed repair in this situation would lead to a fixed flexion deformity from a persistently locked knee.

> ### Note
>
> Kennedy J, Jackson MP, O'Kelly P, Moran R. Timing of reconstruction of the anterior cruciate ligament in athletes and the incidence of secondary pathology within the knee. *J Bone Joint Surg Br* 2010; 92: 362-6. **In this study of 300 patients, the authors found a higher incidence of meniscal tear if surgery was delayed for more than 1 year from injury. Degenerative changes were higher in the group that underwent surgery more than 6 months after the injury compared with those who had earlier surgery.**

The graft placement should ideally be isometric, which prevents deformation of the graft on range of motion (ROM). The knee's centre of rotation is not a fixed point, and hence complete isometry is not possible. The use of double-bundle grafts has been proposed to improve functional outcomes.

The two commonly used grafts are the patellar tendon (bone-patellar tendon-bone graft) and the quadruple hamstring graft. Both provide sufficient strength and adequate fixation. Synthetic ligament

augmentation devices are no longer favoured due to poor long-term results and a high risk of synovitis.

The ruptured stump of the ACL sometimes gives the appearance of a rounded stalk attached to the tibia and is known as a 'cyclops lesion'. This is excised at the time of reconstruction.

The placement of the femoral and tibial tunnels is critical to ensure isometry and avoid impingement of the graft. A notchplasty – clearing the lateral wall of the intercondylar notch – may be needed at the time of reconstruction. The femoral tunnel is located as far posteriorly as possible, with just enough bone posteriorly to avoid a graft blow-out. An alternative is an over-the-top placement of the graft. Here, instead of using the tunnel, the graft is passed over the top of the femoral condyle.

The tibial tunnel is placed in the posteromedial aspect of the footprint of the ACL.

Techniques to reconstruct each band of the ACL individually have been described and experimental data suggest better biomechanics, but clinical differences have not yet been demonstrated.

Fixation of the graft to the bone can be achieved in a variety of ways. Interference screws may be used to compress the cancellous bone of the graft against the cancellous bone of the femoral and tibial tunnels. The screws should be parallel to the graft in the tunnel to maximise the compressed bone. A divergence of more than 15° between the screw and the bone plug can affect the fixation strength.

Bioabsorbable screws are increasingly being used. These allow MR scanning after surgery without the artefact produced by metallic screws.

Femoral EndoButtons can be used in conjunction with the quadruple hamstring graft. The EndoButton is passed retrogradely in the femoral tunnel and sits on the cortical surface of the femur.

Single vs. double-bundle multistranded hamstring grafts

Note

Adachi N, Ochi M, Uchio Y, *et al*. Reconstruction of the anterior cruciate ligament. Single- versus double-bundle multistranded hamstring tendons. *J Bone Joint Surg Br* 2004; 86: 515-20. **This prospective trial randomised 108 patients to single- or double-bundle reconstruction and followed them for 32 months. No differences were seen between the groups in proprioception or in laxity on the KT-2000 arthrometer at 20° and 70° flexion. Notchplasty was required more often in single-bundle reconstruction.**

Note

Ibrahim SA, Hamido F, Al Misfer AK, *et al*. Anterior cruciate ligament reconstruction using autologous hamstring double-bundle graft compared with single-bundle procedures. *J Bone Joint Surg Br* 2009; 91: 1310-5. **A total of 218 patients were randomised to either single- or double-bundle reconstruction. Double-bundle patients had less laxity, but no difference in knee score.**

Complications of ACL reconstruction

Postoperatively, bracing is unnecessary and full weight bearing is allowed. Closed-chain exercises (in which the foot remains in contact with the ground) are recommended. Full recovery can take about 6 months.

Complications of ACL reconstruction include the following:

- Stiffness – anterior placement of the graft leads to impingement in the notch and limits full extension. Excess posterior placement causes impingement of the graft on the posterior cruciate ligament (PCL).
- Tibial and femoral tunnel widening.
- Graft failure – caused by improper positioning, inadequate fixation or repeated injury.
- Patellofemoral (PF) pain or patellar fractures in patients with a bone-patellar tendon-bone graft.

Anterior cruciate ligament injuries in children

ACL injuries are uncommon in children. The incidence is increasing, however, with greater participation in high-level sports.

The cruciate ligaments in children are stronger than the physis. The fibres attach directly to the perichondrium of the articular cartilage (as opposed to in adults, where they attach by Sharpey's fibres).

An MR scan is the gold standard for diagnosis. Associated injuries to the meniscus may be present.

Operative treatment is advised for symptomatic instability and in patients with meniscal tears that require repair. Iatrogenic damage to the growth plate is a concern, and techniques have been developed to minimise the risk.

Posterior cruciate ligament injury

Incidence

PCL injuries are less common than ACL injuries. The prevalence has been reported to be 2-40% in trauma patients with haemarthrosis. More commonly, PCL injuries are associated with injury to the posterolateral corner (PLC).

Mechanism of injury

The common mechanisms are dashboard injury, hyperflexion or hyperextension injury, varus force to the knee and external rotation skiing injury. A hyperflexion force tears the anterolateral bundle, which is taut in flexion. However, the posteromedial bundle escapes injury because it is loose in flexion.

Anatomy

The PCL is intra-articular but extrasynovial, and is covered by synovium anteriorly and on both sides. It has an anterolateral and posteromedial bundle:

- Anterolateral bundle – larger band, taut in flexion, lax in extension.
- Posteromedial bundle – narrow band, lax in flexion, tight in extension.

The PCL runs from the lateral surface of the medial femoral condyle to the posterior edge of the tibia, 1-1.5cm below the edge. On average, it is 38mm long and 13mm wide.

The PCL is the primary restraint to posterior translation of the tibia on the femur. Other restraints are the MCL, the lateral collateral ligament (LCL), and the PLC. The PCL also prevents lateral rotation of the tibia on the femur.

The PLC has three layers:

- Superficial – iliotibial band and biceps femoris.
- Middle – quadriceps retinaculum, PF ligaments and LCL.
- Deep – coronary ligaments, popliteus tendon, Y arcuate ligament and popliteofibular ligament.

The meniscofemoral ligament of Humphrey arises from the posterior horn of the lateral meniscus and runs anterior to the PCL as it inserts on the femur. The ligament of Wrisberg runs posterior to the PCL.

Clinical features

The clinical features depend on the type of PCL injury (Table 3.1).

Table 3.1. Posterior cruciate ligament injuries.

Type of injury	Description
Isolated	Presents with abrasion anteriorly and swelling and bruising in the popliteal fossa, which resolve in 1-2 weeks
	Patients have a firm endpoint on the posterior drawer test
PCL and PLC	Patients are reluctant to flex the knee
	Bruising and swelling are present on the lateral aspect of the knee and around the proximal fibula
	Patients may not have effusion
	Lateral popliteal nerve injury is sometimes associated with this injury
Chronic PCL	Patients have aching around the knee
	Instability is present in only 10-20% of patients
Chronic PCL and PLC	Patients have significant instability and pain

Examination

Several tests may be carried out for PCL injury:

- Posterior sag – the most accurate test:
  - grade 1 – the medial tibial plateau lies less than 1cm anterior to the femoral condyle;
  - grade 2 – the medial tibial plateau lies in the same plane as the femoral condyle;
  - grade 3 – the medial tibial plateau lies behind the femur.
- Posterior drawer test – performed in 90° flexion with the endpoint assessed.
- Reverse Lachman test – performed in 30° knee flexion.
- The dial test – increased external rotation at 30° and 90° of knee flexion indicates PCL and PLC injury. Increased external rotation at 30° flexion only indicates an isolated PLC injury.
- External rotation recurvatum test – passive lifting of the toes with the knees extended. Increased recurvatum and external rotation indicate PLC and PCL injury.
- Reverse pivot shift – with the patient supine, the knee is flexed to 80° and external rotation and valgus are applied as the knee is brought into extension. The tibia is subluxed in the initial position and reduces in 20-30° of knee flexion. This test can be present normally in one-third of the population.
- Gait – varus thrust to the knee may occur.

Investigation

- X-ray – avulsion of the tibial attachment of the PCL is sometimes seen. Full-length standing radiographs are obtained to assess varus deformity in chronic PLC injury.
- MR imaging – the PCL normally has a low signal. In injury, a high signal is seen.
- Arthroscopy – best performed 2-3 weeks after injury to avoid compartment syndrome. A lax lateral compartment with increased opening is evident.

Management

It is important to distinguish acute PCL injuries from those that occurred many weeks prior to presentation. Additionally, the presence of any associated injuries to the PLC will affect treatment.

Most acute PCL injuries heal non-operatively. Bracing in extension is advised for 4 weeks. In the presence of a bony avulsion, good results are achieved with open reduction and internal fixation through a posteromedial approach. An isolated intrasubstance tear does not need surgery.

Chronic PCL injuries are associated with aching, which resolves with bracing and laxity.

Repair of acute PCL and PLC injuries should be performed within 2-3 weeks.

A variety of techniques have been described for reconstruction of the PLC. Usually the anterolateral bundle is replaced. It is possible to replace both bands, but the results are equivocal. An autogenous patellar tendon graft or Achilles tendon allograft is used.

In the Lemaire procedure for LCL, a strip of the iliotibial band attached to Gerdy's tubercle is passed through the femoral tunnel and sutured back onto itself.

Another technique is to use a strip of semitendinosus or tendoachilles allograft passed through a tunnel in the fibular head, and then through a femoral tunnel and sutured onto itself with the knee in 30° flexion and the tibia pulled forward on the femur.

The results of reconstruction are not as good for chronic PCL and PLC injuries compared with ACL injuries.

Postoperatively, the knee is placed in 0-30° flexion for 6 weeks with partial weight bearing. The patient gradually progresses to full weight bearing and quadriceps exercises.

Medial collateral ligament injuries

The MCL is the key restraint to valgus stress. The superficial MCL runs from the medial epicondyle of the femur and attaches to a wide area on the tibia beginning 2cm distal to the joint line. The middle third is thickened to form the deep MCL. The meniscofemoral and meniscotibial ligaments are parts of the medial knee capsule, attaching the medial meniscus to the femur and tibia, respectively.

Injuries to the MCL result from a valgus force applied to the flexed knee.

Clinical features

Injury to individual components of the MCL can be assessed on the basis of localised tenderness. Femoral avulsion will cause pain over the adductor tubercle. Joint-line tenderness indicates a possible medial meniscal injury in association with the MCL injury.

The amount of medial joint opening on valgus stress indicates the degree of MCL injury (Table 3.2). The instability is assessed in 30° of flexion. Valgus stress in full extension is resisted by the cruciate ligaments and the posterior capsule in addition to the MCL, and hence instability in full extension indicates more extensive injury.

The anterior drawer test in external rotation will demonstrate increased forward translation of the tibia. This is more evident if there is associated ACL injury.

Imaging

An MR scan of the knee is diagnostic. The MCL is visualised in the coronal images. (Figure 3.4)

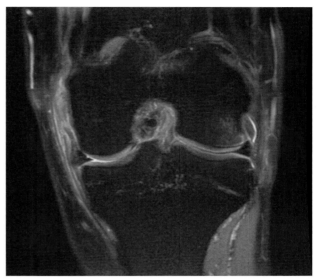

Figure 3.4. Magnetic resonance scan showing avulsion of the medial collateral ligament.

Management

Isolated MCL injuries are managed by full weight-bearing mobilisation with the aid of crutches and an early ROM program to minimise stiffness. Hinged bracing, which allows ROM, can be considered for grade III injuries. Immobilisation in a cast is counterproductive.

Grade	Description
	Table 3.2. Grades of medial collateral ligament injury.
I	<5mm medial joint-line opening on valgus stress in 30° flexion
II	5-10mm medial joint-line opening on valgus stress
III	A complete tear with >10mm medial joint-line opening on valgus stress

MCL injuries with ACL injuries are managed by reconstruction of the ACL when the knee has regained full ROM and non-operative management of the MCL injury.

In chronic MCL injuries resulting in instability, the MCL can be reconstructed using the gracilis or semitendinosus tendons. The femoral attachment of the reconstruction should be isometric with the MCL to avoid stretching the tendons and late recurrent instability.

The patellofemoral joint

The PF joint is subject to substantial forces and the articular surface of the patella is the thickest of any joint in the body. On stair climbing and descent, the forces on the PF joint can be three to five times the body weight.

The patella functions to increase the lever arm of the quadriceps, moving the extensor mechanism further from the centre of rotation of the knee joint. In full extension the patella does not articulate with the trochlea, but comes in contact at about 20° of flexion. The contact point on the patella moves proximally as the knee flexes.

The stability of the patella depends on dynamic and static stabilisers (Table 3.3).

Clinical assessment

The presenting complaint is anterior knee pain. Pain on climbing stairs is likely to be PF in origin. Swelling of the knee, clicking and symptoms of instability can arise from PF joint problems.

Specific features to note on examination are varus or valgus alignment of the leg, recurvatum, gait, patellar tracking, the J sign, the Q angle, patellar mobility and glide. Torsional deformities of the femur and tibia and leg length inequality should also be assessed, as well as foot disorders such as pes planus.

Patellar tracking is assessed on flexion and extension of the knee. The J sign refers to the lateral deviation of the patella towards the end of extension.

The Q angle is the angle between the pull of the quadriceps tendon and the axis of the patellar tendon (Figure 3.5). The first line is drawn from the anterior superior iliac spine to the centre of the patella, and the second from the centre of the patella to the tibial tubercle. The normal Q angle is 8-10° in men and up to 15° in women. A higher angle increases the risk of lateral subluxation of the patella.

Patellar mobility should be less than 50% of the patellar width.

Table 3.3. Dynamic and static stabilisers in the patella.

Dynamic stabilisers	Static stabilisers
Components of the quadriceps femoris	Depth of the trochlear groove
	Shape of patellar facets
	Patellar tendon length
	Quadriceps tendon direction (Q angle)
	Trochlear groove-tibial tubercle distance
	Medial patellofemoral ligament
	Lateral retinaculum

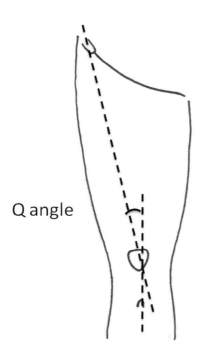

Q angle

Figure 3.5. Measurement of the Q angle.

Radiographic assessment of the patella

Plain radiographs should be taken in the AP, lateral and axial views:

- AP view:
  - alignment of the knee;
  - osteochondral fractures;
  - bipartite patella.
- Lateral view:
  - trochlear dysplasia;
  - patellar height (alta or baja).
- Axial view:
  - for trochlear anatomy;
  - patellar translation or tilt.

A CT scan is helpful in assessing trochlear dysplasia. Lateralisation of the tibial tubercle can be assessed by measuring the distance between the centre of the tubercle and the trochlea (the tibial tubercle trochlear groove distance; Figure 3.6). The distance should be less than 20mm.

An MR scan will demonstrate articular cartilage changes, the patellar retinacula and the extensor mechanism.

The Wiberg classification of patellar shape describes three types (Figure 3.7):

- Type I – the medial and lateral facets are symmetrical and equal in size.
- Type II – the medial facet is smaller than the lateral.
- Type III – the medial facet is markedly smaller than the lateral.

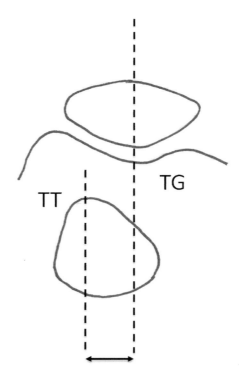

Figure 3.6. Measuring the tibial tubercle trochlear groove distance. The measurement is taken on serial axial images from the centre of the trochlear groove (TG) and the centre of the tibial tubercle (TT).

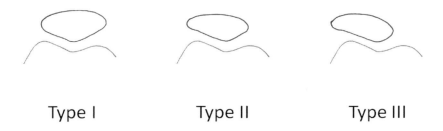

Type I   Type II   Type III

Figure 3.7. Wiberg classification of patellar shape.

Patellar dislocation

Acute patellar dislocation is usually seen in teenagers. The patella may be dislocated laterally as a result of indirect injury. This results in local pain and swelling and painful lateral subluxation of the patella. Generalised laxity should be assessed. Plain radiographs may show avulsion fractures or associated osteochondral fractures. An MR scan will demonstrate the tear in the medial retinaculum and any chondral injury.

Most injuries are managed non-operatively, but acute repair has an increasing number of advocates.

Acute repair of the retinaculum and medial PF ligament is an option in the high-demand athlete.

Osteochondral fractures can be addressed at the same time and fixed back with bioabsorbable screws. A tight lateral retinaculum can be improved with a lateral release. A lateral release will help to correct abnormal patellar tilt, but is not useful in patients with significant patellar shift. Medialisation of the tibial tubercle is considered where there is evidence of a laterally placed tibial tubercle on cross-sectional scanning.

About 20% of patients have recurrent dislocation of the patella. This is seen in patients with predisposing causes (Table 3.4).

Table 3.4. Predisposing causes for recurrent dislocation of the patella.	
Local causes	**General causes**
Femoral trochlear dysplasia	General ligamentous laxity
High Q angle	Ehlers Danlos syndrome
Hypoplasia of the lateral femoral condyle	
Weakness of the vastus medialis	
Patella alta	
A laterally placed tibial tubercle	

Clinical assessment

Patients are assessed clinically:

- Patella tilt test – assesses the tightness of the lateral retinaculum. In normal knees, it should be possible to lift the patella off the lateral femoral condyle.
- Patella glide test – assesses the laxity of the medial retinaculum. In a positive glide test, the patella can be pushed laterally by over 50% of its width.
- Q angle – a higher angle indicates more valgus pull on the patella, which can lead to patellar subluxation.
- Patellar tracking – visual assessment of movement of the patella in the trochlear groove. A patella that moves laterally on knee extension indicates a tight lateral retinaculum (J sign).

Imaging

Patella alta is quantified by the Insall-Salvati index or the Blackburne-Peel index (Figure 3.8).

The Insall-Salvati index is the ratio of the length of the patellar tendon to the diagonal length of the patella on a lateral radiograph. The normal ratio is 1.0, while a ratio of 1.2 indicates patella alta.

The Blackburne-Peel index is the ratio of the length of the articular surface of the patella to the perpendicular distance between the articular surface of the tibia and the inferior pole of the patella. The normal ratio varies from 0.54 to 1.06.

The Blumensaat's line is an anterior extension of the intercondylar notch line on the lateral view. The inferior pole of the patella should be at the level of this line when the radiograph is obtained with the knee at 30° flexion.

The lateral radiograph of the knee and axial view is used to diagnose trochlear dysplasia. The 'crossing sign' indicates a shallow trochlear groove. The MR scan also demonstrates the trochlear groove, the shape of the patella and the condition of the retinacular attachments (Figure 3.9).

a

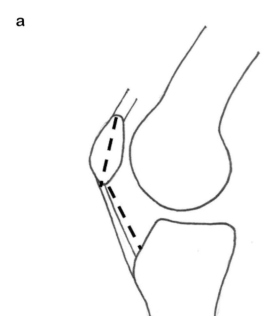

b

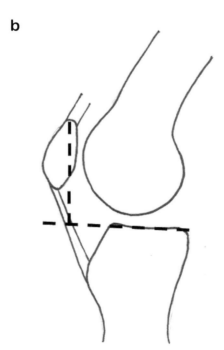

Figure 3.8. Measuring patellar height. (a) The Insall-Salvati index and (b) the Blackburne-Peel index.

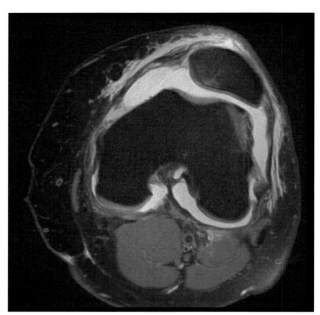

Figure 3.9. A magnetic resonance scan showing tearing of the medial retinaculum following patellar dislocation.

Management

An attempt at non-operative management with strengthening of the vastus medialis muscle is justified in patients with recurrent dislocation. The frequency of dislocation reduces as patients progress beyond the teenage years. Patients who do not respond to non-operative treatment are candidates for realignment procedures.

Realignment of the extensor mechanism can be proximal, distal or combined. Proximal realignment is based on reefing or advancing the medial retinaculum and release of the lateral side. It can be performed in skeletally immature patients with no significant distal malalignment problems.

Proximal realignment using a soft tissue procedure involves advancing the vastus medialis or releasing the lateral retinaculum, or a combination of the two. This is effective if the Q angle is less than 20°. For a higher Q angle, distal realignment is required.

The lateral release is helpful in patients with patellar tilt and clinically demonstrable tightness of the lateral retinaculum. The adequacy of release should be checked to maximise efficacy.

Reconstruction of the medial PF ligament using hamstring tendon is an option where there is attenuation of the medial retinaculum with recurrent instability in the absence of significant malalignment defects. Overtightening of the graft should be avoided.

Distal realignment can involve bony or soft tissue procedures. The bony correction is aimed at medial transfer of the tibial tubercle (Emsllie Trillat). Soft tissue procedures include the Roux-Goldthwait (medial transfer of the lateral half of the patellar tendon) and Galeazzi procedures. Soft tissue procedures can be considered in skeletally immature patients.

Fulkerson tibial tubercle osteotomy translates the tubercle anteriorly and medially. The Maquet procedure is simply anterior translation of the tubercle. It does not correct malalignment, but helps to reduce PF joint reaction force.

Trochleaplasty – an attempt to reconstruct the trochlear groove – is an option for patients with trochlear dysplasia.

Note

Von Knoch F, Böhm T, Bürgi ML, *et al.* Trochleaplasty for recurrent patellar dislocation in association with trochlear dysplasia. A 4- to 14-year follow-up study. *J Bone Joint Surg Br* 2006; 88: 1331-5. Out of 38 patients (45 knees), 93% had radiological correction of trochlear dysplasia but 30% developed degeneration of the PF joint.

In patients with advanced PF degenerative disease, replacement of the PF joint can be considered.

Plica syndrome

Plicae are folds of synovium present normally in the knee. Plicae can occasionally become symptomatic, however, presenting as anterior knee pain or a snapping band in the knee.

On arthroscopy, changes in the articular surface adjoining the plicae should raise suspicion of plica syndrome. In the absence of any changes, the plicae are unlikely to be the cause of symptoms. Arthroscopic resection of symptomatic plicae has a good success rate.

Osteochondritis dissecans

Osteochondritis dissecans is a condition of unknown aetiology affecting the articular cartilage and subchondral bone.

Clinical features

In the early stages, lesions can be asymptomatic. Effusion, generalised tenderness and occasional locking may be present in symptomatic lesions.

Classification

Based on the integrity of the articular cartilage, lesions can be open or closed. The stability of the underlying subchondral bone determines whether the lesion is stable or unstable.

An arthroscopic classification was described by Guhl (Table 3.5).

Site

The classic site is the posterolateral aspect of the medial femoral condyle (70% of patients). The lateral femoral condyle is involved in 20% of patients.

Imaging

Plain radiographs, including tunnel view supplemented with an MR scan, are used to delineate the lesions. The MR scan is particularly helpful to assess the integrity of the overlying cartilage and the viability of the bone bed. Closed lesions have a good prognosis. Younger patients with open physis have a greater potential to heal the lesions and hence a better prognosis.

The presence of a breach in the articular cartilage and displaced lesions indicate a poor prognosis.

Management

Undisplaced, stable lesions (with intact overlying cartilage) are managed non-operatively. A short period of restricted weight bearing while allowing knee flexion is helpful.

Fixation of the fragment is performed for unstable lesions. Displaced lesions can be fixed back if it is

Table 3.5. Arthroscopic classification of osteochondritis dissecans.

Type	Description
A	Intact lesions
B	Lesions showing early separation
C	Partially detached lesions
D	Lesions detached from the bed

Table 3.6. The Beighton score for assessing hyperlaxity.

Finding	Score
Ability to place palms on the floor on bending forward with knees extended	1
Thumbs can touch flexor surface of forearm on passive stretching	2
Knee hyperextension	2
Elbow hyperextension	2
Passive hyperextension of the little finger metacarpophalangeal joints to 90°	2

possible to reduce the fragment anatomically and achieve stable fixation. Excision is recommended for fragments that are unsuitable for fixation.

Hyperlaxity

The Beighton score is commonly used for assessing hyperlaxity (Table 3.6).

The maximum score is 9. A score of 4 or more indicates hyperlaxity. The diagnosis of benign joint hypermobility syndrome takes into account the Beighton score, the presence of arthralgia for more than 3-4 months and several minor factors such as subluxation of joints and the presence of tendonitis, bursitis, abnormal skin striae and marfanoid habitus, among others.

Patellar tendonitis

Patellar tendonitis (also known as jumper's knee) is inflammation of the proximal part of the patellar tendon as a result of overuse.

The underlying process is recurrent microscopic tears of the tendon and degenerative changes. The tendonitis may be associated with PF malalignment, patella alta, tibial torsion or hamstring or rectus femoris tightness.

Four stages have been described:

- Stage I – pain after activity.
- Stage II – pain during and after activity.
- Stage III – pain at rest and activity.
- Stage IV – complete rupture of the tendon.

Management is predominantly non-operative and comprises rest, non-steroidal anti-inflammatory drugs (NSAIDs) and physiotherapy. Open-chain isokinetic exercises should be avoided and appropriate footwear is recommended. Quadriceps and hamstring exercises are helpful in prevention.

Multiple injections of platelet-rich plasma have been shown to have some efficacy in randomised controlled trials. Extracorporeal shock-wave therapy has also had some success.

Note

Filardo G, Kon E, Della Villa S, *et al.* Use of platelet-rich plasma for the treatment of refractory jumper's knee. *Int Orthop* 2010; 34: 909-15. **This study compared the use of platelet-rich plasma with physiotherapy in 15 and 16 patients, respectively. Those given platelet-rich plasma showed a statistically significant improvement on all scores at the end of the injections and further improvement at 6 months.**

Note

Vulpiani MC, Vetrano M, Savoia V, *et al.* Jumper's knee treatment with extracorporeal shock wave therapy: a long-term follow-up observational study. *J Sports Med Phys Fitness* 2007; 47: 323-8. A total of 83 knees underwent four sessions of shock-wave therapy. Improvement was seen in 73%, with a 2-year follow-up.

Surgical debridement of the degenerate tendon is reserved for subjects with persistent symptoms despite adequate non-operative measures.

Prepatellar bursitis

Prepatellar bursitis presents as swelling anteriorly and may be related to a history of trauma or recurrent irritation. Non-operative treatment involves avoidance of the aggravating activity and anti-inflammatory medication. Persistent swelling is treated by excision of the bursa.

Baker's cyst

Baker's cyst is a posterior herniation of the knee synovium, or an enlarged bursa under the semimembranosus tendon or under the medial head of the gastrocnemius. The prevalence follows a bimodal age distribution – the cysts can present in childhood or middle age. Baker's cysts in adults are often associated with intra-articular pathology, while childhood cysts are often bursal enlargements.

A ruptured Baker's cyst can present as a painful swollen calf. It must be differentiated from venous thrombosis.

Cysts in children usually resolve spontaneously. In adults, the intra-articular pathology is addressed. Excision of the cyst is rarely indicated, but can be performed through a posteromedial approach in the supine position.

Snapping knee

A snapping knee can be due to intra-articular or extra-articular causes.

Intra-articular causes include meniscal tears, loose bodies or chondral irregularity in arthritis. Extra-articular causes are usually due to the tendons around the knee joint – the biceps femoris, popliteus or the semitendinosus.

Management is by addressing the underlying intra-articular cause or release of tendons, as appropriate.

Snapping hip

Intra-articular causes of a snapping hip are loose bodies, labral tears, hip subluxation and synovial chondromatosis. Extra-articular causes include movement of the iliotibial band over the greater trochanter, the anterior margin of the gluteus maximus over the greater trochanter or the iliopsoas tendon against the hip capsule.

Management is through physical therapy, steroid injection or surgical release of the tendon. The iliotibial band can be lengthened by Z-plasty.

Shin splints

Also known as medial tibial stress syndrome, shin splints are characterised by pain along the middle and distal third of the medial border of the tibia. There is local tenderness and the symptoms are aggravated by activity.

Plain radiographs are normal, and a Tc-99m bone scan may show increased linear activity along the medial border of the tibia.

Management is largely non-surgical: rest, stretching and a gradual return to activity. Surgical intervention in patients with persistent symptoms involves release of the fascial insertion in the posteromedial border of the tibia. This has a good success rate.

Iliotibial band syndrome

The iliotibial band arises from the fascia of the tensor fascia lata and inserts into the Gerdy's tubercle on the anterolateral aspect of the proximal tibia. The band lies anterior to the lateral femoral condyle in full extension and slips posterior to the condyle at 30° of flexion. Excessive friction between the iliotibial band and the lateral femoral condyle leads to iliotibial band syndrome.

The presenting feature is lateral knee pain on activity. The pain is typically worse on the heel strike. There is local tenderness over the lateral femoral condyle. Pressure with the examiner's thumb over the epicondyle and active knee flexion and extension will reproduce the pain. The Ober test is used to assess tightness of the iliotibial band.

Management of iliotibial band syndrome is based on rest, NSAIDs and stretching exercises. The activity level should be adjusted to avoid aggravating the pain. A lateral heel raise or an orthosis to provide medial arch support may help. Surgical release of posterior fibres of the iliotibial band is an option for persistent symptoms.

Spontaneous osteonecrosis of the knee

As suggested by its name, the cause of spontaneous osteonecrosis of the knee (SONK) is unknown. Possible aetiologies are vascular or trauma. SONK usually affects the medial femoral condyle, but can affect the lateral femoral condyle or the medial tibial plateau.

SONK typically occurs in postmenopausal females, presenting as an acute onset of localised (usually medial) knee pain without pre-existing symptoms of arthritis or significant trauma.

Osteonecrosis of the knee can also occur in patients with steroid and alcohol intake, renal transplantation, Gaucher's disease, systemic lupus erythematosus and coagulation disorders. There are common underlying processes with osteonecrosis of the hip.

Imaging

Plain radiographs are normal in the early stages. Later stages may appear as areas of radiolucency with surrounding sclerosis. Flattening of the condyle may be evident. In due course, these lead to secondary arthritic changes.

A Tc-99m bone scan will show increased local uptake and an MR scan is diagnostic (Figure 3.10).

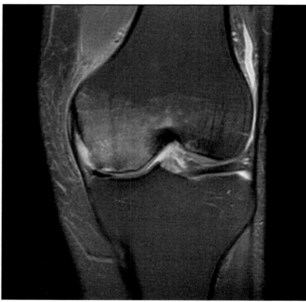

Figure 3.10. Spontaneous osteonecrosis of the knee affecting the medial femoral condyle.

Management

Management is based on the following:

- Offloading the medial compartment with an open-wedge osteotomy.
- Drilling to decompress the condyle.
- Prosthetic replacement. The Oxford group has published results of medial unicompartmental replacement in focal SONK, with similar results to those in arthritic knees.

Note

Langdown AJ, Pandit H, Price AJ, *et al*. Oxford medial unicompartmental arthroplasty for focal spontaneous osteonecrosis of the knee. *Acta Orthop* 2005; 76: 688-92. **This study looked at 29 knees with SONK, 26 with osteonecrosis of the medial femoral condyle and three with osteonecrosis of the medial tibial plateau. The mean follow-up was 5 years. The results in patients with SONK were similar to those in the control group with arthritis.**

Articular cartilage defects in the knee

Articular cartilage has a poor ability to regenerate following injury. The chondrocytes demonstrate a limited cellular response to injury and are unable to migrate due to the collagen matrix.

Management

A variety of techniques have been described to stimulate healing or replace lost cartilage.

Microfracture

Microfracture involves drilling subchondral bone in order to recruit mesenchymal cells. A stable blood clot is essential and the cells differentiate into chondrocytes, which form a fibrocartilage scaffold. Normal hyaline cartilage has type II collagen and the scaffold formed by microfracture has varying amounts of type I, II and III cartilage. The fibrocartilage is unable to withstand physiological loading over a period of time.

Touch weight bearing on crutches for 6 weeks and passive motion are advised postoperatively. Small lesions, age less than 40 years and a relatively short duration of symptoms correlate with a better outcome. The results tend to deteriorate with time.

Mosaicplasty

Mosaicplasty (osteoarticular transfer system) involves harvesting multiple cylindrical plugs of articular cartilage and bone from the knee and transplanting them into a defect in the same knee.

The donor site is the area adjacent to the intercondylar notch and the PF joint. The main disadvantages are donor-site morbidity, limited availability of articular cartilage graft and inadequate stability of the plugs.

Osteochondral allografts

This involves transfer of cadaveric cartilage and subchondral bone to defects. Large defects can be treated with this method, including those with deficient condyles.

The procedure is expensive and technically demanding. There is a risk of disease transmission, incomplete incorporation of the graft and immune rejection.

Autologous chondrocyte implantation

Autologous chondrocyte implantation (ACI) first involves harvesting chondrocytes arthroscopically and culturing them in a laboratory. In a second stage 4-6 weeks later, the chondrocytes are reimplanted by placing them under a periosteal flap sutured around the defect. The second stage is performed as an open procedure.

Note

Brittberg M, Lindahl A, Nilsson A, *et al*. Treatment of deep cartilage defects in the knee with autologous chondrocyte implantation. *N Engl J Med* 1994; 331: 889-95.

The advantage is the formation of hyaline-like cartilage and the results reported show the superiority of ACI/matrix-associated ACI (MACI) over other techniques. Brittberg has demonstrated use of the cultured chondrocytes to treat chondral defects.

Note

Gikas PD, Bayliss L, Bentley G, Briggs TW. An overview of autologous chondrocyte implantation. *J Bone Joint Surg Br* 2009; 91: 997-1006.

Note

Henderson I, Tuy B, Oakes B. Reoperation after autologous chondrocyte implantation. Indications and findings. *J Bone Joint Surg Br* 2004; 86: 205-11. **In this study, 22 out of 135 patients underwent reoperation after ACI. The authors found lifting of 24/31 lesions and detachment of 3/31 periosteal patches. Mechanical symptoms resolved after 2 weeks, and 97% of patients had normal or near-normal visual repair scores. In all, 70% had hyaline or hyaline-like cartilage with good integration with subchondral bone.**

Note

Bentley G, Biant LC, Carrington RW, *et al*. A prospective, randomised comparison of autologous chondrocyte implantation versus mosaicplasty for osteochondral defects in the knee. *J Bone Joint Surg Br* 2003; 85: 223-30. **In this prospective trial of 100 patients randomised to ACI or mosaicplasty, results were excellent in 88% of ACI and 69% of mosaicplasty patients. Arthroscopy at 1 year had a grade I or II appearance in 84% of ACI patients.**

However, the procedure is not without its disadvantages. The periosteal flap is obtained from the distal femur or proximal tibia and some patients develop tissue hypertrophy. The beneficial role of a cambial layer of periosteum is debatable, and most modern techniques rely on an absorbable collagen scaffold. Furthermore, suturing the periosteal flap can damage the surrounding cartilage.

The problems of ACI include postoperative effusion and synovitis, adhesions and arthrofibrosis, hypertrophy of periosteal patch and loosening of the graft complex.

Matrix-associated autologous chondrocyte implantation

In MACI, the autologous chondrocytes are delivered on a bioabsorbable type I or III collagen scaffold. This avoids the problems with periosteal flap harvest required for ACI. The cells are evenly distributed (1 million/cm^2).

Weight bearing is restricted to touch weight for 6 weeks and full weight bearing is allowed after about 3 months.

Hip labral tears

The acetabular labrum is a fibrocartilaginous, triangular structure that extends beyond the midpoint of the femoral head and functions to stabilise the joint. The labrum is deficient inferiorly, where the transverse acetabular ligament substitutes for the labrum and completes the rim.

The labrum has a good blood supply along its peripheral attachment and is avascular at its free edge. Labral tears are most common in the anterosuperior quadrant.

Injuries can be degenerative (50%), traumatic (20%) or idiopathic, and may be associated with chondral damage. Axial and torsion strain on the hip lead to labrum damage.

Traumatic tears of the acetabular labrum are seen in athletes involved in pivoting and hip flexion activities, while degenerate tears of the acetabular labrum are common in patients with dysplastic hips, old Perthes disease or old slipped upper femoral epiphysis.

Labral tears are most often seen in young adults or those in middle age, and present as an insidious onset of pain in the groin. The pain is worse on walking or pivoting activity.

The impingement sign is pain in the hip elicited by flexion of the hip to 90°, adducting and internally rotating. The McCarthy sign is pain on extension of the hip and is elicited by flexing both hips and then extending the affected hip in internal and external rotation.

Differential diagnosis

There are several differential diagnoses for non-arthritic groin pain:

- Acetabular labral tears.
- Femoroacetabular impingement.
- Iliotibial band syndrome.
- Lumbar spine radicular pain.
- Snapping psoas syndrome.
- Avascular necrosis.
- Trochanteric bursitis.
- Stress fracture of femoral neck.
- Femoral hernia.

Imaging

Plain radiographs, CT scanning and a Tc-99m bone scan help rule out other causes. An MR arthrogram has a sensitivity of 92% for labral tears, osteochondral loose bodies and chondral lesions. Hip arthroscopy is the gold standard for diagnosis.

Management

Labral tears can be arthroscopically resected to the stable margin or repaired.

Compared with those with arthritis, patients without arthritis have better results following excision of the tears. Refixation of the labrum is thought to give better results, but the procedure is technically demanding. Both open and arthroscopic repair of labral tears have been described.

Femoroacetabular impingement

Femoroacetabular impingement (FAI) is abutment of the proximal femur against the acetabular rim. This may be due to excess ROM in a structurally normal hip to abnormal morphology of the proximal femur and acetabulum.

Two types of FAI are recognised:

- Cam impingement – seen in young men. A non-spherical part of the femoral head abuts against the acetabulum in flexion and internal rotation. This damages the acetabular cartilage in the anterosuperior area.
- Pincer impingement – more common in middle-aged women. This is due to abnormal contact between the femoral head neck junction and the acetabular rim. The labrum degenerates and becomes calcified. The damage to the acetabular articular cartilage is along a narrow circumferential strip.

Cam and pincer impingement often coexist.

Causes of impingement

Cam impingement is due to a non-spherical femoral head, as seen in Perthes disease, avascular necrosis, a slipped upper femoral epiphysis and malunited femoral neck fractures.

Pincer impingement is seen with a retroverted acetabulum where the anterior margin of the acetabulum abuts against the femoral neck in flexion.

Clinical features

Patients present with groin pain unrelated to trauma. Pain may be worse on activity or on sitting for long periods. Anterior impingement pain can be reproduced with flexion, adduction and internal rotation of the hip. Posteroinferior impingement pain is demonstrated by extension of the hip and external rotation.

Imaging

Plain radiographs may reveal a pistol-grip deformity of the proximal femur on the AP and/or lateral view. Flattening of the femoral head is seen in some patients.

An MR arthrogram has good sensitivity for the detection of labral tears, herniation pits, rim ossification and chondral damage (Figure 3.11).

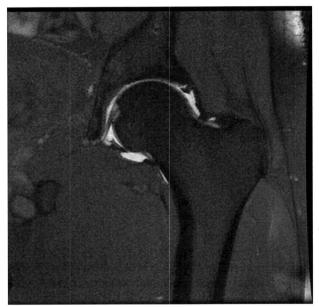

Figure 3.11. A magnetic resonance arthrogram demonstrating a labral tear superiorly.

Management

Non-operative treatment involves NSAIDs and avoiding aggravating activities.

Surgical treatment is aimed at excising the impinging bone. This can be achieved with open or arthroscopic methods.

An open procedure requires dislocation of the femoral head while protecting the medial circumflex femoral artery. Reshaping of the femoral neck is possible to prevent cam impingement. A retroverted acetabulum leads to impingement anteriorly and the anterior rim of the acetabulum can be excised.

Alternatively, a retroverted acetabulum can be corrected by periacetabular osteotomy.

Hip arthroscopy is performed in the supine or the lateral position with traction and image intensifier control. The central compartment is the area medial to the labrum and the peripheral compartment is the area lateral to the labrum.

Labral tears and chondral damage can be debrided with arthroscopy. Labral tears may also be repaired with arthroscopic techniques.

Rupture of the distal biceps tendon

Biceps tendon injuries are most common at the proximal attachment and distal ruptures comprise 3% of all biceps tendon injuries.

The rupture is the result of eccentric loading of the flexed elbow. Swelling and bruising may be present in the cubital fossa. An MR scan differentiates partial rupture from complete rupture.

Non-operative treatment may lead to reduced flexion and supination strength. Athletes and high-demand patients are managed by repair of the tendon to the radial tuberosity by a two-incision technique. The tendon is identified through an anterior incision, while a posterior incision is made to pull the tendon through and attach it.

Potential complications of this procedure are injury to the radial nerve and the risk of radioulnar synostosis.

Partial ruptures can be managed non-operatively, or by reattachment of the tendon to the radial tuberosity.

Lateral epicondylitis

Lateral epicondylitis (tennis elbow) involves the origin of the extensor carpi radialis brevis (ECRB). Repeated microtrauma leads to degeneration in the tendon.

The 'double-lengthening' phenomenon refers to an increase in the length of the sarcomeres of the ECRB on flexion, similar to the length in extension. This can lead to increased eccentric loading in flexion.

Clinical features

The presenting symptom is pain on palpation in the region of the lateral epicondyle. Dorsiflexion of the wrist against resistance elicits pain in the region of the lateral epicondyle. Extension of the middle finger also reproduces the pain. This is due to the insertion of the ECRB on the base of the middle finger metacarpal.

Histologically, hyaline degeneration and angiofibroblastic changes can be seen in the origin of the ECRB.

Management

The majority of patients achieve relief by resting. Recalcitrant situations are managed with steroid injections.

Surgical options include excision of the necrotic tissue, release of the extensor origin, lengthening of the ECRB in the distal forearm and localised denervation of the lateral epicondyle. Approximately 85% of patients benefit from surgery.

Note

Dunkow PD, Jatti M, Muddu BN. A comparison of open and percutaneous techniques in the surgical treatment of tennis elbow. *J Bone Joint Surg Br* 2004; 86: 701-4. In this prospective, controlled trial, 45 patients were randomised to open or percutaneous tennis elbow release. Follow-up was for 12 months. The percutaneous group had better satisfaction, an improved DASH (Disability of Arm, Shoulder and Hand) score, a faster return to work and improved sporting activity.

Chapter 4 Spine and nerve injuries

Spinal anatomy

The main ligaments connecting the vertebrae are the anterior and the posterior longitudinal ligaments, which run along the anterior and posterior aspect of the vertebral bodies. The ligamentum flavum runs between the laminae and the supraspinous and interspinous ligaments connect the spinous processes (Figure 4.1).

Disc disease

The intervertebral disc has a central avascular portion called the nucleus pulposus and a peripheral portion called the annulus fibrosus. The outer third of the annulus has neural innervation, and tears in the annulus can cause backache in degenerative disc disease. The annulus is primarily composed of type I collagen. The nucleus has a proteoglycan matrix with a framework of type II collagen fibres. Fragmentation of the nucleus is considered to be one of the initial events in disc disease, but is largely asymptomatic.

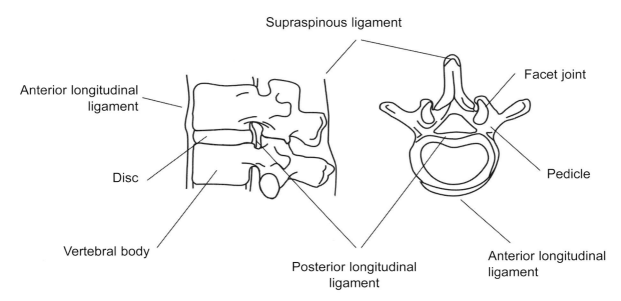

Figure 4.1. Anatomy of the spine.

The lifetime prevalence of low back pain is 80-85%. Most cases of low back pain (90%) will improve within a month of onset, although recurrence is common. In a small percentage of patients (approximately 2%) low backache is associated with radiating pain down the leg (sciatica). Overall, 80% of these patients will recover.

Nomenclature for abnormal discs

There is no standardised nomenclature for disc herniation. One system of classification is described in Table 4.1.

> **Note**
>
> Spitzer WO, LeBlanc FE, Dupuis M, et al. Scientific approach to the assessment and management of activity-related spinal disorders. A monograph for clinicians. Report of the Quebec Taskforce on Spinal Disorders. *Spine* (Phila Pa 1976) 1987; 12(Suppl.): S16-21.

Based on the site of herniation, the extrusion can be central (in the midline posteriorly), posterolateral (the most common form), lateral (foraminal) or far lateral (extraforaminal) (Figure 4.2).

On computed tomography (CT) discography, the tears are graded as follows:

- Grade 0 – no evidence of tear.
- Grade 1 – tear in the inner third of the annulus.
- Grade 2 – tear in the middle third of the annulus.
- Grade 3 – tear in the outer third of the annulus.

The sequence of events in lumbar disc disease is fragmentation of the nucleus followed by annular tears, leading to herniation of the nucleus. Annular tears are associated with backache, and the herniation may cause nerve root symptoms or cauda equina syndrome.

Central and posterolateral herniation involve the nerve root below the level of herniation. For instance, the L4/5 disc will cause pressure on the L5 root as

Table 4.1. A classification system for disc herniation.

Type	Description
Degenerate disc	Deterioration of the internal disc structure, often with loss of hydration and reduced disc height
Bulging disc	Circumferential symmetrical out-pouching of the disc beyond the end plates May be a normal variant
Protruded disc	Focal, often asymmetric extension of the disc beyond the disc space, with a broad connection with the herniated part and the parent disc
Extruded disc	A more extreme extension of the protruding disc, with a narrow or no connection to the parent disc
Sequestration	A subset of the extruded disc, where the disc material is contained by the posterior longitudinal ligament
Migrated disc	The extruded material is displaced above or below the edge of the disc space
Contained disc	Disc herniation where a part of the annulus is intact

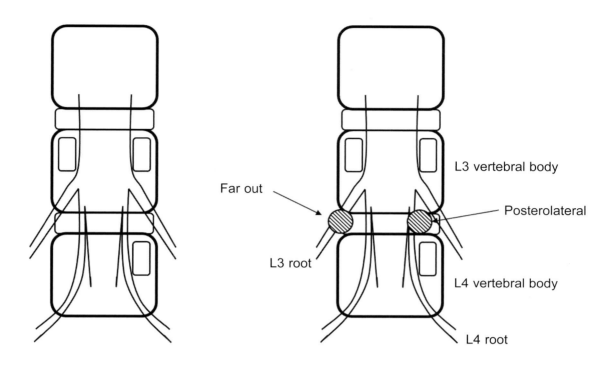

L3 vertebral body

Far out

Posterolateral

L3 root

L4 vertebral body

L4 root

Figure 4.2. Sites of nerve root compression, showing the difference between posterolateral and far-out compression.

the L4 root exits just above the disc. A lateral or far-lateral herniation will press on the root of the same level. For instance, the L4/5 lateral or far-lateral herniation will press on the L4 root (Table 4.2).

The composition of the disc changes with age. Proteoglycan synthesis, chondroitin sulphate, water content and elastin are all reduced, while collagen content increases in the nucleus and annulus. The

Table 4.2. Nerve roots affected by prolapsed discs.			
	L3-4	**L4-5**	**L5-S1**
Posterolateral disc	L4	L5	S1
Far-lateral disc	L3	L4	L5
Pain	Anterior thigh/leg	Posterior leg/front of foot	Posterior/lateral foot
Motor weakness	Quadriceps	Extensor hallucis longus and tibialis anterior	Gastrocnemius
Reflex involved	Knee jerk	Medial hamstring jerk	Ankle jerk
Incidence	3-10%	40-45%	45-50%

loss of water and increase in collagen make the discs stiff. The outer third of the annulus has sensory nerve endings, which may explain the pain of disc disease.

Herniation is a feature of degenerate discs. A normal disc with an annular tear will not herniate because the nucleus is cohesive.

Clinical features

Patients with disc prolapse usually present in the third to fifth decade. Disc prolapse is rare in the young and the elderly.

Degenerative disc disease may cause intermittent low backache over a period of time.

Pressure on the nerve roots results in radicular pain (sciatica). The pain is dermatomal, and radiates from the lower back to the legs. The pain may be worse with coughing, sneezing or sitting for long periods. The sitting position is associated with higher intradiscal pressure compared to standing and lying.

Some patients with radicular pain present without significant backache. Large disc herniations may present as spinal stenosis and can cause cauda equina.

Clinical examination will demonstrate an antalgic gait and lateral curvature in the lower lumbar spine. In posterolateral disc herniation, patients tend to list away from the side of herniation; in axillary presentation, on the other hand, the list is towards the side of herniation. Forward bending may aggravate the radicular pain.

The straight leg raising (SLR) test is valuable, especially in young patients. The deformation of the L5 and S1 nerve roots, at the level of the foramen, is maximal with 35-70° of leg elevation. Reproduction of radicular pain with a leg elevation of 35-70° is highly suggestive of disc herniation.

The cross-over SLR test (Fajersztajn's sign) is elicited by raising the contralateral leg, which causes pain in the affected leg. This is more specific for disc herniation. The SLR test can also be performed by flexing the hip and knee of the affected side to 90° and then extending the knee. This reproduces the radicular pain. Once the pain is elicited, the knee is flexed by a few degrees to relax the stretching of the nerve root. Pressure in the popliteal fossa in this knee position may reproduce radicular pain.

The femoral stretch test is used to check for pressure on the L2-L4 nerve roots. It can be performed in the supine or lateral position. The affected hip is extended, keeping the knee flexed. Reproduction of pain in the front of the thigh and knee is suggestive of femoral nerve root involvement.

A full neurological examination is mandatory. The sensory areas of innervation of lumbar nerve roots are shown in Figure 4.3.

L4 root involvement causes weakness in the quadriceps and loss of the patellar tendon reflex. L5 root involvement causes weakness of the extensor hallucis longus and extensor digitorum longus. S1 root involvement causes weakness of the peronei and the gastro-soleus. The ankle deep tendon reflex will also be weak.

Thoracic disc prolapse is rare and malignancy and infections should be ruled out. Most patients are in their fourth decade and present with cord compression signs and radicular back pain. These are usually below the T8 level.

Patients with cauda equina present with acute onset of perianal sensory loss (saddle anaesthesia), loss of ankle reflex, sensory loss in the L4, L5 or S1 dermatome, weakness of anal tone, urinary retention or overflow incontinence, or a combination of these. Immediate diagnosis and decompression are essential to prevent permanent neurologic deficit.

Imaging

Magnetic resonance (MR) scanning is the imaging modality of choice. The size of the herniation correlates with the improvement following surgery. Large disc protrusions fare better. CT myelography is

a

b

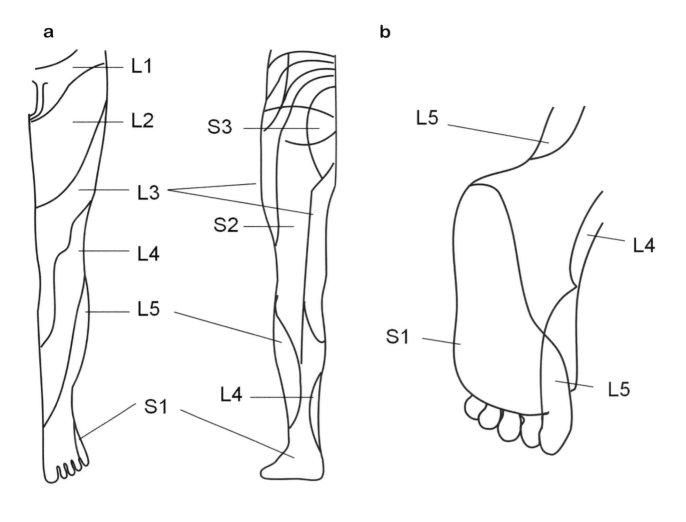

Figure 4.3. Sensory distribution of the lumbar nerve roots.

an option for patients who are unable to have an MR scan.

Differential diagnosis

In the adolescent patient, consider spondylolisthesis, infections and spinal tumours. In the elderly, consider vertebral compression fractures, infections, spinal metastasis, myeloma and primary malignancies.

Management

Non-operative management is appropriate in the initial phase of acute disc herniation. Bed rest for 3-4 days is advised, but longer periods of bed rest do not help recovery.

In the acute phase, non-steroidal anti-inflammatory drugs (NSAIDs) or opioid analgesics are useful. Epidural steroid injection or nerve root blocks are sometimes used to resolve leg pain.

Physiotherapy is helpful in promoting a gradual increase in activity levels.

Most patients (90%) do not have a relapse following an episode of radicular pain. Those with an increasing number of episodes have a poorer prognosis and many will require surgical intervention.

Surgical treatment is open or micro-discectomy and is indicated for patients with unrelenting pain or cauda equina syndrome.

Patients with cauda equina require an urgent MR scan and discectomy. Loss of neurologic function is permanent after 48 hours and decompression should be achieved within 8-12 hours of symptom onset.

Outcomes

A classic paper on the natural history of a herniated disc is by Weber. This study followed 280 patients with lumbar disc herniation proven on myelography. All patients received 14 days of in-patient treatment, followed by randomisation to surgical or non-surgical treatment. Sixty percent of the non-surgical group improved, meaning they would have undergone unnecessary surgery. A 3-month wait before surgery did not compromise the outcome. Symptoms should be allowed to resolve if there is no cauda equina or progressive neurologic deficit. The quality of the surgical result decreases after 12 months of leg symptom onset.

> **Note**
>
> Weber H. Lumbar disc herniation. A controlled, prospective study with ten years of observation. *Spine* (Phila Pa 1976) 1983; 8: 131-40.

A further study found that patients with an uncontained herniated disc had shorter symptoms and better functional outcomes. Sciatica for more than 12 months correlated with a less favourable outcome.

> **Note**
>
> Ng LC, Sell P. Predictive value of the duration of sciatica for lumbar discectomy. A prospective cohort study. *J Bone Joint Surg Br* 2004; 86: 546-9.

A recent prospective randomised study randomised 501 patients to open discectomy or non-operative care. At 4 years, patients receiving surgery had significantly better outcomes. There was a high cross-over between the two study arms.

> **Note**
>
> Weinstein JN, Lurie JD, Tosteson TD, *et al.* Surgical versus nonoperative treatment for lumbar disc herniation: four-year results for the Spine Patient Outcome Research Trial (SPORT). *Spine* (Phila Pa 1976) 2008; 33: 2789-800.

Lumbar disc replacement

Lumbar disc replacement has been proposed as a method to preserve motion at the disc space and minimise adjacent segment disease, which follows immobility of the diseased segment.

The evidence for benefit is debatable, and a recent review found no evidence to suggest better functional outcomes with disc replacement than with arthroplasty.

> **Note**
>
> Resnick DK, Watters WC. Lumbar disc arthroplasty: a critical review. *Clin Neurosurg* 2007; 54: 83-7.

Back pain

Back pain is thought to affect 60-80% people in their lifetime. About 90% of cases are self-limiting and resolve with non-operative measures.

The causes of back pain vary with the age of presentation. In children, the common causes are congenital malformation, spondylolisthesis, infections of the spine and spine tumours such as eosinophilic granuloma, Ewing's sarcoma and neuroblastoma.

In adults, trauma and disc disease are more prevalent, along with Scheuermann's disease and ankylosing spondylitis.

Metastatic tumours and spinal stenosis are common in middle-aged and elderly patients, as are osteopenic fractures and infections.

Waddell's inappropriate signs

In 1980, Waddell and colleagues proposed a set of signs that indicate a non-organic aetiology of back pain:

- Tenderness to a light touch or pinch in a wide part of the lumbar area.
- Non-anatomic deep tenderness in a wide area.
- Pain on axial compression – pressing down on the head of the patient causes pain.
- Pain on pelvic rotation when the shoulder and pelvis are rotated in the same direction.
- Findings disappear when the patient is distracted.
- Non-anatomic voluntary motor release or giving way of muscle groups.
- Non-dermatomal sensory loss.
- A disproportionate verbal or physical response to examination.

The presence of more than three signs is considered to be significant.

> **Note**
>
> Waddell G, McCulloch JA, Kummel E, Venner RM. Nonorganic physical signs in low-back pain. *Spine* (Phila Pa 1976) 1980; 5: 117-25.

Cervical disc disease

Cervical disc disease and nerve compression are seen in the fourth and fifth decades of life and are more common in women.

Compression can be caused by disc prolapse (soft disc) or osteophytes in the uncovertebral joint (hard disc). The C7 root is most often involved.

The presenting features are neck pain, pain in the interscapular region and radiating pain down the arm. This may be accompanied by a sensory and motor deficit. Distribution of sensory and motor changes in dermatomal and myotomal patterns indicates cervical spine involvement, while a deficit in the distribution of specific nerves indicates nerve entrapment syndromes (Table 4.3).

> **Note**
>
> Levin KH, Maggiano HJ, Wilbourn AJ. Cervical radiculopathies: comparison of surgical and EMG localization of single-root lesions. *Neurology* 1996; 46: 1022-5.

Spurling's compression test is helpful in diagnosing cervical spine problems. The head is tilted to the symptomatic side and the neck extended; downward pressure on the head reproduces the pain.

In the shoulder abduction test, radicular symptoms disappear or are reduced on lifting the hand above the head.

Lhermitte's sign is the occurrence of an electric-shock-like sensation radiating down the spine and limbs on flexing the neck.

Table 4.3. Clinical features of cervical nerve root compression.

Disc herniation	Root	Motor involvement	Sensory loss	Pain location	Deep tendon reflex	%
C3-4	C4	None	Shoulder Arm, upper	Neck, upper	Normal	<1
C4-5	C5	Shoulder abduction Elbow flexion	Arm, lateral	Neck; shoulder Scapula Arm, anterior	Biceps Brachioradialis	2
C5-6	C6	Shoulder abduction Elbow flexion Forearm pronation	Forearm, lateral Hand, thumb and second finger	Neck; shoulder Scapula Arm, lateral Hand, lateral	Biceps Brachioradialis Pronator	19
C6-7	C7	Extension Elbow	Forearm, dorsal and lateral Hand, third finger	Neck Shoulder Scapula, medial Forearm, extensor	Triceps	69
C8-T1	C8	Hand, intrinsic	Forearm, medial Hand, fourth and fifth fingers	Neck Scapula, medial Arm, medial Forearm, medial Hand, fourth and fifth fingers	None	9

Imaging

Plain radiographs of the cervical spine may show osteophyte formation and reduced joint space. The herniated cervical discs often have a preserved disc height. MR scanning is the imaging modality of choice for detecting nerve root compression. Foraminal narrowing is better illustrated on a fine-slice CT scan, although a CT myelogram is an alternative for soft tissue imaging if MR imaging is contraindicated.

Management

Non-operative measures include rest, NSAIDs and nerve root blocks. Most patients will improve with these measures, but there is a high incidence of pain recurrence.

Indications for operative interventions are neurological deficit and unremitting pain.

The operation involves decompression of the nerve root/osteophytes, which can be achieved through the anterior (anterior cervical discectomy and fusion) or posterior approach (foraminotomies). Along with decompression, interbody fusion of the involved cervical disc is performed using an iliac crest bone graft or spinal cage.

Ankylosing spondylitis

The common seronegative spondyloarthropathies are ankylosing spondylitis, Behçet's syndrome, psoriasis and inflammatory bowel disease.

Ankylosing spondylitis is a common spondyloarthropathy that is predominantly seen in men. It is related to human leukocyte antigen (HLA) B27, with 90% of patients positive for HLA B27 (HLA B27 is present in 5-10% of the general population). HLA is a surface antigen encoded by the major histocompatibility complex on chromosome 6.

Ankylosing spondylitis causes synovitis of the diarthrodial joints (e.g., costovertebral joints) and inflammation of the fibro-osseous junction of the syndesmotic joints such as intervertebral discs, the sacroiliac joint and pubic symphysis.

The inflammation leads to granulation tissue, bone destruction and formation of fibrous tissue. The calcification of fibrous tissue causes stiffness and syndesmophytes can be seen on radiographs.

Clinical presentation

Most patients present in adolescence with recurrent episodes of back pain accompanied by reduced chest expansion. Thoracic kyphosis develops in due course and spinal movements are grossly restricted. Involvement of the peripheral joints is a late feature and affects the shoulders, hips and knees.

Uveitis and conjunctivitis are seen in about 20% of patients, while other extraskeletal manifestations (pulmonary fibrosis and carditis) are rare.

Imaging

Radiographs in the early stages show sacroilitis, which progresses to fusion of the sacroiliac joint. Spine radiographs demonstrate squaring of the vertebral bodies and formation of syndesmophytes. Ankylosis of the spine gives the appearance of 'bamboo spine' or 'rugger-jersey spine'. Ankylosis of the hips can be seen in late stages.

Management

In the initial phases, the mainstay of treatment is maintenance of activity through physiotherapy and exercises, along with NSAIDs. Surgical intervention is needed in the later stages to correct spinal deformity through a spinal osteotomy, or for joint arthroplasty of the hips, knees or shoulders.

Fractures of the spine in patients with ankylosing spondylitis are often unstable and patients are at higher risk of neurological injury.

Diffuse skeletal idiopathic hyperostosis

Diffuse skeletal idiopathic hyperostosis, also known as Forestier's disease, is a condition of ossification of the ligaments and tendon insertions. It is more common in men.

Rheumatoid cervical spine disease

Involvement of the cervical spine is common in rheumatoid disease. The spine may be affected in various ways:

- Atlantoaxial subluxation.
- Basilar invagination.
- Involvement of the lower cervical spine joint.
- Cervical spine myelopathy.

Atlantoaxial subluxation

Atlantoaxial subluxation is the most common manifestation and is due to a destructive pannus at the synovial joint between the atlas and odontoid process. This leads to destruction of the transverse ligament and anterior subluxation of the atlas on its axis.

The Ranawat classification for clinical presentation is as follows:

- Class I: pain, no neurological deficit.
- Class II: subjective weakness, hyperreflexia and dysaesthesia.
- Class III: objective weakness and long tract signs:
  - IIIA: ambulatory;
  - IIIB: non-ambulatory.

Physicians should maintain a high index of suspicion in patients with upper cervical spine pain. Upper motor neuron signs may be present. Radiographs of the cervical spine are obtained to assess the atlantodens interval (ADI) and the posterior atlas and dens interval (PADI).

Note

Ranawat CS, O'Leary P, Pellicci P, *et al.* Cervical spine fusion in rheumatoid arthritis. *J Bone Joint Surg Am* 1979; 61: 1003-10.

Atlantodens interval

Flexion-extension X-rays of the spine show an increase in the distance between the anterior arch of the atlas and the anterior margin of the odontoid process (Figure 4.4). An increase of 3mm indicates instability and more than 6mm indicates disruption of the alar ligament. Further increases correlate with a high risk of neurological injury.

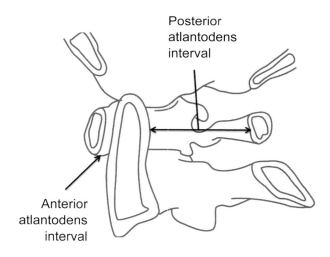

Figure 4.4. Measurement of anterior and posterior atlantodens intervals.

There is a weak correlation between ADI and neurological deficit:

- <3mm – normal ADI.
- >3mm – anterior atlantoaxial subluxation.
- 3-6mm – transverse ligament damage.
- >6mm – alar ligament damage.
- >9mm – surgical intervention (cord compression likely).

Note

Weissman BN, Aliabadi P, Weinfeld MS, *et al.* Prognostic features of atlantoaxial subluxation in rheumatoid arthritis patients. *Radiology* 1982; 144: 745-51.

Posterior atlas and dens interval

The PADI is the distance between the posterior border of the odontoid process and the anterior aspect of the posterior arch of the atlas (Figure 4.4). A normal PADI is more than 14mm, and a space of less than 10mm indicates a risk of neurologic compromise. A minimum of 10mm space is needed for the cord, 2mm for the cerebrospinal fluid and 2mm for the dura.

In studies, a PADI of 14mm or less yielded 97% sensitivity for predicting cord compression and paralysis.

Predictors of recovery:

- Ranawat classification.
- Preoperative PADI (≤10mm, poor chance of recovery; ≥14mm, significant motor recovery).
- Subaxial diameter (<14mm, less chance of recovery).

Note

Boden SD, Dodge LD, Bohlman HH, Rechtine GR. Rheumatoid arthritis of the cervical spine. A long-term analysis with predictors of paralysis and recovery. *J Bone Joint Surg Am* 1993; 75: 1282-97.

Management

Surgical treatment of atlantoaxial subluxation is indicated when the ADI is more than 6mm or the PADI is less than 14mm, in the presence of neurologic impairment or instability.

The indications for surgery are shown in Table 4.4.

Table 4.4. Indications for surgery in patients with atlantoaxial subluxation.

Asymptomatic	Ranawat class I	Ranawat class II or III
PADI <10mm (MR scan)	PADI <12mm	Medically fit
PADI 10-14mm + pannus on MR scan	PADI >12mm + pannus on MR scan	Includes some IIIb patients
ADI >8mm		
ADI = atlantodens interval; MR = magnetic resonance; PADI = posterior atlas and dens interval		

Stabilisation can be achieved by posterior fusion between C1 and C2 (Gallie/Brooke's technique) or with a transarticular screw (Magerl technique) or Harm's fusion.

Basilar invagination

Basilar invagination is cranial migration of the dens. Diagnosis is based on measurement in radiographs. An occiput to C2 fusion is performed to stabilise this. Further anterior decompression may be required through a transoral odontoidectomy.

Involvement of the lower cervical spine joint

In the lower cervical spine, rheumatoid disease involves the facet joint and the uncovertebral joints. This can lead to subluxation, which is managed by posterior fusion with lateral mass screws (Roy-Camille or Magerl techniques).

Cervical spine myelopathy

Cervical spine compression can be present in patients with rheumatoid disease because of pressure on the cord from the bony instability of rheumatoid pannus.

Torticollis

Torticollis (from the Latin torti meaning twisted and collis meaning neck) is a condition where the head is tilted to one side and the chin is elevated and turned to the opposite side.

Torticollis can be congenital or acquired. Congenital causes are Klippel-Feil syndrome and congenital muscular torticollis. Acquired causes may or may not be related to the cervical spine (Table 4.5).

Congenital muscular torticollis is the result of contracture of the sternomastoid muscle on one side. The contracture may be related to intrauterine pressure, as this condition is often associated with a breech presentation and dysplasia of the hip.

The deformity is obvious by the age of 1-2 years and the sternomastoid muscle feels hard and fibrotic. The heat tilt leads to asymmetric development of the face.

Table 4.5. Acquired causes of torticollis.

Related to the cervical spine	Not related to the cervical spine
Trauma: atlantoaxial subluxation	Contractures of the neck
Inflammatory conditions: rheumatoid arthritis and ankylosing spondylitis	Paralysis of the superior oblique muscle resulting in compensatory head tilt
Infections: pyogenic, tubercular and sometimes following upper respiratory tract infection (known as Grisel's syndrome)	Posterior fossa tumours
Tumours: osteoid osteoma causing painful torticollis	

Congenital muscular torticollis is managed by division of the lower end of the muscle (unipolar release) and rarely by division of both the lower and upper ends (bipolar release), followed by stretching exercises.

Klippel-Feil syndrome is a failure of segmentation resulting in multiple fused cervical vertebrae. The classic triad of a low posterior hairline, short webbed neck and restricted cervical movements is seen in less than half of patients. The syndrome is associated with congenital scoliosis, renal aplasia, Sprengel's deformity, congenital heart disease and brain-stem abnormalities.

Scoliosis

Scoliosis is lateral curvature of the spine associated with rotational malalignment. On the basis of Hueter-Volkmann law, the compressive forces restrict growth while tensile forces increase growth. This leads to progression of the deformity.

Aetiology

Scoliosis has several possible aetiologies:

- Genetic.
- Tissue deficiency – fibrous dysplasia, Marfan syndrome, Duchenne muscular dystrophy.
- Vertebral growth abnormality theory – anterior spinal growth outpaces posterior growth, leading to buckling of the vertebral column.
- Disorders of the brain or spinal cord – syringomyelia, Chiari malformation.
- Melatonin deficiency in chicks leads to scoliosis.

Based on its aetiology, scoliosis can be idiopathic or secondary. Secondary causes of scoliosis include congenital malformations, neuromuscular disorders, degenerative diseases, trauma, tumours, infections and improper posture.

Examination

Specific features to discuss in the history are family history, growth spurt, menstrual history and pain. The age of onset and rate of progression should be noted, along with the presence of any neurological symptoms. The family history is relevant and should be documented.

Examination includes the following:

- General – neurofibromas, café-au-lait spots, axillary freckling, spinal cord dysraphism (tuft of hair, naevus, skin dimple), cavus feet, Ehlers-Danlos syndrome.
- Trunk – symmetry is determined by the level of the shoulders, the waist crease, the level of the iliac crest and the prominence of the loin.

- Balance and rib deformity – a rib hump is the major cause of cosmetic disability. The balance of the curve is determined by the relationship of the occiput to the sacrum.
- Limb length.
- Correction of curve on bending forward and side bending – a plumb line from the vertebra prominens demonstrates decompensation of the curve.
- Neurologic examination – to check abdominal reflexes and rule out syrinx.
- SLR – reduced in hamstring tightness due to spondylolisthesis or a spinal tumour.
- Sitting and standing heights.
- Neuromuscular scoliosis – balanced curves have a square pelvis while unbalanced curves have a tilted pelvis.
- Sitting patient – sit the patient on the edge of the bed and assess head control and sitting ability.

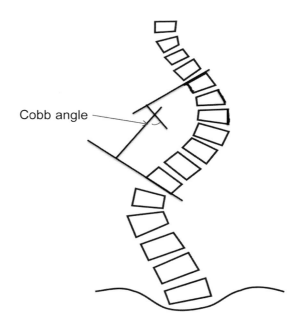

Figure 4.5. Measurement of the Cobb angle.

Investigation

X-rays

A standing AP view is the standard radiograph to assess the deformity. Side bending and lateral views are obtained if surgery is being considered.

The Cobb angle is measured and the Risser sign graded. The superior and inferior end vertebrae are identified for measurement of the Cobb angle. The end vertebrae are those that are tilted maximally towards the concavity of the curve being measured. A line is drawn along the superior end plate of the superior end vertebra and the interior end plate of the inferior end vertebra. The angle between these lines, or the perpendiculars drawn to these lines, is the Cobb angle (Figure 4.5).

The Risser sign is based on appearance and progressive fusion of the iliac apophysis. The fusion progresses from lateral to medial and the iliac crest is divided into four segments. Grade 0 is when the apophysis has not appeared, while grades 1-4 indicate the segments where the apophysis is visible. In grade 5, the entire apophysis is fused.

The triradiate cartilage and X-rays of the wrist can be used to estimate bone age.

Peak height velocity (PHV) is thought to be a more accurate assessment of maturity than the Risser sign and, consequently, a better indicator of curve progression. The average PHV is approximately 8cm/year in girls and 9.5cm/year in boys.

MRI

MR imaging is indicated for all preoperative patients, for left thoracic curves and in patients with painful scoliosis.

In boys, a bone scan is used to screen for painful scoliosis, while a single-photon emission CT (SPECT) scan is useful for detecting spondylolysis.

Idiopathic scoliosis (a curve >10°) is found in 0.5-3% of the adolescent population. Curves of greater than 30° are present in 0.3%.

Classification

Scoliosis is commonly classified based on the age diagnosis is made: early onset (<10 years) or late onset (>10 years of age). The alveoli are not fully developed before the age of 4 years and a deformity before the age of 5 years seriously limits pulmonary function.

Idiopathic scoliosis can be of three types, based on the age at which the curve is noticed.

- Infantile, <3 years of age.
- Juvenile, 3-10 years.
- Adolescent, >10 years.

Infantile scoliosis

Infantile scoliosis is more common in boys and typically presents as thoracic curves, convex to the left. It can be associated with mental retardation, developmental dysplasia of the hip, congenital heart problems and plagiocephaly.

It has been suggested that scoliosis may be preventable if infants are laid prone. Infants tend to lie on the right side, causing plastic deformation of the thorax.

> **Note**
>
> Wynne-Davies R. Infantile idiopathic scoliosis. Causative factors, particularly in the first six months of life. *J Bone Joint Surg Br* 1975; 57: 138-41.

Infantile curves can be progressive or resolving. Resolving curves are usually detected before 1 year of age. There are no compensatory curves, and these curves are associated with plagiocephaly (intrauterine moulding defect).

The rib-vertebral angle difference (RVAD) is an important measurement in scoliosis (Figure 4.6). A line is drawn perpendicular to the apical vertebral endplate. Another line is drawn from the mid neck to the mid head of the convex rib and concave rib. The RVAD is the difference in angles between the two sides. If the convex rib head overlaps the vertebral body, or if the angle is more than 20°, there is a high chance of curve progression.

> **Note**
>
> Mehta MH. The rib-vertebra angle in the early diagnosis between resolving and progressive infantile scoliosis. *J Bone Joint Surg Br* 1972; 54: 230-43.

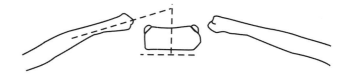

Figure 4.6. Measurement of the rib-vertebral angle difference.

Management

Treatment of infantile scoliosis is indicated if the RVAD is more than 20° and there is a rigid curve on examination.

Bracing is advised for small, flexible curves and can be a thoracolumbosacral or cervicothoraco-lumbosacral orthosis (Milwaukee brace). The brace is continued until the curve has been stable for 2 years.

A cast can be applied for children who are too young to brace. The cast is changed every 2-3 months.

Surgical treatment involves short anterior and posterior fusion to prevent a crankshaft phenomenon of the structural curve only. Subcutaneous growth rods may be considered.

Juvenile scoliosis

Juvenile scoliosis usually presents as a right thoracic curve and is more common in girls. For the diagnosis of scoliosis, the curve should be more than 10° on standing AP radiographs.

About two-thirds of these curves are progressive. Progression occurs in 100% of cases where the curve is more than 20°.

An MR scan is indicated for patients with a left thoracic curve, pain, neurological deficit or rapid progression.

Management
For curves less than 20°, a standing PA X-ray is obtained every 4-6 months. A 10° increase in the RVAD indicates curve progression. Bracing is advised if the curve progresses by 5-7° on follow-up. Bracing is also advised for curves between 20° and 40°, while curves of more than 40° require operative treatment. Observation to check for curve progression continues until skeletal maturity.

A Milwaukee brace or thoracolumbosacral orthosis is given for curves with an apex below T8. The brace is worn for 22 out of 24 hours. If the curve improves after 1 year, bracing is reduced gradually to night-time wear.

In the crankshaft phenomenon, solid posterior fusion stops growth of the posterior elements, but the vertebral body continues to grow. This anterior growth causes the vertebral bodies to bulge laterally towards the convexity, leading to recurrence of the rib hump and loss of correction.

Moe advised using a subcutaneous Harrington rod without fusion in juvenile scoliosis. Surgery is required every 6 months to lengthen the construct, before final fusion.

The amount of shortening as a result of fusion is calculated by the following formula:

$$\text{Shortening} = 0.07 \text{ cm} \times \text{no. of segments fused} \times \text{no. of growth years remaining}$$

If the child is older than 9-10 years then combined anterior and posterior fusion is often needed. Anterior release with fusion and no instrumentation is performed along with posterior multihook segmental instrumented fusion.

Growing rod treatment has been used for early-onset scoliosis, but has a high complication rate related to implant and wound problems.

> **Note**
>
> Bess S, Akbarnia BA, Thompson GH, et al. Complications of growing-rod treatment for early-onset scoliosis: analysis of one hundred and forty patients. *J Bone Joint Surg Am* 2010; 92: 2533-43.

Adolescent scoliosis

Adolescents present with lateral curvature plus rotation. Lordosis or hypokyphosis is seen in the dorsal region.

The aetiology may be genetic (there is a high concordance in monozygotic twins) or hormonal (related to growth hormone).

Overall, 2-3% children younger than 16 years have curves of more than 10°, but only 10% need treatment.

Probability of progression
The probability of progression is indicated by several features:

- A 5° increase in the Cobb angle over 1 year.
- Rapid growth in girls prior to their first menses.
- Risser sign 0, 36-68% will progress; Risser sign 4, 11-18% will progress.

- A double curve; single thoracic curves progress more than single lumbar.
- Curve magnitude (20% of 20° curves progress vs. 90% of 50° curves).

Overall, 3% of curves resolve (usually if <11°).

Imaging
The following radiographs should be taken:

- Standing PA radiograph (reduced radiation to breast), including iliac crest and cervical spine.
- Spot lateral of the lumbosacral junction to check for listhesis.
- Stagnara lateral view – corrects for rotational malalignment.
- Side bending only if considering surgery or bracing.

Assessment of skeletal maturity
Skeletal maturity should be assessed:

- Clinical assessment of secondary sexual characteristics.
- Risser sign.
- Bone age at hand and wrist.
- Maturation of vertebral ring apophysis.
- PHV.

PHV is based on serial measurement of height. It is 8cm/year in girls and 9.5cm/year in boys. Growth stops 3.6 years after PHV in 90% of people, and also indicates cessation of curve progression.

Curve measurement
The curve can be measured with the Cobb angle and vertebral rotation. Nash and Moe recommended measuring the distance of the pedicle from the centre of the vertebra.

Note
Nash CL Jr, Moe JH. A study of vertebral rotation. *J Bone Joint Surg Am* 1969; 51: 223-9.

A Perdriolle torsionmeter measures rotation on an AP X-ray.

Sagittal balance should also be measured. A vertical line drawn from the dens passes anterior to the thoracic spine, posterior to the lumbar spine and through the posterosuperior corner of the S1 vertebral body. In a positive sagittal vertebral axis, the line passes anterior to the body of S1; in a negative axis, the line passes posterior to S1.

Lumbar lordosis should be 20-30° more than thoracic kyphosis to maintain sagittal balance. Thoracic kyphosis is measured from T4 or T5, and 14° (±8°) is added to the figure for kyphosis from T1 to T4 or T5. T1 is not normally seen on the lateral spine view.

Lumbar lordosis is mostly in the disc. L5 and S1 cause 60% of lumbar lordosis cases. The thoracolumbar junction is normally straight.

Curve patterns
Ponseti and Friedman have identified five types of curve pattern, with a sixth added by Moe:

- Single major lumbar curve – apex between L1 and L4. Causes an asymmetric waist line and prominent hip.
- Single major thoracolumbar curve – apex at T12 or L1. Causes disbalance and severe cosmetic disability.
- Combined thoracic and lumbar curves (double major curves) – usually well balanced.
- Single major thoracic curve – convex right. Produces prominence of ribs on the convex side and elevation of the shoulder causing cosmetic deformity.
- Single major high thoracic curve – causes an unsightly deformity due to an elevated shoulder. Curves from C7 to T5.
- Double major thoracic curve – a short upper thoracic curve from T1 to T6 and a lower curve from T6 to L1. The upper curve is convex to the left. Deformities are not severe.

Management

Initial treatment is often with observation. X-rays of the spine are regularly obtained to document curve size and progression.

Curves of less than 20° in skeletally immature patients are examined every 6-12 months. In skeletally mature patients, curves of less than 20° do not need follow-up. In skeletally mature patients with curves of 30-40°, yearly X-rays are performed for 2-3 years and then every 5 years.

Curves of more than 20° in skeletally immature patients should be X-rayed every 3-4 months. If curve progression is more than 5° during 6 months, orthosis is advised.

Curves of over 30-40° in skeletally immature patients are treated with an orthosis. A Milwaukee brace will improve curves by 50% within 6 months, but the results of bracing are the same as no bracing after 5 years.

Other braces are the Boston underarm brace and Wilmington brace. Patient adherence is a problem. Patients may be more likely to adhere to part-time brace wear (16 hours), but this is less effective in preventing curve progression.

Surgery is indicated by the following:

* An increasing curve in a growing child.
* Over 50° deformity in a mature patient.
* A curve of more than 40-50° in a skeletally immature patient.
* Uncontrolled pain.
* Thoracic lordosis.

Cotrel-Dubousset instrumentation allows distraction and compression on the same rod. A rod rotation manoeuvre is performed to translate the apex of the curve to a normal position.

Anterior release and fusion is performed for curves over 75°.

Anterior disc excision increases disc flexibility and bone graft leads to stable fusion. Anterior vertebral body screw fixation and anterolateral rod constructs can be used, but an iatrogenic flat back should be avoided.

For children with aggressively progressive curves, a subcutaneous rod and limited fusion at the proximal and distal hook sites is an option. Sequential distraction should be performed every 6 months and the patient protected with a brace throughout. Formal fusion is eventually performed.

The treatments for various curve types are shown in Table 4.6.

Outcomes

Harrington rods provide 48% coronal correction on long-term follow-up. These are no longer in use in most centres.

The Cotrel-Dubousset instrument gives 61% coronal plane correction.

An anterior lumbar approach gives 67-98% correction, but maintaining lumbar lordosis is a challenge.

Anterior thoracic correction is comparable with posterior correction, but has a higher incidence of rod breakage.

Congenital scoliosis

Several abnormalities of vertebral shape cause deviation, which leads to congenital scoliosis. These can cause isolated scoliosis, kyphosis or lordosis, or a combination of the three.

Examination

It is easiest to examine the child dressed in a nappy, sitting on a parent's lap and facing the parent.

Note:

* The size of the child.
* Alertness level.
* Head and neck control.
* Nourishment.

Table 4.6. Treatments for different curve types.

Curve	Treatment
Right thoracic curve	Posterior instrumentation and fusion
	Distal hook – one level above the stable vertebra
	Multiple hooks or sublaminar wires on concave side
	Can also do anterior correction – fuse all vertebrae within the Cobb angle
Right thoracic, left lumbar	Usually thoracic is primary
	Can fuse only the thoracic, but avoid decompensation
	Trunk may decompensate to left if the lumbar curve is 45-50° and only the thoracic is corrected
	If both are instrumented, extend fusion to L3 or L4 or up to the stable vertebra
Double thoracic – elevated left shoulder	Correct both curves
	An elevated right shoulder means an isolated right thoracic curve
Left lumbar – isolated fusion of the lumbar curve	Limited anterior fusion is more effective in controlling rotation
	Posterior fusion with pedicle screws is acceptable

- Comfort.
- Palpate the spine.
- Deformity – note the number of curves.
- Shape of head – plagiocephaly, plagiothorax.
- Bat ear, wry neck or adducted hip.
- Sternomastoids (examine for stiffness).
- Short neck and low hair line.
- Sprengel's deformity – the height of the scapula.
- Use of all muscle groups.
- Leg lengths and hip range of motion.
- Lower-limb wasting, signs of spinal dysraphism.

X-ray:

- Asymmetric size or number of pedicles.
- Absent rib.
- Unsegmented bar.

Natural history:

- Thoracic curves progress the most.
- Multiple hemivertebra indicate a poor prognosis.
- Block vertebra do not require surgery – progress is less than 1°/year.
- Hemivertebra progress at 1-2.5°/year.

- An unsegmented bar progresses at 6-9°/year.
- An unsegmented bar with contralateral hemivertebra progresses at more than 10°/year.

Management

Regular radiographic follow-up is needed. Brace treatment is not very effective.

Preoperative evaluation includes an ultrasound of the genitourinary tract and MR imaging of the spine.

It may be possible to correct the curve, but this can cause neurologic damage. A safe approach is to fuse *in situ*.

Treatment options are as follows:

- Posterior fusion.
- Anterior fusion.
- Partial fusion, hemiepiphysiodesis – fuse only on the convex side.
- Hemivertebra excision – for lower lumbar vertebrae with truncal decompensation.

Neuromuscular scoliosis

The neuromuscular causes of scoliosis include cerebral palsy, Duchenne's muscular dystrophy, syringomyelia, Marfan syndrome, myelodysplasia and polio.

The onset of deformity is early and it is generally severe and progressive. Cerebral palsy is associated with a long C curve, while curves in neurofibromatosis often involve few vertebrae.

Bracing is commonly needed and surgical stabilisation of curves should be performed to prevent progression. The principle of surgery is multiple-level long fixation and fusion to the pelvis.

In neurofibromatosis, the vertebral foramen is widened and there is scalloping of the vertebrae, pencilling of the ribs and cervical kyphosis.

Postural scoliosis

Postural scoliosis is non-structural and is not associated with rotational malalignment. It may be a result of leg-length discrepancy or of a painful lesion in or adjacent to the spine.

Scheuermann's disease

Scheuermann's disease is kyphosis of the spine. For the diagnosis, at least three adjacent vertebrae must be wedged by 5° each.

The normal sagittal curvature of the thoracic spine is 20-40°. Two types of Scheuermann's disease are recognised:

- Type I – lower thoracic.
- Type II – lumbar Scheuermann's or apprentice kyphosis.

Type II is more commonly seen in athletic adolescent boys and with heavy lifting. There is no increased kyphosis, but severe endplate irregularity and Schmorl's nodes.

Aetiology

The aetiology of Scheuermann's disease is unknown. It is not related to osteonecrosis of the apophysis, disc herniation or a persistent anterior vascular groove.

Mechanical factors include tight hamstrings, which prevent anterior pelvic tilt.

Incidence

The incidence varies from 1% to 8%. The age of presentation is 8-12 years, and the usual presentation is with pain and deformity.

Natural history

Pain is present in 50% of patients and gradually subsides with skeletal maturity. It is debated as to whether the deformity causes disabling back pain.

Management

A brace is advised for kyphosis of less than 65°, if there is growth remaining.

The indications for surgery are controversial and depend on the patient's choice. Surgery may be indicated for kyphosis of more than 75° with pain.

Posterior Harrington compression instrumentation produces good initial correction, but this is lost over time.

Anterior disc excision, fusion and instrumented posterior spinal fusion improve the correction and prevent late loss of correction. This is indicated if the patient has severe kyphosis of more than 75° or more than 50° kyphosis on an extension lateral radiograph. Fusion from T3 to L2 is generally necessary.

Junctional kyphosis at the superior and inferior end of the fusion is seen with all instrumentations. To avoid this, correction is limited to 50% of the initial deformity.

Spinal stenosis

Spinal stenosis is a narrowing of the spinal canal, leading to compression of the neural elements. The stenosis may be localised to one level or diffuse.

Classification

Spinal stenosis can be congenital or acquired. Causes of congenital stenosis are idiopathic narrowing of the spinal canal or achondroplasia causing developmental stenosis.

Acquired causes include degenerative changes, Paget's disease, tumours, and infections. Spinal stenosis can also occur following trauma and surgery.

Depending on anatomic location within the spinal canal, stenosis can be central, in the lateral recess or foraminal (Figure 4.7). Central is in the region of the

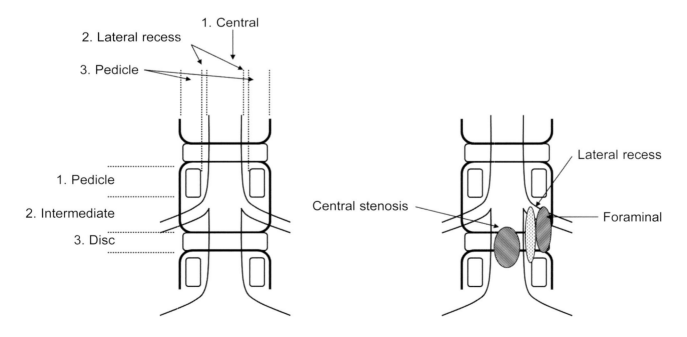

Figure 4.7. Diagrammatic representation of the types of canal stenosis.

intervertebral disc. The lateral recess is the region lateral to the dural sac and the longitudinal line along the medial border of the pedicles. Foraminal is in the region of the pedicles. This is based on the grid pattern whereby each level is divided into three segments from the cephalad to the caudad: pedicle, intermediate and disc. In the coronal plane, there are five zones: one central zone, two lateral recesses and two pedicle zones.

Pathology

Degenerative changes in the facet joints with osteophyte formation cause narrowing of the spinal canal. The inferior articular process causes central canal narrowing, while the superior articular process causes narrowing of the lateral recess and the intervertebral foramen. Cyst formation in the synovial joints contributes to narrowing and activity-related pain.

Central stenosis leads to compression of the dural sac and the cauda equina, while lateral and foraminal stenosis cause pressure on the nerve root. Facet hypertrophy, congenital narrowing of the canal, spondylolisthesis, central disc herniation, trauma and surgery can lead to central spinal stenosis. Lateral stenosis is predominantly due to disc protrusion, facet hypertrophy or ligamentum flavum hypertrophy.

Clinical features

Spinal stenosis causes neurogenic claudication symptoms that are worse with standing, activity or extension of the lumbar spine. The pain radiates to the thigh or leg and may be associated with sensory symptoms such as burning or numbness. Flexion of the spine, sitting and lying tend to relieve the symptoms.

Patients with lateral stenosis have more night pain, but better walking ability compared to those with central stenosis.

Vascular claudication can mimic neurogenic claudication. Associated signs of vascular insufficiency – skin changes and weak pulses – point to a vascular cause. Standing makes the pain worse in neurogenic claudication, but relieves it in vascular claudication. Riding a stationary bicycle with the spine flexed will exacerbate the pain from vascular causes, but not neurogenic pain.

Imaging

Plain radiographs of the lumbar spine are helpful in diagnosing coexisting scoliosis and degenerative spondylolisthesis. A CT scan will provide good osseous detail and MR scans provide soft tissue delineation. Myelography is invasive and is less frequently employed. The use of electromyography and somatosensory evoked potentials is limited to differentiation of neuropathy from spinal compressive lesions.

Management

The symptoms of spinal stenosis can be non-progressive and may resolve with time. Non-operative treatment is therefore considered in the first instance. The mainstays are NSAIDs, physiotherapy, bracing, activity modification and epidural steroid injections.

Operative treatment is aimed at decompression and can be achieved by removing the lamina and ligamentum flavum at the affected level. The nerve roots are decompressed up to their exit from the neural foramen. Total laminectomy should be avoided. Medial facetectomy is helpful in lateral recess stenosis to remove the part of the facet joint causing pressure on the nerve root.

More limited resection techniques have been described. These involve removal of the anterior part of the lamina, foraminotomies, multiple laminotomy, partial laminectomy or laminoplasty. Soft stabilisation with interspinous spacers offers an alternative in both central and foraminal stenosis. Limited decompression is effective in patients where the involved level can be accurately diagnosed on the basis of clinical examination and imaging.

The early results of decompression are generally good, but symptoms may recur in the long term.

Spondylolisthesis is a complication of laminectomy where posterior fusion is not performed and can result in an unsatisfactory outcome. Removal of single facet joints may not significantly compromise spinal stability, but removal of both facet joints is an indication for concomitant fusion, although this is not universal practice. The use of internal fixation avoids progression of spondylolisthesis after laminectomy. Patients with scoliosis and spinal stenosis should be managed by concomitant stabilisation to prevent deformity progression.

Spine infections

Spine infections can broadly be classified into pyogenic (bacterial) or non-pyogenic (commonly tubercular).

Pyogenic osteomyelitis of the spine

Bacterial spread to the spine is along the end arteriole in the region of the vertebral end plate. These are low-flow vessels and bacterial seeding leads to destruction of the end plate and involvement of the intervertebral disc. The destruction and collapse of the disc is one of the first signs of the disease. The infection spreads to adjacent discs through the posterior spinal arterial anastomoses. The spread of infection along Bateson's venous plexus is unlikely.

Risk factors
Immune deficiency is a risk factor for the development of vertebral osteomyelitis. Smoking, diabetes, malignancy, irradiation, intravenous drug abuse and trauma can predispose to infection. It is more common in older people and prevalence is equal in men and women.

Infective organisms
Staphylococcus aureus is the most common organism causing pyogenic osteomyelitis. Gram-negative infections are increasingly common, with the spine secondarily infected from the genitourinary tract, chest or foot ulcers. Infecting organisms include *Escherichia coli* and *Pseudomonas*, *Proteus* and *Enterococcus* species. MRSA is on the increase.

Clinical features
The first symptom is back pain. This may be pain at night and associated with muscle spasm, causing hip flexion or torticollis depending on the site of infection. The lumbar spine is the most common site of infection.

Infection in the spine can lead to abscesses and tracking of the infection along the tissue planes. Cervical epidural abscesses are often anterior and can track into the mediastinum causing pressure symptoms. Lumbar and dorsal spine abscesses are usually posterior.

Approximately 15-20% patients have neurological deficit. Various causes of neurologic deficit are pressure on the neural structures from pus, scar tissue, an extruded disc, vertebrae or oedema. Ischaemic damage to the cord from septic emboli or phlebitis can also cause neurologic deficit.

Differential diagnosis
Pyogenic osteomyelitis of the spine must be differentiated from granulomatous osteomyelitis, primary and secondary neoplasms, degenerative disease, trauma, osteoporotic vertebral fractures and multiple myeloma.

Vertebral discitis can produce localised pain and restricted movements in the back in young patients. Patients are typically not systemically unwell and radiographs show a reduced disc height.

The erythrocyte sedimentation rate and C-reactive protein level are elevated in acute infections and serve as a marker to response to treatment. They are non-specific, however, and elevation of these markers by itself does not imply infection. Blood cultures are useful, if positive, to identify the responsible organism, but a negative blood culture has a poor predictive value.

Imaging
The first sign on plain radiographs is diminution of the joint space, which may appear 2-4 weeks after the onset of infection. In addition, osteolysis and haziness of the end plate may be seen. Obliteration of the psoas shadow indicates a possible abscess. A prevertebral shadow or widened mediastinum may appear in patients with a paraspinal abscess.

Destruction of the intervertebral disc space is a late feature of malignant disease and generally indicates an infective process.

A gallium-67 scan is more sensitive and specific than the Tc-99m scan. It is positive earlier than the Tc-99m scan in infection and the return to normal is also quicker following treatment. SPECT scanning increases the accuracy.

An MR scan is the modality of choice. Gadolinium enhancement is useful in differentiating postoperative scarring from acute infection changes. Significant oedema in the bone is evident in T2-weighted images.

CT-guided biopsy is useful to obtain tissue and fluid for cultures and identification of the organism. Antibiotic therapy diminishes the positivity of samples. Histology should be obtained routinely along with cultures from the tissue samples. Cultures are performed for aerobes, anaerobes, mycobacteria and fungi.

Management
The aim of treatment is to maintain spinal stability and eradicate infection. The management of spinal infections can be surgical or non-surgical.

The trend of inflammatory markers – erythrocyte sedimentation rate and C-reactive protein level – is useful to monitor response to treatment. An adequate immune system and age less than 60 years are associated with an improved prognosis.

Non-surgical treatment is aimed at correcting malnutrition, initiating appropriate antibiotics and using an orthosis to prevent deformity and control pain.

The indications for surgical intervention are as follows:

- Failure of response to non-surgical treatment.
- Acute onset of neurologic deficit.
- Management of spinal instability.
- Systemic sepsis.
- Formation of a paraspinal or epidural abscess.

Surgery achieves debridement of the infected tissue, decompression and reconstruction. Reconstruction can be performed with an iliac crest bone graft, fibular graft, allograft or instrumentation. Anterior instrumentation achieves good debridement, but carries the risk of persistent infection due to direct contact between the metalwork and the infected tissue. Debridement of infected tissue from an anterior approach, with posterior instrumentation, is an option.

Granulomatous osteomyelitis

Mycobacterium tuberculosis is the predominant organism responsible for granulomatous infection of the spine. This has been widespread in developing countries and is staging a resurgence in developed countries in immune-compromised hosts.

Pathology
Tuberculous osteomyelitis can affect the peridiscal, anterior, posterior or central part of the vertebral column. This is based on the site of initial infection in the spine.

The peridiscal site is the most common place for the initial infection. The infection begins in the vertebral metaphysis, spreading to the adjacent vertebra under the anterior longitudinal ligament. This leads to destruction of the vertebral ends, without disc destruction. The central type causes destruction of the centre of the vertebral body and collapse. The anterior type tracks under the anterior longitudinal ligament and scallops the anterior margins of multiple adjacent vertebrae. The posterior type is rare and involves the posterior elements only.

Paraspinal abscess formation can be seen in tubercular osteomyelitis. Epidural abscess is a particularly serious complication that can lead to paralysis within 3-4 days of onset. It requires urgent treatment through decompression – either from the anterior approach or via a laminectomy.

In tuberculous osteomyelitis the thoracic spine is involved more often than the lumbar spine, and the disc spaces are preserved until the late stage of the disease. This helps to differentiate it from pyogenic infection.

Candida, *Aspergillus* and *Actinomyces* species can all cause granulomatous infections.

Diagnosis

The diagnostic work-up for granulomatous infections is similar to that for pyogenic infection. The white cell count is often normal. Cultures for acid-fast bacilli may take up to 8 weeks.

X-ray imaging shows localised osteopenia of two adjacent vertebrae, which is an early sign. In later stages, vertebral collapse may be evident. Paraspinal abscesses are sometimes seen.

A nuclear scan has a high false-negative rate. An MR scan with gadolinium enhancement is useful in differentiating abscess cavities from granulation tissue. CT-guided biopsy and polymerase chain reaction are the modalities of choice for a definitive diagnosis.

Management

The treatment mainstay of tubercular spinal infection is antitubercular drugs. The most commonly used drugs are rifampicin, isoniazid, pyrazinamide and ethambutol. The duration of treatment is 6-9 months.

Table 4.7. Classification of spondylolisthesis.	
Type	**Description**
I	Congenital/dysplastic: • Facets are malaligned or improperly developed (axially or sagittally oriented) • The cranial vertebra displaces anteriorly, but the integrity of the ring is maintained • Underlying cause in 25% of patients • Symptoms include tight hamstrings • Neurologic signs such as paraesthesia or cauda equina may be present because the canal is closed
II	Isthmic/spondylotic: • Defect in the pars interarticularis • Neurologic sequelae are less common than in type I • May present by the age of 5-6 years or at adolescence • This is the most common type and comprises 50% of patients with spondylolisthesis • Symptoms are low back pain, tight hamstrings and possibly irritation of the fifth nerve root
IIA	Lytic/fatigue pars fracture
IIB	Elongated but intact pars
IIC	Acute fracture of pars
III	Degenerative: • Due to loss of disc/structure integrity or facet joints • Accounts for 20% patients
IV	Traumatic: • Traumatic disruption of facets allowing anterior slip • Results from a severe traumatic event
V	Pathologic: • Destruction of the pars/pedicle/facet by tumours or Paget's disease

Bracing may be needed to control deformity.

Surgery (in addition to medical treatment) is indicated where there is neurologic involvement, lack of response to medical treatment, a large abscess or signs of spinal instability.

Spondylolisthesis

Spondylolisthesis is anterior translation (slipping) of a vertebra caused by a defect in the pars interarticularis. It is a common cause of low backache in adolescents.

The defect in the pars is most commonly due to a stress fracture from repeated hyperextension stresses.

Classification

Spondylolisthesis is classified with the Wiltse and Newman classification (Table 4.7).

Note

Wiltse LL, Newman PH, Macnab I. Classification of spondylolysis and spondylolisthesis. *Clin Orthop Relat Res* 1976; 117: 23-9.

Imaging

Plain radiographs show the lesion in 80% patients. Oblique views of the lumbar spine improve the sensitivity and the classic sign, the defect in the pars, is known as the 'Scottie dog' sign.

Radiographs should be obtained in the standing position to assess the degree of slip and the slip angle.

Spondylolisthesis can be graded with the Meyerding system. Five grades of slip are described based on anterior translation of the posterior border of the vertebra in relation to the posterior border of the vertebra below. The translation distance is measured in relation to the AP dimension of the vertebra below.

- Grade I – less than 25% slip.
- Grade II – 25-50% slip.
- Grade III – 50-75% slip.
- Grade IV – 75-100% slip.
- Grade V – more than 100% slip (known as spondyloptosis).

In grade V, the posterior border of the vertebra above displaces anterior to the anterior margin of the vertebra below.

Other measures are the percentage of slip (related to the upper border of S1), the lumbar index, sacral inclination, sagittal pelvic tilt and slip angle (Figure 4.8).

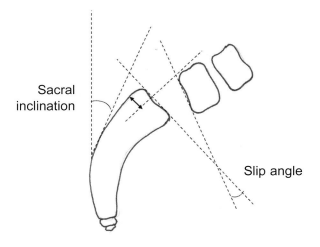

Figure 4.8. Measurement of severity of slip by percentage of slip, slip angle and sacral inclination.

The slip angle is the angle between the lower border of the vertebra above and the upper border of the vertebra below. Normally the gap between the vertebra is wider anteriorly, making the slip angle positive. In spondylolisthesis the gap is wider posteriorly, making the angle negative.

Serial radiographs are helpful to document progression. Changes of less than 10% are not considered significant because of errors in radiographs.

> **Note**
>
> Rothman RH, Simone FA, Eds. *The Spine*, 2nd edn. Philadelphia: WB Saunders, 1982.

Investigation

Spondylolisthesis is investigated with the following:

- Selective nerve root blocks for L5, caudal block.
- Discography.
- Bone scan – to distinguish an acute (increased uptake) from a longstanding pars defect.
- CT scan – for planning.
- MR imaging – to identify the nerve roots, disc and other congenital anomalies such as a tethered cord.

Non-surgical treatment

Isthmic
In children:

- Asymptomatic – yearly X-rays are taken, but no activity modification is needed.
- Symptomatic – stretching exercises for the hamstrings are recommended.

In adults, a stretching program and weight control is advised. Nerve root blocks can be considered for radicular pain caused by narrowing of the foramen.

Dysplastic

In children, there is a high incidence of neurologic complications and most require surgery. A study looking at conservative treatment examined the use of a soft thoracolumbar brace in 23 children and adolescents with a pars defect. A high signal in the adjacent pedicle on a T2 MR scan and early-stage defect on CT correlated with better healing potential.

> **Note**
>
> Sairyo K, Sakai T, Yasui N. Conservative treatment of lumbar spondylolysis in childhood and adolescence: the radiological signs which predict healing. *J Bone Joint Surg Br* 2009; 91: 206-9.

In adults, tight hamstrings and low back pain can be managed non-operatively. Cauda equina, however, requires an urgent operation.

Management

Non-surgical treatment
During the acute phase, it is generally agreed that conservative management should be attempted before surgical intervention. Many studies support the non-surgical approach.

Wiltse *et al* demonstrated that 12 of 17 young patients diagnosed with spondylolysis showed osseous healing with conservative treatment and no surgery.

> **Note**
>
> Wiltse LL, Widell EH Jr, Jackson DW. Fatigue fracture: the basic lesion is inthmic spondylolisthesis. *J Bone Joint Surg Am* 1975; 57: 17-22.

Early diagnosis is important for a good prognosis in bone healing. Ciullo and Jackson studied gymnasts and found that the longer symptoms were present before treatment, the more likely surgical intervention became.

Note

Ciullo JV, Jackson DW. Pars interarticularis stress reaction, spondylolysis, and spondylolisthesis in gymnasts. *Clin Sports Med* 1985; 4: 95-110.

During the acute phase of rehabilitation for patients with spondylolysis, the focus is on reducing pain. Instruction in posture and biomechanics with activities of daily living can help to protect the injured pars, thus reducing symptoms and preventing further injury. A period of rest for an average of 2-4 weeks can provide beneficial effects by modulating pain, decreasing inflammation and decreasing the risk for further progression of a pars stress reaction to a frank fracture.

Applying ice to the injured area for 20 minutes three to four times a day, in conjunction with gentle range of motion exercises and stretching of the quadriceps and hamstring muscles, is strongly advised. Activity modification is recommended. The patient is advised to stop the activity or sport that evokes the back pain for an average of 2-4 weeks. In particular, the patient should avoid any activities involving hyperextension.

Indications for the use of a brace are lack of symptom improvement by 2-4 weeks, the presence of a true fracture or spondylolisthesis, the need for pain control and lack of patient adherence with activity restrictions.

The risk factors for progression of slip are female sex, young age, high slip angle, high-grade slip, a dome-shaped sacrum and high sacral inclination.

Note

Seitsalo S, Osterman K, Hyvärinen H, *et al*. Progression of spondylolisthesis in children and adolescents. A long-term follow-up of 272 patients. *Spine* (Phila Pa) 1991; 16: 417-21.

Surgical treatment

Surgical treatment is indicated in most patients with high-grade slip ($\geq$2), progressive slip, an associated neurologic deficit or unremitting back and leg pain.

Pars interarticularis repair is indicated if the disc is normal on MR imaging, pain is arising from the defect, low back pain is increased by extension and pain relief is obtained with injection of the pars.

Ideal candidates for direct repair of the pars defect are those with early lesions, with lysis but no listhesis, and with the lytic defect between L1 and L4. L5 lytic defects have been reported to yield less predictable results because many L5 defects arise from a developmentally weakened and elongated pars.

Surgical techniques generally employ debridement of the lytic defect, application of large amounts of autogenous iliac crest cancellous bone graft and tension band wiring or screw fixation from the cephalad portion of the posterior element to the free-floating caudal fragment.

Fusion *in situ* procedures are performed in patients with low-grade spondylolisthesis that remains symptomatic despite non-operative measures or those with high-grade listhesis but acceptable sagittal balance. Decompression and fusion are indicated when severe neurologic signs of compression are present, such as radiating leg pain, numbness and weakness, with corresponding imaging studies demonstrating nerve root or thecal sac compression.

Reduction is indicated to prevent the complications of slip progression, pseudarthrosis and cosmetic deformity associated with *in situ* fusion; hence, reduction of high-grade slips is often performed. Reduction (closed or open) serves to correct lumbosacral kyphosis and diminish the sagittal translation seen in high-grade slips. For more severe slips, instrumented fusion from S1 to L4 is recommended. It may be difficult to place a pedicle screw in the L5 pedicle.

In spondyloptosis (grade 5 slip), an attempt is made to improve the slip angle and fuse L4 to S1; alternatively, a vertebrectomy may be indicated.

Gaines procedure is to anteriorly remove L5 and fuse L4 to S1 posteriorly as a second stage. This has a high complication rate, with 25% iatrogenic neurological deficit.

General complications of surgery include pneumonia, urinary tract infections, deep vein thrombosis, pulmonary embolism and infection.

Further complications are as follows:

- Surgical approach:
  - epidural scarring;
  - nerve root injury;
  - dural tear;
    - great vessel injury;
    - bowel injury;
    - injury to the ureter;
    - injury to the hypogastric plexus and genitofemoral nerve.
- Related to fusion:
  - pseudarthrosis;
  - graft extrusion or subsidence;
  - accelerated degeneration of adjacent discs;
  - donor-site morbidity.
- Related to the metalwork:
  - implant failure;
  - misplaced/fracture of pedicle screws;
  - nerve root injury.

Chapter 5 Foot and ankle

Hallux rigidus

Structural hallux rigidus refers to degenerative arthrosis of the first metatarsophalangeal joint (MTPJ). It is differentiated from functional hallux limitus by having a painful fixed reduction in joint motion, even when non-weight bearing. Other clinical features include a prominent 'dorsal bunion' and synovitis, particularly dorsolaterally. The incidence is one in 45 adults over the age of 65 years, but it commonly affects much younger patients.

There are various causes:

- Trauma.
- Functional hallux limitus.
- A long first metatarsal.
- Gout.

The earliest radiographic sign may be a depression in the dome of the metatarsal head. Radiographs may also show osteophyte formation and a reduction in the joint space. Lateral osteophytes are often responsible for the symptoms. The severity of hallux rigidus is determined by the radiographic appearance.

Classification

- Grade I – mild to moderate osteophyte formation, but the joint space is preserved.
- Grade II – moderate osteophyte formation with joint space narrowing and subchondral sclerosis.

- Grade III – marked osteophytosis and joint space reduction, including the inferior aspect of the joint.

Management

Conservative measures include non-steroidal anti-inflammatory drugs (NSAIDs), an adequate toe box, a rigid or rocker-bottom sole, Morton's extension splint (a stiff foot plate with an extension under the great toe) and steroid injection.

Surgical options are cheilectomy, fusion or resection and replacement arthroplasty (grade III).

Cheilectomy

Cheilectomy may be used for grade I or II hallux rigidus. The aim is to eliminate dorsal impingement and achieve 70° of dorsiflexion. This involves resection of the proliferative bone and removal of 30% of the metatarsal head and the lateral osteophytes flush with the shaft.

Cheilectomy may be combined with dorsiflexion osteotomy of the metatarsal in young, active patients in order to avoid fusion. Osteotomy alone may be used in patients who lack dorsiflexion and do not have dorsal impingement.

Fusion

Fusion is used in cases of advanced arthritis and failed cheilectomy (grade III).

A standard medial or dorsomedial approach to the MTPJ is used. After releasing the capsule dorsally and plantarly, osteophytes are excised. The surfaces of the metatarsal and phalanx are prepared using congruent reamers down to bleeding subchondral bone. Small holes are drilled in the MTP surfaces to promote bony ingrowth. A guide wire is inserted just distal to the flare of the proximal phalanx and the position is checked with a foot plate or X-ray. The optimal position of fusion is 10° dorsiflexion in relation to the floor (25° in relation to the first metatarsal) and 10° of valgus. Reduction in valgus puts increased strain on the interphalangeal joint (IPJ) and can result in arthritis. Cannulated 4mm screws or a fusion plate can be used for fixation.

Specific complications are malunion, non-union, IPJ degenerative disease developing after the fusion and hardware problems. Excessive dorsiflexion will cause the IPJ to rub in the shoe and the joint may begin to claw. Insufficient plantar flexion will cause lateral roll-off or a vaulting gait.

Resection and replacement arthroplasty

There has been limited success with joint replacement and this is reserved for less active individuals. Interposition arthroplasty is useful in higher-demand patients and both should be considered when the adjacent sagittal plane joints are also affected by degeneration. Keller's resection arthroplasty is associated with shortening, deformity, instability and reduced push-off, and is rarely performed today.

Hallux varus

Hallux varus is medial deviation of the hallux. It can be congenital, but is most commonly due to previous hallux surgery. The muscle imbalance can be caused by resection of the lateral sesamoid, abductor hallucis or lateral slip of the flexor hallucis brevis. Excessive medial eminence resection, medial tightening of the capsule and lateral positioning of the metatarsal head following osteotomy can also cause it.

Patients present with deformity or painful rubbing from their footwear. Symptomatic flexible deformity is treated by extensor hallucis longus (EHL) transfer to

the base of the proximal phalanx under the intermetatarsal ligament. This can be combined with fusion of the IPJ. If the deformity is fixed or is associated with arthritis of the MTPJ, fusion of the first MTPJ is advisable and is the most reliable procedure for all types.

Rheumatoid foot

Foot involvement is common in rheumatoid arthritis. The forefoot is most commonly involved and usually presents with hallux valgus and claw toes (see later). The initial pathology is related to synovitis, which leads to incompetence of the joint capsules and collateral ligaments. Soft tissue contracture and MTP dislocation lead to claw toe deformity. Plantar fat-pad atrophy and migration can cause metatarsalgia.

In the early stages, forefoot involvement presents with metatarsalgia and painful bunions. Separation of the toes with synovitis leads to the 'daylight' sign. Callosities develop beneath the metatarsal heads and the dorsal aspect of the lesser toes and tips of the distal phalanges. The final feature of forefoot involvement is splaying of the metatarsals due to weakening of the transverse metatarsal ligaments.

Hindfoot involvement commonly occurs in the subtalar joint. Disruption of the interosseous ligament can lead to progressive hindfoot valgus deformity. Damage to the posterior tibial tendon occurs secondarily to synovitis and increased strain. This leads to tibialis posterior dysfunction and loss of longitudinal arch height.

Vasculitis can present as skin ulceration, digital ischaemia, rheumatoid nodules and mononeuritis multiplex.

Early radiographic features are soft tissue swelling, widening of the joint space and osteopenia. Later, marginal bony erosions, joint space narrowing and subchondral cysts are seen. In advanced disease, bony ankylosis, fragmentation, subluxation, dislocation and deformity appear on radiographs.

Management

Conservative management

Conservative management comprises optimal medical therapy, physical therapy, corticosteroid injection and orthotic support. Extra-deep, light-weight, soft shoes can be used to accommodate forefoot deformities. When no fixed deformity is present, a UCBL (University of California Biomechanics Laboratory) insert may be used for mid- and hindfoot pain. An in-shoe orthosis or custom ankle-foot orthoses (AFOs) can be used when instability and mid- or hindfoot deformities develop.

Surgical management

In the early stages, surgical options are synovectomy and soft tissue reconstruction. However, most patients present to the orthopaedic clinic with advanced disease and require formal reconstruction with either resection arthroplasty or arthrodesis. Multiple procedures can be performed on one foot, but concomitant bilateral procedures are best avoided.

The most common pattern of forefoot deformity is hallux valgus with clawing of lesser toes and the most common procedure is therefore forefoot arthroplasty. The goals of forefoot surgery are to provide pain relief, restore the plantar fat pad in a more proximal position, restore alignment of the toes, unload the metatarsal heads and provide a stable first MTPJ.

The treatment of choice is fusion of the first MTPJ and excision arthroplasty of the lesser metatarsal heads. Keller's arthroplasty may be used to address the deformity of the first MTPJ in low-demand patients. An alternative to excision of the metatarsal heads is the Stainsby procedure. This involves resecting the proximal phalanx through the neck. It is important to release and reduce the plantar plate; when all the toes are dislocated, they may all need to be released before reduction is possible.

Medical management remains the mainstay of treatment, and as a result patients often have reduced immunity and poor wound healing. Rheumatoid arthritis patients frequently have severe deformity and thus the soft tissues (and also the neurovascular bundle) can be very stretched after reduction. It may be preferable to do a 2/3 and 3/4 web-space incision, rather than four separate but close incisions. If all toes are dislocated, many specialists advocate a single transverse incision, which can then be left to granulate.

The current advice is to operate without stopping methotrexate and even anti-tumour necrosis factor agents. These therapies have a long half-life and it can be difficult for the patient to manage if they are discontinued.

Surgical management of midfoot involvement entails fusion of the involved joints. This can be performed as an *in situ* fusion if there is no deformity. When a larger deformity is present, fusion is performed in the corrected position.

When hindfoot involvement is isolated to the subtalar, a subtalar fusion will suffice. When the patient has significant hindfoot varus or valgus deformity with involvement of the talonavicular and calcaneocuboid joints, triple arthrodesis is the preferred surgical treatment. In patients with subtalar and ankle degeneration, subtalar fusion and ankle replacement can result in excellent function. Rheumatoid arthritis patients do very well with ankle arthroplasty.

Subtalar fusion

In subtalar fusion, the incision is made from the tip of the fibula to the base of the fourth metatarsal. The sural nerve lies 1-2cm beneath the distal tip of the fibula and should be protected, as should the extensors, which lie anteriorly, and the peroneal tendons, which lie posteriorly.

The extensor digitorum brevis (EDB) tendon is exposed, freed from its insertion and reflected distally. Dissection is kept subperiosteal to avoid damage to the neurovascular bundle, which enters approximately 1.5cm medial and distal to the anterior process of the calcaneum. The EDB is delivered out of the sinus tarsi, and the fibro-fatty contents of the sinus tarsi are removed.

The calcaneocuboid joint, which is found just distal to the anterior beak of the calcaneus, is identified. The talonavicular joint lies superior and medial to the calcaneocuboid joint. The neck of the talus is identified and the extensor tendons are elevated off the neck. A retractor is inserted over the neck and under the extensor tendons, which helps to retract the neurovascular bundle. Another retractor is placed deep to the peroneal tendon and around the calcaneus at the level of the subtalar joint.

The lateral process of the talus can be removed for better exposure of the posterior facet. The joint capsule of the talocalcaneal joint is incised and a laminar spreader is inserted into the sinus tarsi to expose the entire subtalar articulation.

Articular cartilage and subchondral bone of the subtalar joint is excised. All of the articular cartilage must be removed from the anterior, middle and posterior facets, but excessive bone resection is avoided as this will decrease the subtalar joint height and disrupt the articular relationship of the talonavicular joint. Additional bone can be removed to correct fixed valgus or varus deformity.

The joint is held in a corrected position and can be stabilised with two or three 6mm cannulated screws or staples. A variety of configurations have been described.

Flat foot

Loss of the normal medial longitudinal arch leads to pes planus or flat foot. This can be broadly classified as congenital and acquired. The congenital variety is usually seen in children and the acquired variety in adults. The causes of both varieties are listed in Table 5.1.

A key discriminator is whether the foot is fixed or flexible. In children, a fixed flat foot points to a tarsal coalition or congenital vertical talus that requires specialist assessment. In adults, it points to a late stage with fixed, degenerative changes that invariably require major bony fusion surgery.

Clinically the main distinction is between the following:

- Feet with a low arch, but no rotation into planovalgus. This is almost always clinically irrelevant, but the patient or parents may require reassurance that it is a normal appearance.
- Flexible, overpronated feet without any other pathology (e.g., arthritis, muscular imbalance, tendinopathy). Here the arch reappears and the

Table 5.1. Causes of flat foot.		
Congenital		**Acquired**
Normal variant/generalised ligamentous laxity		Trauma – fractures of the talus, os calcis or midfoot resulting in post-traumatic osteoarthritis of the mid- or hindfoot
Congenital vertical talus		
Tarsal coalition – may present in adolescence as the midfoot ossifies or in adulthood as a flat foot with degenerative change		Rupture or stretching of the tibialis posterior tendon
		Mueller-Weiss syndrome (avascular necrosis of the navicular)
Accessory navicular		
Spina bifida		Rheumatoid arthritis
Cerebral palsy		Diabetes – Charcot neuropathic foot
		Neuromuscular disease (e.g., polio)

heel moves into varus on tiptoe or when the great toe is dorsiflexed (Jack test), as the plantar fascia tightens. Reassurance that this is a normal variant may be all that is required.

- Overpronated feet with evidence of tibialis posterior tendinopathy.
- Stiff, overpronated feet. These may be simple flexible feet that have stiffened with age, or they may have developed arthritis or muscle imbalance.
- Arthritic flat feet may require investigation to identify a rheumatological diagnosis. Treatment is directed at controlling the arthritis and protecting the foot against deforming forces with an orthosis (either in-shoe or external devices).
- Neuromuscular flat feet may particularly occur in myelomeningocele or spastic cerebral palsy. Orthoses, usually external devices such as knee-AFOs, may protect against further deformity and give support to allow walking. Some of these patients will need soft tissue procedures, tendon transfers or hindfoot fusions (usually triple fusions to prevent and treat progressive deformity).

Clinical assessment is aimed at identifying the severity of symptoms, and particularly whether there is associated pain. Flexibility is also assessed and the underlying cause of the deformity identified.

Radiographic analysis is based on standing anteroposterior (AP) and lateral views.

In standing lateral views, there is normally a straight-line relationship between the talus and first metatarsal. In a flat foot, this relationship is lost and either the talonavicular or naviculocuneiform joint sags. A C-shaped line created by the outline of the talar dome and the inferior margin of the sustentaculum tali can be seen.

The talocalcaneal angle is measured in standing AP views. If the angle is more than 35° then heel valgus is said to be present. AP views also show the degree of talonavicular uncoverage and subluxation indicative of an advanced deformity. Oblique views are preferred for showing calcaneonavicular tarsal coalition. If tarsal coalition is suspected, the extent and severity is assessed with either computed tomography (CT) or magnetic resonance imaging (MRI) (for fibrous coalition).

Management

A flexible flat foot rarely requires treatment. If symptomatic, physiotherapy in the form of gastrocnemius stretching is useful, as the gastrocnemius is often tight. Orthotics can help to correct flexible deformity (e.g., when medial pain and lateral impingement are present). They are used to accommodate and support a fixed deformity in midfoot degeneration, but by this stage only about 50% of patients will show some improvement.

Indications for surgery are a painful rigid flat foot, a painful uncontrolled or deteriorating flexible flat foot and a neuromuscular flat foot. A neuromuscular flat foot, especially in cerebral palsy associated with tendoachilles contracture, can be treated with subtalar fusion before midfoot breakdown occurs. Once a midfoot break (i.e., midfoot abduction) occurs, triple arthrodesis is required. Hypermobile syndrome does not respond well to soft tissue surgery.

Treatment options are fusion of the involved joints (subtalar, triple fusion or midfoot joints) for fixed deformity. Reconstruction – for example, flexor digitorum longus (FDL) transfer, medial calcaneal osteotomy, spring ligament reefing and lateral column lengthening – is reserved for flexible deformities.

Posterior tibial tendon dysfunction

The tibialis posterior is an invertor of the foot that originates in the deep posterior compartment of the leg. It has a complex insertion, with the main bulk of the tendon inserting to the navicular tuberosity. In addition to the navicular, the tendon has multiple slips that insert on the cuboid, cuneiforms and bases of the second, third and fourth metatarsals. It functions as a dynamic stabiliser of the longitudinal arch and resists hindfoot valgus.

Table 5.2. Strom and Johnson/Myerson classification of posterior tibial tendon dysfunction.

Stage	Description
1	Tendon tenosynovitis and/or degeneration No deformity Medial foot pain Able to perform a single limb heel raise, heel goes into varus 'Too many toes' sign negative No ankle deformity or arthritis
2	Tendon degeneration and elongation Flexible and reducible pes planovalgus, hindfoot in equinus Medial and/or lateral pain Weakness with single limb heel raise, no or weak inversion of hindfoot 'Too many toes' sign positive No ankle deformity or arthritis
3	Tendon degeneration and elongation Fixed, irreducible pes planovalgus deformity Medial and/or lateral pain Unable to perform single limb heel raise, no inversion of hindfoot 'Too many toes' sign positive No ankle deformity or arthritis
4	Degeneration and elongation Fixed irreducible pes planovalgus deformity Medial and/or lateral pain Unable to perform single limb heel raise, no inversion of hindfoot 'Too many toes' sign positive Ankle deformity or arthritis, talus has started to go into valgus

Posterior tibial tendon dysfunction has been described as a 'hidden epidemic', and recent evidence suggests that its incidence is as high as 6% in women over the age of 40 years. Early diagnosis and treatment is the key to preventing morbidity.

There is an area of hypovascularity 1cm distal to the medial malleolus that could be the reason for tendon failure here. The common causes and factors associated with tendon dysfunction are deterioration of a longstanding flat foot, trauma, inflammatory arthritis (rheumatoid and seronegative arthritis), diabetes and obesity.

Diagnosis

The initial clinical presentation is with pain and tenderness medially along the course of the tendon. The pain is aggravated by resisted active inversion. There may be evidence of an objective weakness of inversion. Later, a planovalgus attitude of the foot develops with flattened longitudinal arches and the classic sign of 'too many toes' when viewed from behind the patient.

A positive single heel raise test is the best method for clinically evaluating functional loss resulting from tibialis posterior dysfunction. When the patient stands on the ball of the toe, the heel should move into a varus position. If the patient is unable to perform this fully then the test is positive. In late stages, when there is calcaneal impingement against the fibula, lateral heel pain is experienced by the patient.

Classification

The Strom and Johnson/Myerson classification is shown in Table 5.2.

Investigation

Plain X-rays are useful in excluding causes such as trauma, coalition and Mueller-Weiss syndrome. They are also useful in determining the presence and extent of degeneration. Degenerative changes of the subtalar and ankle joint will be seen with advancing stages of the disease.

Radiological signs of deformity are useful in surgical planning. They include talocalcaneal divergence due to heel valgus and talonavicular sag due to the planus. On weight bearing, the talus plantarflexes in the lateral view. The talometatarsal angle, which is normally 0° in the lateral radiograph, is negative.

In the weight-bearing AP view, there is talar head uncoverage and an increase in the angle between the longitudinal axis of the talus and calcaneus. Sclerosis and collapse of the lateral half of the navicular suggest Mueller-Weiss syndrome, especially if the talonavicular joint is not uncovered, as would be expected with the degree of deformity.

MRI is the best modality to assess the tendon pathology, particularly in the initial stages.

Management

Flexible deformity
Flexible deformities that are correctable to a plantigrade position can be treated conservatively or with joint-sparing surgery.

Management includes analgesics, shoe adaptations and weight reduction. The mainstay of non-surgical treatment is a suitable orthotic device (e.g., a UCBL-type device). This provides correction of hindfoot valgus and ankle loading and produces a demonstrable improvement in gait parameters. AFO-type braces have also been used successfully. The crucial part of conservative management is that close observation is maintained. If the foot does not respond or deteriorates then surgery needs to be considered. If the foot is left uncontrolled, progression to fixed deformity and degeneration mandates bony fusion surgery rather than soft tissue reconstruction and joint salvage.

Tenosynovectomy is useful in early disease (stage 1, prior to rupture) if symptoms do not settle with conservative measures. Part of the flexor retinaculum is preserved to prevent subluxation of the tendon. The tendon sheath is opened and the diseased tissue is removed. The flexor retinaculum is not closed. Early synovectomy of the tendon sheath relieves discomfort and may delay rupture of the tendon.

FDL transfer is performed for stage 2 disease when there is almost full inversion at the subtalar joint. If the subtalar joint cannot be brought into nearly full inversion then FDL transfer is contraindicated; in this case, subtalar fusion is considered. The flexor hallucis longus or the tibialis anterior can also be used for transfer instead of the FDL. Tendon transfer must be combined with a medialising osteotomy of the calcaneum in order to protect the transferred tendon from the biomechanical abnormalities that led to the much stronger tibialis posterior tendon to fail. The calcaneum is translated about 1cm and fixed with one or more screws. The osteotomy is made 1cm posterior and parallel to the peroneal tendons. The realignment neutralises the eversion force of the Achilles tendon, but gastrocnemius tightness is common and may need to be addressed.

Multiple deformities often need to be addressed at the same time to give a plantigrade foot. Myerson has advocated for a more complex classification system that identifies and manages all the separate issues that are present. For instance, a supinated forefoot is a common feature of longstanding pes planovalgus; if this is fixed then a Cotton osteotomy of the medial

Table 5.3. Motion available following isolated arthrodesis.			
	ST fusion	CC fusion	TN fusion
ST motion	-	90%	10%
CC motion	50%	-	-
TN motion	25%	70%	-
CC = calcaneonavicular; ST = subtalar; TN = talonavicular			

cuneiform may be required. A midfoot break with abduction is also common and can require correction with a lateral column lengthening.

Fixed deformity

Fixed deformities require surgical intervention, although a trial of accommodative orthotics may be helpful. Arthrodesis is advisable in advanced disease (stages 3 and 4). This usually requires a triple fusion, although a more limited fusion is occasionally possible. Table 5.3 shows the outcomes following isolated arthrodesis.

Concomitant Achilles tendon lengthening is often required to correct equinus deformity. Pantalar fusion is advised in cases of severe deformity and arthritis involving the tibiotalar joint, although triple arthrodesis with ankle replacement is an option. This is more complex and can only be performed in the presence of minor talar tilt, but does provide better gait function.

Management summary
- Stage 1:
  - conservative (orthotics – medial arch support, medial heel wedge, UCBL, AFO);
  - tendon sheath divided and synovitis excised.
- Stage 2:
  - FDL transfer to the tibialis posterior tendon;
  - plus calcaneal shift with or without tendo-Achilles lengthening;
  - plus spring ligament reconstruction.
- Stage 3:
  - fusion of degenerate and deformed joints.
- Stage 4:
  - pantalar fusion.

Diabetic foot

Fifteen percent of people with diabetes will sustain a foot ulcer in their lifetime, and approximately 20% of diabetic admissions are due to foot problems. The main pathologies are vasculopathy and neuropathy.

Neuropathy, particularly sensory neuropathy, is the most common cause of foot complications in diabetic patients. However, autonomic neuropathy affecting sweating plays a key role in aetiology and progression. This causes drying of the skin, leading to fissuring and finally ulcers.

Motor involvement is less common than sensory neuropathy. The intrinsic muscles of the foot are involved initially, resulting in atrophy. This causes the plantar fat pad to shift and the plantar fascia to shorten. This, in turn, leads to cavus deformity of the foot and clawing of the toes. The combined effect of these changes is less plantar protection of the bony prominences, callus formation and subsequent ulceration. Isolated neuropathy can involve the common peroneal nerve, resulting in foot drop. This leads to ulceration of the tips of the toes.

The sensory neuropathy is progressive from distal to proximal, beginning with a stocking distribution in the feet. An inability to perceive a 5.07 Semmes-Weinstein monofilament is a key finding, as this is associated with loss of protective sensation and hence a high risk of ulceration in the feet.

Peripheral vascular disease occurs in about 70% of people who have had diabetes for more than 10 years. Both small and large vessels are involved. In addition, people with diabetes have poor cellular defence because of changes in white-cell phagocytic mechanisms.

Another complication of neuropathy in diabetic patients is Charcot arthropathy (see later).

The risk factors for major complications in the diabetic foot are:

- A history of previous ulceration.
- A long duration of diabetes.
- Poor metabolic control.
- Poor foot care.
- Ill-fitting shoes.
- Deformity.
- A tight Achilles tendon (which increases forefoot overloading).

Examination

The initial physical examination should include an assessment of foot deformities, skin and ulcers, as well as a neurological examination for neuropathy.

Vascular examination involves measurement of the ankle-brachial pressure index and absolute toe pressures. The normal value of the ankle-brachial pressure index is 1, and the minimum required for

healing is 0.45. The absolute toe pressure is normally 100mmHg and the minimum required for healing is 40mmHg. In addition, a transcutaneous oxygen measurement of toes greater than 40mmHg is predictive of healing. Doppler scans and MR arteriograms can also be used to assess the vascular supply.

Plain radiographs will show the severity of deformities and any evidence of osteomyelitis or Charcot arthropathy. MRI is very useful in assessing abscesses and soft tissue involvement. A white blood cell labelled or dual-image Tc scan is more sensitive and specific for osteomyelitis than standard bone scans.

Ulcer classification

Ulcers are assessed for their location, size and depth. Diabetic ulcers used to be classified according to Wagner but the more recent University of Texas system (Table 5.4) has modified this to include the presence of infection and ischaemia and provides a more useful validated system.

Note

Wagner FW Jr. The diabetic foot. *Orthopedics* 1987; 10: 163-72.

Table 5.4. University of Texas classification of diabetic foot ulcers.

Stage	Grade 0	1	2	3
A	Pre- or post-ulcerative lesion completely epithelialised	Superficial wound, not involving tendon, capsule or bone	Wound penetrating to tendon or capsule	Wound penetrating to bone or joint
B	Infected	Infected	Infected	Infected
C	Ischaemic	Ischaemic	Ischaemic	Ischaemic
D	Infected and ischaemic	Infected and ischaemic	Infected and ischaemic	Infected and ischaemic

Note

Armstrong DG, Lavery LA, Harkless LB. Validation of a diabetic wound classification system. The contribution of depth, infection, and ischemia to risk of amputation. *Diabetes Care* 1998; 21: 855-9.

Management

The basic principles of diabetic foot treatment are as follows:

- Education and prevention.
- Footwear modification.
- Glycaemic control.
- Treatment of preulcerative sites.
- Broad-spectrum antibiotics for secondary infection.
- Abscess drainage and debridement.
- Limited amputation or surgical resection.

The primary goal in the treatment of diabetic foot ulcers is to obtain wound closure. A multidisciplinary approach should be employed because of the multifaceted nature of foot ulcers and the numerous comorbidities that can occur in these patients. Rest, elevation of the affected foot, pressure relief and appropriate footwear are the essential components of treatment.

A total-contact cast is used for the optimal management of neuropathic ulcers. In patients with

Grade	Lesion	Treatment
	Table 5.5. Wagner classification.	
0	No open lesions; may have deformity or cellulitis	Extra-depth shoes Custom-moulded pressure relief insoles Serial examinations
1	Superficial diabetic ulcer (partial or full thickness)	Debridement of the ulcer Total-contact cast if vascularity is satisfactory Cast changes weekly in the initial stages and then every 2 weeks until healing is complete
2	Ulcer extension to ligament, tendon, joint capsule or deep fascia without abscess or osteomyelitis	Debridement Total-contact cast
3	Deep ulcer with abscess or osteomyelitis	Debridement Total-contact cast
4	Gangrene localised to a portion of the forefoot or heel	Partial amputation if ischaemia is present Vascular surgery consultation to decide if vascular reconstruction is possible Debridement and total contact cast
5	Extensive gangrenous involvement of the entire foot	Major amputation Consider arterial bypass for the healing of a below-knee amputation

Table 5.6. Risk of amputation based on the University of Texas classification.

Stage	Grade			
	0	1	2	3
A	0%	0%	0%	0%
B	12.5%	8.5%	28.6%	92%
C	25%	20%	25%	100%
D	50%	50%	100%	100%

diabetic foot infections, non-operative treatment is indicated if there is no systemic sepsis. Cultures from ulcers are usually unreliable. Surgical debridement is indicated for all patients who appear to have acute toxicity. A mainstay of ulcer therapy is debridement of all necrotic, callus and fibrous tissue.

Table 5.5 outlines the management of diabetic ulcers based on Wagner grades, while Table 5.6 shows the risk of amputation based on the University of Texas classification.

Hallux valgus

Hallux valgus is a medial deviation of the first metatarsal joint and lateral deviation and/or rotation of the hallux, usually with medial soft tissue enlargement of the first metatarsal head.

Hallux valgus affects 1% of adults, with a higher incidence in women. The incidence increases with age, with rates of 3% in persons aged 15-30 years, 9% in those aged 31-60 years and 16% in those older than 60 years. There is also a genetic predisposition, with evidence to suggest familial tendencies.

The aetiology of hallux valgus includes genetic factors, biomechanical factors (e.g., footwear), arthritic conditions (e.g., rheumatoid arthritis), neuromuscular diseases (e.g., cerebral palsy, Charcot-Marie-Tooth disease [CMTD]) and hypermobility syndromes (e.g., Ehlers-Danlos syndrome, Down's syndrome).

In hallux valgus there is pronation of the hallux and the MTPJ may become incongruent. A congruent joint is usually stable, but lateral subluxation of the base of the proximal phalanx occurs with incongruence. The medial joint capsule gradually becomes attenuated while the lateral capsule becomes contracted. The transverse metatarsal ligament maintains the position of the sesamoid complex in relation to the second metatarsal. This results in sesamoids subluxing from the first metatarsal head and crystal erosion. The abductor hallucis moves toward the plantar aspect and accentuates the pronation deformity. Callus formation occurs under the lesser toes, secondary to eventual first ray insufficiency.

Medial tension causes the medial collateral ligaments to pull on the dorsomedial aspect of the first metatarsal head, causing bone proliferation. Remodelling also occurs laterally in addition to medially, as evidenced by an increase in the proximal articular set angle or structural remodelling of the cartilage. Therefore, without correction of biomechanical factors, excessive pronation continues, with propagation of the deformity.

Clinical presentation includes deformity, shoe pressure, pain over the bunion, swelling and metatarsalgia. Lesser toe problems include MTPJ instability, pain, claw toes, transfer metatarsalgia and calluses over the heads of metatarsals.

Physical examination includes a sitting and standing evaluation and gait observation. Range of motion of the metacarpophalangeal joint and IPJ and any hypermobility of the first metatarsocuneiform joint must be assessed. The plantar aspect is assessed for keratosis. The lesser toes are assessed for any deviation, metacarpophalangeal joint instability, pain and clawing. It is very important to assess the passive correction of the hallux and motion of the MTPJ following correction of the deformity. The arch of the foot and any tightness of the heel are also assessed. Finally, a neurovascular assessment is carried out.

Radiography continues to be the standard means with which to assess joint pathology and measure angular deformity. Weight-bearing AP, lateral oblique and lateral projections are routinely used. The AP projection is used to determine the intermetatarsal angle, metatarsus adductus angle, hallux valgus angle, distal metatarsal articular angle, hallux valgus interphalangeus, first metatarsal length, sesamoid position, first MTPJ condition and medial metatarsal head enlargement. Figures 5.1 and 5.2 show angles in the foot X-rays.

If lateral subluxation of the proximal phalanx on the metatarsal head is present then the joint is incongruent, meaning that the proximal phalanx can

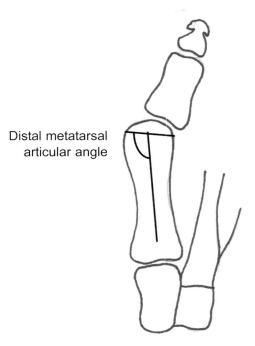

Distal metatarsal articular angle

Figure 5.2. The distal metatarsal articular angle.

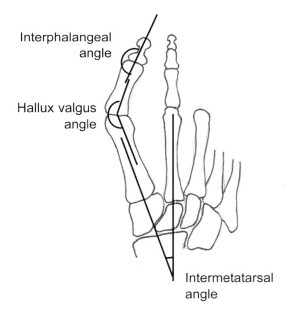

Interphalangeal angle

Hallux valgus angle

Intermetatarsal angle

Figure 5.1. Angles in hallux valgus on a dorsoplantar foot X-ray.

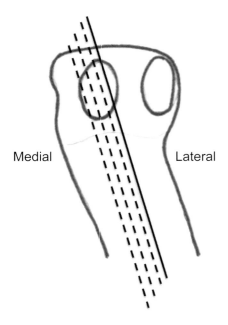

Medial   Lateral

Figure 5.3. Measurement of sesamoid subluxation.

be rolled medially on the metatarsal head to correct the deformity.

The lateral projection is used to determine the first metatarsal sagittal plane position and the presence of dorsal exostosis or osteophytes. The lateral oblique projection is useful to evaluate the presence of dorsomedial exostosis. The sesamoid axial view can be used to detect any lateral subluxation of the sesamoids out of their respective grooves (Figure 5.3), erosion of crista and sesamoid-metatarsal joint-space degenerative changes.

The normal angles in hallux valgus are summarised in Table 5.7.

The hallux valgus and intermetatarsal angles are used to quantify the severity of hallux valgus (Table 5.8).

Table 5.7. Normal angles in hallux valgus.

Angle	Location	Importance	Normal
Hallux valgus interphalangeus	Long axis of the proximal phalanx and distal phalanx	Degree of deformity at interphalangeal joint	<8°
Hallux valgus angle	Long axis of the proximal phalanx and first metatarsal	Degree of deformity at metatarsophalangeal joint	<15°
Intermetatarsal angle	Long axis of the first and second metatarsal	Increased in metatarsus primus varus	<10°
Distal metatarsal articular angle	Long axis of the metatarsal, with a line through the base of the distal articular cartilage cap of the first metatarsal	Increased offset predisposes to development of hallux valgus	<100°

DMAA = distal metatarsal articular angle

Table 5.8. Classification of severity of hallux valgus based on the hallux valgus and intermetatarsal angles.

	Hallux valgus angle	Intermetatarsal angle
Mild	<30°	<13°
Moderate	30-40°	13-20°
Severe	>40°	>20°

Management

The mainstay of treatment is non-operative management in the form of patient education, footwear modification and tendo-Achilles stretching. Operative treatment is indicated if conservative methods fail.

The goals of surgery are to relieve symptoms, restore function and correct the deformity. The clinician must consider the patient's history, physical examination and radiographic findings before selecting a procedure. On occasion, the final procedure is determined intraoperatively when the physical appearance of the joint, bone and tissue can be observed directly.

The following features of surgical repair allow successful correction of the deformity:

- Establishment of a congruous first MTPJ.
- Reduction of the intermetatarsal angle.
- Realignment of the sesamoids underneath the metatarsal head.
- Restoration of the ability of the first ray to bear weight.
- Maintenance or increase of the first MTPJ range of motion.

The specific procedures used will vary depending on the surgeon's preference, the nature of the deformity and the particular needs of the patient. The main surgical goal is to reposition the first metatarsal head over the sesamoids using the simplest method possible. Distal chevron osteotomy with lateral translation of 5mm may correct mild and moderate deformities.

With severe deformities where more lateral translation is required, a scarf osteotomy is used. Both chevron and scarf osteotomy can achieve satisfactory correction and allow immediate weight bearing without a cast.

A scarf osteotomy is a metaphyseal osteotomy of the first metatarsal. This is a very flexible osteotomy and can be modified to correct many common problems. The flat osteotomy plane means that immediate postoperative weight bearing is possible

without a cast. Some surgeons use it as their only (or main) procedure for hallux valgus.

Hallux valgus interphalangeus can be corrected with an Akin osteotomy when the great toe touches the second after a standard procedure. Increased distal metatarsal articular angle (DMAA) can be corrected with either a distal chevron or scarf osteotomy.

In general, it is safe to perform a distal osteotomy for an intermetatarsal angle of up to 12° and a proximal or scarf osteotomy above this.

If the patient has severe osteoarthritis then either fusion or Keller's arthroplasty can be performed, based on the physical demand. In a patient with rheumatoid arthritis, fusion of the first MTPJ provides a stable post.

Surgical technique

Access to the first MTPJ and to the osteotomy site is obtained from a medial longitudinal incision on the first ray from the middle of the distal phalanx to the first tarsometatarsal joint. A lateral release is initially performed through a first space incision. The adductor hallucis tendon and the lateral capsule of the first MTPJ are exposed. The deep peroneal nerve and its branches are protected with retractors.

A partial lateral capsulotomy is performed and the sesamoid-metatarsal ligament released. A Macdonald elevator in the first MTPJ is useful to identify and tense the sesamoid-metatarsal ligament for incision. The adductor tendon is released from the proximal phalanx, taking care not to damage the flexor hallucis brevis.

A medial longitudinal incision is deepened to the capsule of the first MTPJ and the metatarsal shaft. The plantar part of the capsule is partially exposed to facilitate later double-breasting. The capsule is opened longitudinally and the medial eminence exposed. The eminence is excised with a power saw in line with the medial surface of the metatarsal. The joint is inspected and its alignment relative to the metatarsal shaft (DMAA) assessed.

The longitudinal cut is made first. It starts about 1cm proximal to the tarsometatarsal joint where the metatarsal starts to flare out – about 2mm above the junction of the superior and inferior surfaces. The osteotomy runs distally parallel with the ground to 2-3mm short of the articular surface. The osteotomy plane runs downward parallel to the inferior surface of the metatarsal. It may be best to first cut the medial surface completely to establish the line.

Transverse cuts are then made from the ends of the longitudinal cut to the lateral surface, taking care to cut down in the same plane as the main cut. Lengthening can be achieved by directing the cuts more distally, but it is usually easier to physically translate the distal fragment distally.

The distal fragment is carefully separated and translated laterally by a combination of pushing the head and pulling the shaft fragments. DMAA can be corrected by rotating the distal fragment. The metatarsal can be shortened if necessary to allow full correction of a stiff MTPJ, or to take some tension out of a degenerate joint, by removing a slice from each transverse cut. The downwards translation of the head allows more shortening than is the case with some other osteotomies. Alternatively, length can be gained by translating the distal fragment distally.

The osteotomy is fixed with two cannulated headless screws. Mini-fragment cortical screws can be used and are cheaper than headless screws, but patients sometimes find the screw heads uncomfortable. The medial spike is trimmed off and any necessary rounding is performed. The capsule is repaired to restore soft tissue tension. A double-breasting technique may be used. Once the correction is completed, or earlier if more convenient, the degree of residual hallux valgus in the phalanx can be assessed. If necessary, an Akin osteotomy can be added.

Charcot arthropathy

Charcot arthropathy is a severe destructive process affecting the bone architecture and joint alignment in people who lack protective sensation. The most common cause is diabetes, although about 10% of Charcot patients have other causes such as spina bifida, leprosy, hereditary motor/sensory neuropathy, post-traumatic sensory deficits and alcoholic peripheral neuropathy.

Charcot arthropathy can occur with or without neuropathic ulceration. In those with diabetes it typically arises in the fifth and sixth decades of life, and can occur alongside a relatively normal vascular examination. Charcot arthropathy probably begins with either a recognised traumatic incident or multiple episodes of microtrauma. Care must be taken with foot and ankle injuries (even if fracture is not present) in patients with diabetes.

Injury to the joint is followed by rapid destruction of the joint surfaces and demineralisation. There is osteoclast overactivity, bone vascular shunting and bone breakdown.

The joint destruction and demineralisation may lead to deformity, skin pressure and ulceration. Healing begins after a few weeks, and there is usually bony union with joint incongruity and deformity in a few months.

Charcot arthropathy is often said to be painless, but pain is in fact very common – although it may be less than expected from the degree of arthropathy and deformity.

Classification

Eichenholtz has described three stages of Charcot arthropathy.

Stage 1: fragmentation or destruction stage
This process may last as long as 6-12 months. The bone fragments, the joint(s) become unstable and, in some cases, the bone is completely reabsorbed. This stage is clinically identified by significant swelling, erythema and a warm foot.

Stage 1 Charcot arthropathy can be confused with infection and the distinction may be very difficult. MRI can be helpful, and white-cell-labelled bone scans may be more reliable. The increased availability of positron emission tomography scanning offers hope of improved accuracy.

As the bones and joint are affected, fractures and instability develop and the joints can dislocate or shift in relation to each other. This can lead to severe deformity of the foot and ankle. Most often the midfoot joints are affected. The result is a very flattened foot, which is wider where the normal foot narrows in the arch. Bony prominences often develop on the plantar surface of the foot and are risk factors for subsequent ulceration.

Stage 2: coalescence
During this stage the acute destructive process slows and the body tries to begin healing. The swelling and heat begin to disappear.

Stage 3: resolution/consolidation
The swelling and erythema resolve. There may be residual instability.

Radiographs
In the early stages, plain radiographs show bone fragmentation. There may be joint subluxation or dislocation. Later on, resorption and coalescence of fragments occur. Periosteal new bone formation with sclerosis may be seen. In the final stage of resolution, remodelling occurs with smoothing of bone edges and reduction of the sclerosis.

Brodsky classification
The Brodsky classification describes the site of destruction:

- Type 1 – tarsometatarsal and lesser tarsus.
- Type 2 – peritalar.
- Type 3a – ankle; type 3b, posterior calcaneum.
- Type 4 – multiple sites.
- Type 5 – forefoot.

Management

Management in the early and acute phase is non-weight bearing followed by a total-contact cast. This allows even distribution of pressure and supports areas of softening and collapse. Orthotic management is the mainstay of treatment if the residual deformities are minimal and can be braced. In severe deformities, a combination of osteotomy (particularly of a 'rocker-bottom' deformity),

arthrodesis and soft tissue release can be performed once bone scans show that the disease process has settled.

Amputation may be required if ulceration and deep infection are present.

Lesser toe disorders

Commonly encountered lesser toe problems include deformities (claw toe, hammer toe and mallet toe), metatarsalgia, Morton's neuroma, Freiberg's disease, MTPJ instability and bunionette.

Deformities

These are usually associated with first ray deformities and insufficiencies causing the second toe to elevate or drift. Footwear is the most common and important factor in the development of lesser toe deformities.

Deformities may be flexible or fixed. Full passive correction can be achieved in flexible deformities, but not in fixed deformities. This is a key discriminator because fixed deformities require bony correction.

Claw toes
Claw toes are characterised by hyperextension of the MTPJ and flexion of the IPJs, and are due to imbalance of the intrinsic and extrinsic muscles. A neuromuscular pathology is suspected if all of the lesser toes are involved. Clawing in the second or third toes only is unlikely to be from a neuromuscular cause. Other causes include rheumatoid arthritis, previous foot compartment syndrome and a cavus foot deformity. Most, however, are idiopathic.

Deformities are initially flexible, becoming fixed as the disease advances. The plantar plate is placed under stretch, whereas the dorsal capsule becomes inflamed and contracted. The toe begins to sublux dorsally and results in downward pressure on the metatarsal head; this causes metatarsalgia, further damaging the plantar tissues. Eventually the plantar plate can rupture altogether and the toe dislocates dorsally.

Conservative management of claw toe deformities is similar to that of other lesser toe deformities. These include accommodative footwear, protective padding and strapping. In the early stages, taping the toe down and stretching can settle the synovitis and prevent a worsening deformity. Intra-articular steroids can also help, but carry a small risk of accelerating the deformity.

Surgery is considered when conservative management fails to control the symptoms. Addressing the first ray pathology is very important when treating lesser toe deformities and should be included whenever the first ray is symptomatic.

MTPJ deformity is addressed by extensor digitorum Z-lengthening, EDB release and dorsal capsulotomy. For flexible deformities, Girdlestone flexor to extensor tendon transfer of the FDL is useful but the toe can become stiff and swollen. Fixed flexion deformity of the IPJ is addressed by resection arthroplasty or fusion of the proximal IP joint (PIPJ). Severe deformities require temporary stabilisation with K-wire for 4-6 weeks, with taping and physiotherapy beyond that to reduce the risk of recurrence.

Hammer toes

Patients with hammer toes have an abnormal flexion posture of the PIPJ and a compensatory extension of the distal IP joint (DIPJ). The second toe is most commonly affected. There is no rotational deformity as in curly toes. If conservative measures fail then milder deformities are treated with flexor tenotomy or flexor to extensor transfer. In severe deformities, resection arthroplasty of the PIPJ is necessary, with or without DIPJ fusion.

Mallet toes

In mallet toes there is an isolated flexion deformity of the DIPJ. The underlying pathology is a spastic FDL. The involved digit may be elongated. Surgically, smaller deformities are treated with flexor tenotomy alone. For more severe deformities, however, tenotomy alone is associated with a high rate of recurrence. In these patients, resection arthroplasty or fusion of the DIPJ is advisable. This may be combined with flexor tenotomy. Amputation of the distal phalanx is reserved for very severe deformities involving the nail.

Crossover toe

Crossover toe describes a deformity in which the second toe lies dorsomedial relative to the hallux. This is caused by rupture of the collateral ligament and disruption of the plantar plate. There may be attrition of the lateral capsule and first dorsal interosseous tendon. The medial structures, such as the capsule, collateral ligament, lumbricals and interosseous tendon, become tight and contracted. The deformity may be initially correctable passively. As the disease advances, the deformity becomes fixed.

Conservative treatment consists of strapping to the third toe and accommodative footwear. In mild deformities, surgical correction consists of soft issue release of the medial structures, extensor tendon and dorsal capsule. Flexor to extensor tendon transfer can be performed to stabilise the toe. Alternatively, the EDB tendon can be used as a dynamic stabiliser.

In severe deformities, resection arthroplasty or metatarsal shortening osteotomies are advised. It is important to address the hallux deformity as well because the recurrence rate is high, especially in the presence of a deforming force from a deviated hallux.

Metatarsalgia

Metatarsalgia is a symptom rather than a diagnosis. It is pain in the plantar aspect of the lesser metatarsal heads.

Causes include the following:

● First ray insufficiency – when the first ray deviates medially it is associated with elevation and pronation of the first metatarsal, resulting in load transfer to the lesser metatarsals.
● MTPJ synovitis and instability.
● Morton's neuroma.
● Freiberg's disease.
● Stress fracture.
● Prominent metatarsal head fibular condyle.
● Restricted ankle movement causing forefoot overload.

Metatarsophalangeal joint synovitis and instability

Instability and synovitis of the lesser MTPJs is a common cause of forefoot pain. The typical patient is a middle-aged woman with hallux valgus. This is due to mechanically induced synovitis with damage to the plantar plate.

On examination there is puffiness around one or more MTPJs, divergence of the toes and tenderness around the joint, especially under the plantar plate. The fat pad under the metatarsal heads deteriorates with age. In patients with severe overload this deterioration is accelerated, resulting in easily palpable and painful metatarsal heads. Patients may have associated hallux valgus, hammer toe, crossover toe deformity and instability, subluxation or dislocation of the MTPJ.

Conservative measures of management include NSAIDs, functional taping to limit dorsiflexion, steroid injection and footwear modification. Steroid injection risks causing complete rupture of the capsule and plantar plate, increasing the deformity. The metatarsalgia becomes less responsive to conservative measures with dislocation of the joint.

When subluxation is not severe then synovectomy, extensor tenotomy, dorsal capsulotomy and immobilisation in the corrected position for 6 weeks is advised. For severe deformities, in addition to the above procedure the collateral ligaments and plantar plate are released, as they can become reattached in a dislocated position. Any associated hammer toe deformity is also corrected with proximal IP resection arthroplasty. The MTPJ is stabilised with flexor to extensor transfer and K-wire fixation of the joint in flexion for 4 weeks. Irreducible dislocations can require metatarsal neck osteotomy and holding the toe in the corrected position with K-wires for 4 weeks.

Overload and plantar keratosis

The second toe is most often affected with overload under the second metatarsal head. This is evidenced by a plantar keratosis on the skin overlying the second metatarsal head. It is particularly common if there is a defunctioned first metatarsal due to medial drift or a long second metatarsal. Diffuse plantar keratosis suggests that the overload is affecting all the metatarsals; this is particularly common in pes cavus.

A discrete intractable plantar keratosis can be due to a plantar wart (*Verruca plantaris*). These can be very painful and the lesion under the skin is often larger than what is visible on the surface. Plantar warts can be identified by a dark discolouration due to capillaries and can be very large. They are easily treated with liquid nitrogen, but occasionally require excision.

Other causes of a discrete intractable plantar keratosis include a prominent metatarsal head fibular condyle. This is best viewed on a sesamoid-view X-ray and is especially common on the fourth metatarsal. Treatment is with condylectomy if it fails to settle with orthotics. The medial sesamoid is often subject to overload; again, this can be treated very successfully with accommodative insoles. If this fails, the superior half can be removed to decompress and elevate the sesamoid. Sesamoidectomy is associated with a high risk of complications, including pain and deformity.

Pedobarography can be helpful in orthotic design and modification, and in surgical planning. The fourth and fifth metatarsals (the so-called lateral column) are mobile, and the risk of transfer metatarsalgia to them is therefore low if the second and third metatarsals have been addressed. The second and third metatarsals are reasonably immobile, and therefore if the second metatarsal is addressed in isolation there is a risk of transfer metatarsalgia. Operating on an asymptomatic metatarsal is controversial and it is more important to be sure preoperatively that this is not already overloaded.

Surgery to the metatarsal neck is commonly performed using a Weil osteotomy. This aims to shorten and elevate the metatarsal head. Swelling and stiffness are common. Other risks include recurrence, nerve or vessel injury and deformity.

Morton's neuroma

Morton's neuroma consists of degenerative and fibrotic changes in the common digital nerve near its bifurcation. There may be similar changes in adjacent unaffected nerves. Suggested causes are entrapment by the deep transverse metatarsal ligament or metatarsal heads, tethering of the third space nerve by the anastomotic branch between the medial and lateral plantar nerves, traction on the nerve by hindfoot valgus, interdigital bursitis and forced toe dorsiflexion in high-heeled shoes.

Symptoms most commonly occur in middle-aged women (78% of cases are in women). The third interdigital space is most often involved, then the second. Symptoms in the fourth space are rare and should make one doubt the diagnosis, while symptoms in the first space are virtually unknown.

Diagnosis

Diagnosis is primarily based on history and examination. Patients complain of pain, burning and tingling down the interspace of the involved toes. The pain is usually made worse by walking in high-heeled shoes with a narrow toe box and is relieved by rest and removing the shoe. The pain will radiate to the toes or vague pain may radiate up the leg. This condition can be very non-specific.

The whole foot should be examined, looking for any other factors likely to produce metatarsalgia. Patients may have local tenderness and swelling in the intermetatarsal space. There may be reproduction of pain or, less reliably, a Mulder's click on metatarsal compression. Local anaesthetic injection into the affected space may relieve symptoms and support the diagnosis.

Standing AP and lateral and oblique forefoot films should be obtained if other forefoot pathology is suspected. Ultrasounds and MRIs can be used if the clinical situation is atypical. Ultrasound-guided injections and pain monitoring increase the diagnostic accuracy.

Management

Conservative measures of management are footwear modification, NSAIDs and local steroid injection. Footwear modification is by avoiding high heels and narrow toe boxes. Metatarsal bars and pads placed proximally to the painful area decompress the nerve by widening the intermetatarsal space during weight bearing. Local steroid injection brings initial pain relief in about 80% of patients, but the recurrence rate is high (50%).

Surgical management is indicated if conservative measures fail to adequately relieve symptoms. Contraindications are poor circulation, diabetes mellitus, reflex sympathetic dystrophy, atypical symptoms and personality disorders.

The standard operation is a digital neurectomy, which is most often performed through a dorsal approach (although a plantar incision has also been advocated). The nerve is divided 2-3cm proximal to the bifurcation and excised. The deep transverse metatarsal ligament may be wholly or partially released. Surgery has a success rate of 80%. Recurrent symptoms can be caused by inadequate resection of the nerve, recurrent neuroma formation and an initial wrong diagnosis.

Surgery for Morton's neuroma

A dorsal approach is preferred to prevent a tough, painful scar on the plantar aspect. The incision starts at the proximal portion of the involved webspace, coursing 3-4cm proximal to the interspace parallel to the metatarsal shafts, not to the extensor tendons. The incision is kept directly in the mid-line of the webspace in order to avoid damage to the digital nerves.

A self-retaining retractor is then placed between the metatarsals to put tension on the transverse ligament. The ligament is divided to visualise the common digital nerve. Applying digital pressure from the plantar surface of the web helps to locate the common digital nerve. The nerve is isolated from the accompanying vascular bundle. If it is difficult to identify the common digital nerve, the proper digital nerve can be identified near the appropriate phalanx and then followed proximally.

The dissection is carried proximally into the interspace and the common digital nerve is isolated 3cm proximal to the bifurcation. The plantar digital cutaneous nerve should be transected 3cm proximal to the transverse ligament or to the neuroma. Digital nerves distal to the bifurcation are then transected, including all the plantar branches.

Freiberg's disease

Freiberg's disease is an 'infraction' of the dorsal part of one of the lesser metatarsal heads. It is a condition of young adults, occurring during puberty, mostly in girls. Repetitive trauma with micro-fractures is one attributed cause. Two-thirds of lesions occur in the second metatarsal, and a quarter in the third. The metatarsal head partially collapses, with later degenerative changes in the joint. The inferior part of the head is normally well preserved.

Gauthier and Elbaz described five stages:

- Stage 0 – subchondral fracture.
- Stage 1 – osteonecrosis without deformation.
- Stage 2 – deformation by crushing of the osteonecrotic segment.
- Stage 3 – cartilaginous tearing.
- Stage 4 – arthrosis.

Patients present with pain in the forefoot localised to the head of the second metatarsal. The pain is aggravated by high heels. There may be localised swelling and a limited range of movement in the involved MTPJ, as well as signs of synovitis.

Radiographs initially show sclerosis of the epiphysis and widening of the joint space. Subsequently, the epiphysis becomes fragmented with formation of bone spurs, giving the appearance of osteoarthritis. In late stages the metatarsal head becomes irregular, widened and flattened.

Initial management includes proper footwear with a metatarsal bar or pad and limitation of activity for 4-6 weeks. For more troublesome joints, a steroid injection, local anaesthetic and immobilising the foot in a short-leg walking cast for 4 weeks can help resolve symptoms.

Failure of conservative measures is an indication for surgery. Surgical options are debridement with excision of osteophytes, debridement with dorsiflexion osteotomy, metatarsal shortening osteotomy, interposition arthroplasty and joint replacement.

Bunionette (Tailor's bunion)

The bunionette deformity is a prominence of the fifth metatarsal head, usually with medial deviation of the fifth toe. This is associated with a wide fifth metatarsal head, lateral bowing of the fifth metatarsal shaft, an increased angle between the fourth and fifth metatarsal shafts and an increased incidence of hallux valgus. When bunionette is associated with hallux valgus and metatarsus primus varus, the deformity is called splay foot. There is usually pain over the lateral aspect of the MTPJ. Almost 50% of patients have bilateral bunionettes.

Three distinct types have been described by Coughlin:

- Type 1 – large, wide metatarsal head.
- Type 2 – lateral metatarsal shaft bowing.
- Type 3 – increased fourth/fifth metatarsal angle (intermetatarsal angle >8°).

Besides cosmetic concerns, patients usually complain of pain over the prominent fifth metatarsal head, difficulty in finding comfortable shoes and rubbing between the fourth and fifth toes. General widening of the forefoot is often seen on examination. The deformity may be associated with hallux valgus, hammer toes and congenital curly toes.

Initial treatment is conservative and consists of shaving the symptomatic callus and footwear modification. A metatarsal pad or plantar pressure-relieving orthosis is advised if there is coexisting pes planus or if the callosity is plantar. Surgical options include distal, basal and diaphyseal osteotomies, such as the reverse scarf osteotomy. Proximal osteotomy is avoided because of the tenuous blood supply. As a general guide, Coughlin type 1 deformities are treated with head shaving, type 2 with a distal or diaphyseal osteotomy and type 3 with a proximal diaphyseal osteotomy.

Plantar heel pain

Causes of plantar heel pain include the following:

- Plantar fasciitis.
- Calcaneal stress fracture.
- Calcaneal periostitis.
- Loss or instability of the heel pad.
- Entrapment of Baxter's nerve should be considered when the pain is resistant to treatment.

Plantar fasciitis

This is the most common cause of heel pain and can affect both the active and sedentary adult population. Micro-tears at the origin of the plantar fascia are the likely pathology. These incite an inflammatory and repair process, which, if healing fails, becomes a chronic plantar fasciitis with a downgrading of the inflammatory process.

The typical presentation is with pain and tenderness under the medial aspect of the heel at the attachment of the fascia. Typically this is worst on the first step in the morning, improving as the day goes on and then often becoming more painful towards evening. Some patients have more weight bearing than first-step pain. The pain may radiate across the heel or down the plantar fascia. Patients may have symptoms suggestive of a spondyloarthropathy such as ankylosing spondylitis. Some patients have pain and tenderness of the abductor hallucis due to entrapment and inflammation of the first branch of the lateral plantar nerve. Plantar 'spurs' seen on lateral X-rays are not relevant as they lie on the lateral part of the calcaneum away from the attachment of the fascia.

Plantar fasciitis will resolve with conservative management in most patients. This includes NSAIDs, cushioned heel inserts, Achilles tendon stretching, night splints, steroid injections and shock-wave treatment. Resistant cases are treated with release of the medial third of the plantar fascia with spur resection. Complete plantar fascia release leads to a slight flattening of the arch and may produce pain in

the lateral column of the foot. Neurolysis of the first branch of the lateral plantar nerve by release of deep fascia of the abductor hallucis is beneficial if nerve entrapment is suspected.

Calcaneal stress fracture

Calcaneal stress fracture results from multiple compressive loads and weight-bearing activities and is most often seen in military recruits. Symptoms include pain and swelling on both sides of the heel and exquisite tenderness to palpation on the lateral and medial aspects of the heel.

Plain radiographs may not become positive for 2-4 weeks. A lateral radiograph may show an area of increased density perpendicular to trabecular stress lines through the posterior aspect of the calcaneus (from the posterior-superior surface to the anterior-inferior surface). Bone scans can be useful in those with acute symptoms and negative radiographs. MRI is more specific and sensitive in the diagnosis.

Management involves reducing activity and a cast or brace immobilisation until the symptoms have resolved and bone healing is evident on radiographs. This takes approximately 4-8 weeks.

Posterior heel pain

Common causes of posterior heel pain are as follows:

- Retrocalcaneal bursitis.
- Haglund's deformity.
- Achilles tendonitis (insertional or non-insertional).
- Paratenonitis.
- Inflammatory arthritis like rheumatoid arthritis, ankylosing spondylitis, psoriatic arthritis and Reiter's syndrome.

The aetiology is multifactorial, and includes poor lower-extremity alignment and training errors.

Paratenonitis

When the paratenon is inflamed, the whole area is diffusely swollen and tender and crepitation may be felt when the tendon glides. This typically occurs in distance runners and is worth identifying, as an injection of saline with or without local anaesthetic can rapidly resolve the condition.

Non-insertional Achilles tendinosis

Non-insertional tendinosis occurs approximately 2-6cm proximal to the insertion of the tendon and a tender fusiform swelling can be palpated. Non-insertional Achilles tendinosis generally responds well to conservative treatment, NSAIDs, heel-cord stretching with an eccentric strengthening programme and bracing. Heel lifts and very occasionally a short period of immobilisation in a walker, followed by gradual mobilisation, can be helpful. Steroid injections into or around the Achilles tendon may provoke rupture and should generally be avoided. There is plenty of anecdotal evidence, however, that steroid injections can offer good relief of symptoms.

Resistant cases are treated surgically by excision of the inflamed paratenon and debridement of the pathologic areas of tendon, followed by repair. If more than 50% of the tendon is involved then flexor hallucis longus tendon transfer is a very successful procedure.

Insertional Achilles tendonitis

Insertional Achilles tendonitis is an enthesopathy with tenderness localised to tendon insertion. Pathologies include attritional changes, tendinosis, intratendinous ossification and a bony spur. The pain is related to contact between the posterior calcaneus and the Achilles tendon, and there can be progressive enlargement of the bony prominence of the heel. Localised calcification within the Achilles tendon can be a cause of insertional tendonitis.

Conservative management is the mainstay of treatment. NSAIDs, ice, heel lifts, silicone pads and stretching are the conservative measures, but are less successful than in non-insertional tendinosis. Surgical treatment is by excision of heterotopic bone and the degenerative part of tendons, and re-anchoring or repair of the tendon if more than 50% of the tendon is involved.

Retrocalcaneal bursitis and Haglund's deformity

Retrocalcaneal bursitis presents with anterior pain (deep to the tendon), with pain on palpation of the soft spot. It can occur alone or with tendinosis. When it occurs in isolation, a steroid injection can be very useful in resolving the pain.

Haglund's deformity is a normal variant and is a prominence of the posterior superior calcaneal tuberosity. Retrocalcaneal bursitis is due to inflammation of the bursa along the anterior surface of the Achilles tendon. It is most common in women and is related to footwear, rigid heels or heel counters.

Patients present with posterolateral heel prominence, deep posterior heel pain, fullness of the tendon and increased pain with dorsiflexion of the ankle. Conservative management is similar to that for Achilles tendonitis, and consists of NSAIDs, heel-cord stretching, footwear adjustment and raising the heel out of the shoe with a heel insert, which shifts the contact against the heel.

Surgical treatment consists of debridement of the inflamed retrocalcaneal bursa and excision of the Haglund's prominence. The excision must be kept proximal to the Achilles insertion. A lateral approach is easier, but care must be taken to avoid the sural nerve. A medial incision may also be used. In this case, a vertical incision is made 1cm anterior and parallel to the medial border of the Achilles tendon, and down onto the calcaneus. Then the posterior calcaneal tuberosity is removed, and the Achilles tendon is debrided and reattached using bone anchors. The Achilles tendon is dissected subperiosteally at the insertion of the Achilles tendon and about 50% of the tendon is elevated. The calcaneal prominence is then removed. The average size of fragment removed is 3cm long, 3cm wide and 6mm thick. The ankle is subsequently immobilised for 4-6 weeks.

'Pump bump' refers to the bony prominence that is found at the back of the heel distal to the tendon insertion. Management includes padding the area, but it occasionally needs to be shaved down.

Pes cavus

Pes cavus describes a foot with an abnormally high longitudinal arch that does not flatten with weight bearing. The forefoot is plantarflexed, which is most marked in the first ray causing apparent pronation of the forefoot. The hindfoot is usually in dorsiflexion (calcaneus), although in some neuromuscular conditions, such as CMTD, the gastrocnemius/soleus complex becomes tight or shortened and the hindfoot goes to equinus. The heel may be neutral, but more often lies in varus creating a cavovarus foot.

A cavovarus foot is considered pathological until proven otherwise, but in particular beware the unilateral pes cavus.

The causes of cavus foot are as follows:

- Neuromuscular (from proximal to distal):
  - cerebral palsy;
  - multiple sclerosis;
  - Friedreich's ataxia;
  - spinal cord tumour;
  - syringomyelia;
  - tethered cord;.
  - myelodysplasia;
  - poliomyelitis;
  - Guillain-Barré syndrome;
  - muscular dystrophy.
- Congenital.
- Residual talipes equinovarus.
- Arthrogryposis.
- Trauma.
- Fibrosis post-compartment syndrome.
- Peroneal palsy.
- Fracture malunion.
- Burn contracture.

Charcot-Marie-Tooth disease (hereditary sensory motor neuropathy)

CMTD is the most common inherited neuropathy, affecting 1 in 2,500 people. CMTD has different genetic variants with variable expressivity and clinical picture. The most common foot presentation in CMTD is the cavovarus deformity. Some patients may present with muscle cramps, recurrent ankle sprains and difficulty with gait. The upper extremities are involved in as many as two-thirds of patients with peripheral neuropathy. It is important to note, however, that up to 20% of patients show no demonstrable sensory loss at presentation. Upper-limb involvement tends to be milder than lower-extremity involvement, and becomes clinically symptomatic as the patient ages. Later, intrinsic-minus hands develop with clawing of the fingers and atrophy of the small muscles of the hand.

Type 1

Type 1 CMTD is inherited as an autosomal dominant disease. There is hypertrophic demyelination and slow nerve conduction.

Patients with type 1 CMTD have a defect in the gene encoding peripheral myelin protein-22 on chromosome 17. Clinical presentation is most common during the second decade of life. This is a progressive neuropathy in which both motor and sensory nerve function are affected. Distal muscle groups are involved first with weakness (lower limbs first), loss of reflexes and atrophy. Sensory loss occurs later in the disease course, although vibratory sense can be affected early. Type 1 CMTD may be associated with scoliosis and hip dysplasia.

Type 2

Type 2 CMTD (neuronal form) is infrequently seen. Patients have an axonal neuropathy with relatively normal nerve conduction. The inheritance pattern is variable. Onset is delayed until the second or third decade of life. The reflexes are normal and there is more profound distal lower-extremity weakness than encountered in type 1. A characteristic stork-leg appearance, caused by atrophy of the distal third of the quadriceps and hamstrings, is frequently seen. Some patients develop a calcaneovalgus deformity.

Cavovarus deformity

The underlying pathology in the development of cavovarus deformity in CMTD is muscle imbalance. The tibialis anterior and peroneus brevis weaken early on in the disease course. This may be due to their relatively small cross-sectional area compared with their antagonists. The weakness results in plantar flexion of the first ray, resulting in hindfoot varus through the tripod effect (i.e., with a plantar flexed first ray and mobile lateral rays). For the foot to remain plantigrade, the heel must roll into varus in order to get the lateral metatarsals on the ground.

In the early stages of the disease the hindfoot is flexible. Deformities of the hindfoot involve malposition of the talus and calcaneus, with the latter inverted into a varus position. In later stages the plantar flexed position of the first ray eventually becomes rigid, which forces the heel to remain in varus and fixes the hindfoot in varus.

When deformities become rigid, neither weight bearing nor passive manipulation fully corrects the foot. The degree of rigidity is classically elicited by the Coleman block test, which confirms whether the hindfoot deformity is forefoot driven. The test is performed by placing a block under the lateral column of the foot and allowing the first metatarsal to drop. This eliminates the need for hindfoot varus. If the hindfoot is flexible, the varus will correct.

Management

Because of the progressive nature of the disease, surgical management is preferred to conservative measures such as braces. In general, the treatment comprises two soft tissue releases (plantar fascia, tendo-Achilles), two tendon transfers (peroneus longus to brevis, EHL to first metatarsal or 'Jones procedure') and two osteotomies (lateralising

calcaneal osteotomy, dorsiflexion osteotomy of the first metatarsal).

Plantar fascia release (Steindler release) is the first procedure considered, though this is seldom performed in isolation. A medial plantar approach is used to transect the plantar fascia and the fascia investing the abductor hallucis. The contracted intrinsic muscles are also released. The Achilles tendon can be released to correct the equinus.

The deforming force of the peroneus longus can be countered by transferring the longus to brevis. The clawed hallux is managed by transferring the EHL to the first metatarsal; this also increases the dorsiflexion power. This procedure can be combined with fusion of the IPJ of the big toe (Jones procedure). Clawing of lesser toes may need extensor tendon lengthening, MTPJ capsulotomies and resection of the head and neck of the proximal phalanges.

A lateralising or lateral closing wedge osteotomy of the calcaneum will help to shift the weight-bearing axis slightly medial to the midline of the calcaneum. This converts it to a stabilising force and protects the stretched lateral ligaments.

A first metatarsal osteotomy is performed to correct plantar flexion deformity of the first ray. The second and third metatarsal can also be corrected if required.

Advanced fixed deformities are corrected by osteotomies and fusion of the midfoot or hindfoot, depending on the deformities (e.g., triple fusion). Management is described as 'à la carte' because the procedures are selected according to the needs of the individual foot – for example, the most severe toe clawing may be asymptomatic and can therefore be left.

Ankle arthritis

Ankle arthritis is uncommon compared with arthritis of other weight-bearing joints, possibly because it has the largest contact area. Rare and common causes are listed in Table 5.9. Disorders that cause bleeding into the joint (e.g., haemophilia, pigmented villonodular synovitis) can also cause ankle arthritis.

Table 5.9. Causes of ankle arthritis.

Common	Rare
Post-traumatic arthritis	Septic arthritis
Inflammatory or systemic arthropathy (e.g., rheumatoid arthritis, psoriatic arthropathy, gout)	Primary osteoarthritis
	Chronic instability
	Ochronosis
	Polyostotic fibrous dysplasia

Clinical symptoms can be due to mechanical block or inflammation. Inflammatory changes cause swelling, pain and stiffness, especially in the morning. Mechanical symptoms are due to anterior osteophytes causing impingement, particularly on dorsiflexion. Osteophytes develop first in the anterior tibia, with a 'kissing lesion' subsequently developing in the talus. The pain due to impingement may be relieved by high heels.

Pain and tenderness in the anterior joint line with dorsiflexion (Molloy impingement test) suggest anterior impingement. Some patients complain of locking or giving way. This may be due to a loose body or reflex inhibition of the supporting muscles. Other joints are often involved in patients with arthritic ankles, which may affect the surgical option and likely outcomes.

Investigation

Preliminary investigation includes a standing AP and lateral radiograph of the ankle. This can show narrowing of the joint space, spurs and loose bodies and malalignment. The surrounding joints can also be seen and may have a bearing on the management strategy, especially if degenerate. A CT scan is useful where there is loss of bone stock due to trauma, infection and so on. An MRI is useful to assess the extent of talus osteonecrosis.

Management

Conservative management is advised if the symptoms are mild. This comprises NSAIDs, disease-modifying drugs for the specific treatment of inflammatory arthropathy, splints, braces, boots and local steroid or hyaluronic acid injections. Adding a rocker-bottom orthosis to the shoe will improve transition throughout the stance phase.

Surgery is an option where non-surgical treatment has failed to control the patient's symptoms and the patient's activities of daily living are seriously affected. A wide range of surgical options are available: arthroscopic debridement, arthrodesis, arthroplasty, arthroscopy, osteotomy and joint distraction.

Arthroscopic debridement

Arthroscopic debridement is useful when the joint is reasonably well preserved, especially if the main problem is impingement from synovitis, spurs or loose bodies. Arthroscopic debridement for impingement has a 75% success rate at 5 years in the presence of spurs, but only 50% with loss of joint space. In severely degenerated ankles there is a small risk of worsening pain due to the increased movement.

Arthrodesis

Arthrodesis is the mainstay of treatment for advanced symptomatic arthritis of the ankle. It can be performed with an open technique or arthroscopically. Prior to ankle arthrodesis, it is beneficial if the patient is given the option of wearing either a below-knee cast or Cam walker. A good candidate for ankle arthrodesis is a patient with documented ankle arthritis who has obtained pain relief from a Cam walker. Cigarette smoking increases the risks of ankle non-union by at least three times, and may affect wound healing after any procedure.

Compression arthrodesis using internal fixation is popular. The ankle should be held in a neutral position with regard to varus/valgus and plantar/dorsiflexion, as well as in slight external rotation. The talus should be directly beneath the tibia. AP translation should be avoided, but a slight medial translation is acceptable. A variety of approaches have been described. A lateral approach excising the fibula is quite popular.

Arthroscopic arthrodesis

Arthroscopic arthrodesis requires a correctable deformity, or less than 10° varus or valgus malalignment. The main advantages are reduced postoperative pain and a high rate of rapid union. This is particularly useful in patients with a poor vascular supply, poor soft tissue envelope and bleeding disorders.

One of the disadvantages of ankle fusion is that adjacent joints have accelerated wear. Radiological studies have shown that the majority of patients develop degeneration in the long term, although not all are symptomatic.

> **Note**
>
> Fuchs S, Sandmann C, Skwara A, Chylarecki C. Quality of life 20 years after arthrodesis of the ankle. A study of adjacent joints. *J Bone Joint Surg Br* 2003; 85: 994-8.

> **Note**
>
> Coester LM, Saltzman CL, Leupold J, Pontarelli W. Long-term results following ankle arthrodesis for post-traumatic arthritis. *J Bone Joint Surg Am* 2001; 83-A: 219-28.

Ankle replacement

Early prostheses did not reproduce the biomechanics of the ankle well and had a very high failure rate. Second-generation prostheses have reported success in more than 90% of patients. Ankle replacement is advisable in patients with bilateral disease or rheumatoid arthritis, and when other joints around the ankle are involved.

The latest evidence suggests superior pain relief at 2 years. The failure rate for revision arthroplasty is high and most such patients will require a tibiotalocalcaneal fusion.

> **Note**
>
> Saltzman CL, Mann RA, Ahrens JE, *et al*. Prospective controlled trial of STAR total ankle replacement versus ankle fusion: initial results. *Foot Ankle Int* 2009; 30: 579-96.

Distraction arthroplasty

In distraction arthroplasty, a distraction force is applied with an external fixator frame. Joint movement is possible through the hinges in the fixator. This technique is not very popular because of the long periods required in the fixator and less than optimal improvement.

Osteotomy of the distal tibia

Realignment is an option if the joint is reasonably well preserved. However, the results are not uniformly reproducible.

Ankle instability

Chronic ankle instability is a result of ankle ligament sprain. Patients present with pain, stiffness, swelling, locking, giving way or repeated sprains. Tenderness is usually maximal over the lateral ligament, often in the anterior talofibular ligament only. A few patients will also have localised tenderness over the deltoid ligament, which tends to indicate more complex injuries. Tenderness or swelling over the Achilles, peroneal or tibialis posterior tendons should be identified.

There is an association between ankle instability and peroneal tendon instability: the patient will usually complain of snapping or giving way over the peroneal tendons, and instability is maximal on plantar flexion/eversion.

Investigation

Ankle instability is demonstrated with the anterior drawer and tilt tests. The anterior drawer test should be performed with the ankle in 20° plantar flexion. The tibia may be pushed posteriorly against a fixed foot or the foot drawn forwards. The characteristic positive sign is a 'suction sign' as the synovium is sucked into the joint, drawing the skin inwards in the lateral gutter. In many patients, however, there is no suction sign but the talus can obviously be drawn anteriorly more than on the other side.

The talar tilt test is conventionally performed by tilting the hindfoot and looking for a suction sign or asymmetrical movement. It should be performed with the ankle plantigrade. Palpation of the talar neck will help in differentiating between movement in the ankle and the subtalar joint.

There are three common presentations of chronic ankle instability:

- Pain.
- Pain and instability symptoms.
- True mechanical instability.

Functional instability is a subjective sensation of giving way. Mechanical instability is excessive laxity of the lateral ligament complex. Clinically, the anterior drawer test is positive.

Radiologically, instability may be demonstrated with the anterior drawer or talar tilt test. Absolute displacement of more than 10mm or a difference of more than 3mm compared with the opposite side is considered positive radiographic evidence on an anterior drawer stress radiograph. A talar tilt stress radiograph should show a difference of more than 10° compared with the opposite side to be positive.

Management

Conservative treatment consists of peroneal strengthening and proprioceptive rehabilitation. This is particularly useful in functional instability. Ankle braces can also be used. Surgery is advised if symptoms persist, although generalised hypermobility is a contraindication for surgery. Patients with mechanically stable ankles and other intra-articular problems generally have good results with arthroscopic surgery.

The most commonly performed surgical procedure is anatomic reconstruction. Originally described by Bostrum and modified by Gould, this consists of detachment, shortening and reinsertion of the attenuated anterior talofibular and calcaneofibular ligaments, with reinforcement using the extensor retinaculum.

Non-anatomic surgical techniques are rarely used as these procedures are extensive and can cause excessive stiffness.

Osteochondral lesions of the ankle

The aetiology of non-traumatic osteochondral lesions of the ankle is unknown, but it may be related to a primary ischaemic event. Non-traumatic lesions can be familial. The majority of osteochondral lesions occur after a definite injury, but some have no clear history of injury. Most lesions occur on the talus, but about 10% occur on the tibial plafond, often as 'kissing lesions' with a talar defect. Only 50% of lesions are visible on plain radiographs.

Talar lesions usually occur in two distinct regions:

- Medial lesions constitute 70% of talar lesions. These lesions are deep and cup-shaped. About 50% of cases have a history of injury.
- Lateral lesions constitute 30% of lesions and are almost always associated with injury. These wafer-shaped superficial lesions are more likely to displace.

Medial lesions tend to be posteromedial, and lateral lesions anterolateral.

Classification

Osteochondral lesions were classified by Berndt and Harty in 1959 (Table 5.10 and Figure 5.4) and by Hepple and colleagues in 1999 (Table 5.11). Cheng and colleagues developed the arthroscopic staging system shown in Table 5.12.

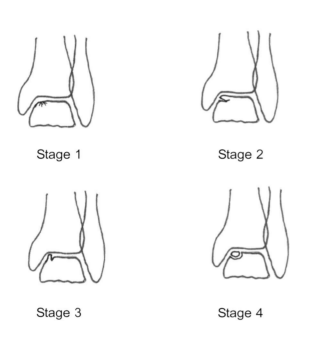

Stage 1   Stage 2

Stage 3   Stage 4

Figure 5.4. The Berndt and Harty classification of osteochondral lesions of the talus.

Note

Berndt AL, Harty M. Transchondral fractures (osteochondritis dissecans) of the talus. *J Bone Joint Surg Am* 1959; 41-A: 988-1020.

Note

Hepple S, Winson IG, Glew D. Osteochondral lesions of the talus: a revised classification. *Foot Ankle Int* 1999; 20: 789-93.

Table 5.10. Berndt and Harty classification of osteochondral lesions of the ankle.	
Stage	**Description**
1	Subchondral fracture
2	Partially detached fragment
3	Detached but undisplaced fragment
4	Displaced fragment

Table 5.11. Hepple and colleagues' classification of osteochondral lesions of the ankle.	
Stage	**Description**
1	Articular cartilage damage only
2	Cartilage injury with underlying fracture
2a	Cartilage injury with underlying fracture and oedema
2b	Cartilage injury with underlying fracture but no oedema
3	Detached (rim signal) but undisplaced fragment
4	Displaced fragment
5	Subchondral cyst formation

Table 5.12. Cheng and colleagues' arthroscopic staging system.

Grade	Description	Stability
A	Smooth and intact, but soft or ballotable	Stable
B	Rough surface	Stable
C	Fibrillation/fissuring	Stable
D	Flap present or bone exposed	Unstable
E	Loose, undisplaced fragment	Unstable
F	Displaced fragment	Unstable

Most patients have an inversion injury to the lateral ligamentous complex. Patients typically present with chronic ankle pain along with intermittent swelling, locking, weakness, stiffness, instability and giving way.

Investigation

Patients usually have tenderness in the joint. This can be localised, giving a clue as to the site of the lesion, or diffuse. Lateral lesions often have tenderness in the angle between the tibia and fibula, while medial lesions may have medial talar dome tenderness in plantar flexion. Anterolateral lesions may be tender when the anterolateral ankle joint is palpated with the joint in maximal plantar flexion, while tenderness behind the medial malleolus in dorsiflexion may indicate a posteromedial lesion. Occasionally a loose body may be palpable. There may be swelling or synovitis, and 30-50% of patients have ligament injuries. The anterior drawer and talar tilt tests for instability may be positive.

Plain films will show about half of all lesions and will also show other fractures, spurs and joint narrowing. Isotope bone scanning will show an area of increased activity at the site of an osteochondral lesion of the ankle, but has been largely superseded by MR and CT. MRI findings include areas of low signal intensity on T1-weighted images, which suggest sclerosis of the bed of the talus and indicate a chronic lesion. T2-weighted images reveal a rim that represents instability of the osteochondral fragment.

Management

Conservative management of osteochondral lesions of the talus should initially be attempted. This includes an initial period of immobilisation, followed by physical therapy.

Surgical treatment depends on a variety of factors, including patient characteristics (e.g., activity level, age, degenerative changes) and lesions (e.g., location, size, chronicity). Small symptomatic lesions are treated by loose-body removal, with or without stimulation of fibrocartilage growth (microfracture, curettage, abrasion or transarticular drilling). Larger lesions can be treated with fixation and bone grafting. More recently, mosaicplasty and autologous chondrocyte implantation have been used successfully.

Outcomes of surgery

Curettage has a success rate of around 80%. The addition of drilling gives even better results.

Lesions that fail to settle or recur may be considered for further reconstructive surgery by bone and/or cartilage grafting. Osteochondral plug grafts can be harvested from the intercondylar notch of the femur or the non-weight-bearing surface of the talus. The success rate for this procedure is reportedly as high as 94%. Autologous cultured chondrocyte grafts also give a high success rate.

Lower-limb amputations

Most limb amputations are of the lower extremities. Foot and ankle amputations may be secondary to trauma, tumour, infection or congenital deformity. Trauma is the most common cause in younger age groups and peripheral vascular disease in older patients.

Common amputations in the foot and ankle are Syme's, Boyd-Pirogoff, Lisfranc and Chopart amputations. All need adequate prosthetic foot and socket support because of the remaining short lever arm available.

A toe filler can be used for phalangeal and distal metatarsal amputations. Slightly proximal amputations such as toe disarticulation need a silicone boot.

Syme's amputation

The most common indications for Syme's amputation are infection and limb deficiencies. A patent posterior tibial artery is needed for satisfactory healing of the flaps. Syme's amputation includes ankle disarticulation, removal of malleoli and anchoring the heel pad to the weight-bearing surface. The malleoli are resected flush with the joint and the fat pad is fixed to the residual bone.

Boyd-Pirogoff amputation

Boyd-Pirogoff amputation provides a more solid stump because it preserves the function of the plantar heel pad. In this procedure, a portion of the calcaneus is left and fused to the tibia. Boyd-Pirogoff amputation

can also be chosen for salvage after an unsuccessful Lisfranc or Chopart amputation.

Lisfranc amputation

Lisfranc amputations are performed through all of the tarsometatarsal joints except the second, which should be osteotomised to preserve the stability of the medial cuneiform.

Chopart amputation

Chopart amputation removes the fore- and midfoot, saving the talus and calcaneus. This is an unstable amputation and is not performed for ischaemia. Chopart amputation can result in equinovarus deformity.

Transmetatarsal amputation

Complete transmetatarsal amputations lead to a good functional result if the maximum length can be maintained to aid the terminal stance phase. Muscular balance between the dorsiflexors and plantarflexors of the foot is well conserved if a length of 3-4cm can be kept. If necessary the dorsal extensors can be sutured to the flexors, but only if the stumps do not have to be shortened by more than 1cm.

The amputation levels of each metatarsal shaft should mimic the natural shape of the metatarsal bones. The amputation level should thus be more proximal laterally than medially. The recommended difference in the remaining length of metatarsal stumps from medial to lateral is 2mm between adjoining metatarsals. In order not to harm the Lisfranc ligament, a minimum of 3cm of the second metatarsal base should be maintained.

Toe and ray amputations

There is little disability from toe amputations. The big toe is amputated distal to insertion of the flexor hallucis brevis.

Isolated second toe amputations are performed distal to metaphyseal flare of the proximal phalanx. This acts as a buttress and prevents the development of hallux valgus. Resections of one or more rays cause narrowing of the foot and late equinus deformity.

The first metatarsal ray may be amputated with only moderate loss of foot function.

Foot and ankle orthosis

Foot and ankle orthoses can correct deformities, including distal deformities presenting from abnormal proximal joints. In addition, they transfer the weight proximally, augment muscle weakness and control motion.

The UCBL orthosis used for tibialis posterior insufficiency was introduced to control hindfoot valgus and midfoot pronation.

An AFO controls the joints of the foot and ankle and is a term used for a variety of designs. There are several different varieties:

- Posterior leaf-spring AFO – for patients requiring dorsiflexion assist for ground clearance in the swing phase.
- Solid ankle AFO – immobilises all the joints of the foot and ankle (e.g., in patients with paralysis or polio).
- Clamshell – an anterior shell is used to control the anterior portion of the leg (e.g., for pseudarthrosis of the tibia or fracture bracing).
- Floor-reaction AFO – used in patients with weak quadriceps and in those with spastic diplegia with tight gastrocnemius to improve crouch gait.
- Patellar tendon-bearing AFO – used to axially unload the foot, this is effective in treating diabetic and other neuropathic ulcers.

A Charcot restraint orthotic walker uses contact plastic technology. It is very effective in the treatment of Charcot foot.

Foot and ankle prosthesis

Commonly used designs for foot and ankle prostheses are the single-axis foot, solid ankle cushion heel and dynamic response foot.

The single-axis foot has an ankle hinge that provides dorsiflexion and plantar flexion. The dynamic-response foot additionally provides inversion and eversion, which are useful on uneven surfaces.

Chapter 6 Hand

Extensor tendon injury

Anatomy

The dorsum of the wrist and hand contains 12 main extensor/abductor tendons. These tendons run in six dorsal compartments under the extensor retinaculum.

The location of an extensor tendon injury is described in zones in relation to the wrist and finger joints (Table 6.1).

Table 6.1. Fascial compartments of the dorsum of the wrist (radial to ulnar).

Zone	Level
I	Distal interphalangeal joint
II	Middle phalanx
III	Proximal interphalangeal joint
IV	Proximal phalanx
V	Metacarpophalangeal joint
VI	Metacarpals and carpal bones
VII	Extensor retinaculum

Extensor tendons derive vascularity from three sources:

- Muscular arteries – proximal to the dorsal retinaculum.
- Synovial diffusion and mesotendons – under the dorsal retinaculum.
- Arterial branches from the paratenon – distal to the dorsal retinaculum.

Diagnostic pitfalls

Two factors should be considered when examining an extensor tendon injury:

- The extensor digitorum communis tendons are also cross-connected to their adjacent neighbours by tendon slips called juncturae tendinum. An injury that divides an extensor tendon proximal to these juncturae will still allow active extension of the affected finger from an adjacent extensor tendon pulling through the juncturae.
- A proximal interphalangeal joint (PIPJ) can still be actively extended via the lateral bands even if the central slip is completely divided.

Extensor tendon repair

The method of repair differs according to the zone of the tendon injury.

Proximal to the middle of the proximal phalanx (zones IV-VII), the tendon is oval or cylindrical. A multistrand (4-6) 4/0 non-absorbable grasping or locking core suture can be used. This can be supplemented by a circumferential 6/0 monofilament suture.

Distal to the middle of the proximal phalanx, the central slip is flattened. The lateral bands and their common tendon to the distal phalanx are also flattened and ribbon-like. A non-absorbable 4/0 or 5/0 suture is used as a continuous running suture. The joint must be immobilised for 4 weeks postoperatively either with transarticular wire or a splint.

Repair tips to consider are as follows:

- Lacerations to the extensor digitorum communis tendons (especially distal to the juncturae tendinum) cause minimal retraction.
- Lacerations to the extensor pollicis longus tendons proximal to the metacarpophalangeal joint (MCPJ) are likely to cause retraction to Lister's tubercle. A separate incision at that level is often needed to retrieve the proximal tendon.
- A round-bodied non-cutting needle should be used, otherwise the needle will slice the tendon and possibly the core sutures.

Management of closed tendon avulsions

Mallet finger (zone 1)
Mallet finger is an avulsion of the extensor digitorum longus from the base of the distal phalanx. This can be either a pure tendinous avulsion, or with a bone fragment.

If no fracture is present, the distal interphalangeal joint (DIPJ) should receive continuous hyperextension splinting for 6-8 weeks.

A dorsal distal phalanx avulsion fracture without subluxation can be ignored, irrespective of its size. Treatment is the same as with no fracture: continuous hyperextension splinting for 6-8 weeks. An X-ray must be taken in the splint. If the distal phalanx is subluxed in a palmar direction then the DIPJ is reduced in extension and held with a transarticular wire for 4 weeks and then a splint for a further 2 weeks.

Boutonnière deformity (zone III)
The Boutonnière deformity is described as a flexion deformity of the PIPJ and hyperextension of the DIPJ. It is rare for an acute central slip avulsion to present with a classic Boutonnière deformity. The deformity tends to develop in the weeks and months following injury.

The components of Boutonnière deformity are:

- Disruption of the central slip.
- Attenuation of the triangular ligament.
- Palmar migration of the lateral bands.

In the acute setting a central slip avulsion can be diagnosed by the following findings:

- Tenderness over the central slip insertion.
- Palmar dislocation (diagnosed clinically or radiologically) of the PIPJ (for this to happen, the central slip must have detached).
- The Elson test – hold the PIPJ at 90°. Resist PIPJ extension by holding the middle phalanx. If the central slip is intact the lateral bands are not recruited and the DIPJ remains floppy. If the central slip is detached the DIPJ firmly extends.

Treatment of acute Boutonnière deformity is as follows:

- Closed injuries are managed by splinting the PIPJ in extension, allowing active DIPJ flexion for 6 weeks.
- Open injuries require open repair.

Treatment of chronic Boutonnière deformity is as follows:

- If the joints are stiff, the first step is therapy with or without surgical release of the PIPJ.
- If the joints are mobile, any scarring is excised and direct reattachment is performed. The lateral bands are mobilised.
- Reconstructive options are Y-V advancement and a Littler reconstruction.

Flexor tendon injuries

Flexor tendon nutrition

Vascular supply

The vascular supply to the flexor tendons mainly comes from the vincula on the dorsal surface of the tendons. The digital artery splits into four transverse branches along its course. Two branches are for the profundus tendon and two for the superficialis tendon. Both tendons have avascular segments over the proximal phalanx and the flexor digitorum profundus (FDP) has an additional avascular segment over the middle phalanx.

Synovial fluid diffusion

When the digit is flexed and extended, a pumping mechanism known as imbibition moves the fluid into tendon interstices through rigid conduits on the surface.

Flexor tendon healing

Tendon healing occurs through the action of fibroblasts. There is an intrinsic and extrinsic healing process. Extrinsic healing leads to more adhesion formation.

Tendon healing has three phases:

- Inflammatory phase (3-5 days after repair) – in this phase, the strength of repair depends on the strength of the sutures and minimally on the fibrin clot.
- Fibroblastic or collagen-producing phase (begins on day 5, lasts for 3-6 weeks) – fibroblasts proliferate, collagen is produced and new capillaries form. The tendon loses strength in the first 5-21 days.
- Remodelling or maturation phase (lasts for 6-9 months) – fibres become longitudinally oriented and stronger.

Biomechanics

Five annular (A1-A5) and three cruciate pulleys (C1-C3) prevent bowstringing of the tendon on flexion (Figure 6.1).

A1, A3 and A5 overlie the MCPJ, PIPJ and DIPJ, respectively. A2 and A4 arise from the periosteum of the proximal and middle phalanx, and are critical for mechanical function. Cruciate pulleys are thin and collapse to allow annular pulleys to approximate each other during digital flexion.

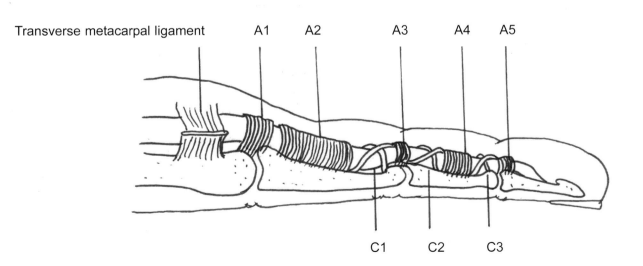

Figure 6.1. Flexor tendon pulleys.

Table 6.2. Zones of flexor tendon injury.

Zone	Location
I	Distal to insertion of the flexor digitorum superficialis tendon
II	Flexor tendon sheath
III	Lumbrical muscles
IV	Carpal tunnel
V	Distal portion of forearm
In the thumb	
T1	Distal to the A2 pulley
T2	Between the A1 and A2 pulley
T3	Proximal to the A1 pulley

Zones of injury

The location of a flexor tendon injury is described in zones (Table 6.2 and Figure 6.2).

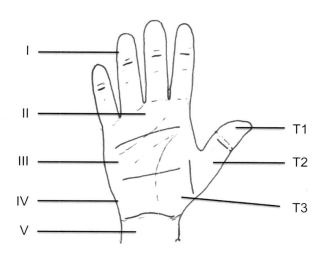

Figure 6.2. Zones of flexor tendon injury.

Avulsion of the flexor digitorum profundus tendon

Avulsion of the FDP tendon usually occurs in athletes. The tendon avulses as the object being grasped (e.g., an opponent's shirt) is pulled out of the hand. The forced extension thus occurs during maximal contraction of the FDP. The ring finger is most commonly affected.

Classification systems (e.g., Leddy and Packer) classify avulsion of the FDP tendon according to the level of proximal retraction:

- Type I – the tendon end retracts into the palm.
- Type II – the tendon end retracts to the level of the PIPJ and rests against the A3 pulley.
- Type III – avulsion of a large bony fragment; A4 and A5 pulleys prevent retraction.

Flexor tendon repair

The following principles apply to flexor tendon injury repair:

- Repair is not an emergency and delayed primary repair has better results.
- It is better to repair both the flexor digitorum superficialis (FDS) and FDP if both are cut.
- Badly contaminated wounds or wounds with skin loss should not be sutured primarily.
- Associated fractures should be stably fixed and primary repair performed.
- If there is concern regarding infection, repair should be delayed for a few days.

Wound extension

Adequate exposure is needed to assess the extent of the injury, retrieve the tendons and perform the repair. The most common incision is a 'zigzag' or Brunner incision.

Retrieval of tendon ends

Tendon ends retract and need to be retrieved with minimal damage to the tendon. Retrieval methods include the following:

- Proximal to distal milking of the tendon.
- Reverse Esmarch bandage.
- Skin hook – can be used to pull the tendon if the end is visible in the sheath.
- Infant catheter – a proximal incision is made and an infant catheter is passed from the distal wound through the sheath and retrieved from the proximal wound. The tendon is sutured to the catheter and the catheter is then pulled distally.

Once retrieved, the tendon can be transfixed through a pulley using a hypodermic needle.

Repair

- Core suture (4 or 6 strands) – a 4-0 braided polyester suture is most commonly used with a non-cutting needle. It is used as a grasping suture, which can be locked at the grasping site (Savage repair) or unlocked (Kessler). All strands should be kept under a similar tension and knots should be located outside the repair site if possible. If a repair fails, it is usually at the knots. Partial lacerations of less than 60% do not need a core suture.
- Peripheral epitendinous suture – a peripheral epitendinous suture enhances the strength of repair by 10-50% and reduces gaps. A 6-0 monofilament suture is used with a non-cutting needle.
- Tendon sheath – there is no definite advantage to repairing the sheath, although it may improve synovial nutrition and act as a barrier to external adhesions. However, it may also cause narrowing and restrict gliding.
- Pulleys – the A2 and A4 pulleys must be preserved as a minimum. If the repair is likely to catch on the pulley entrance, pulleys may be vented (partially divided) facing the repair.

Zone I repair

In zone I injuries, only the FDP is cut. The A5 pulley may have to be opened to find the distal stump. If the distal stump is too short (<1cm), reattachment is performed directly to the bone. The osteoperiosteal flap is elevated and parallel oblique holes are drilled with a 1.2mm K-wire through the distal phalanx, exiting through the nail. A straight needle 3-0 suture is placed in the proximal tendon end and pulled out through the bone holes. The suture is then tied over a button on top of the nail.

Zone II-V repair

Zone II-V repair involves standard repair of the FDS and FDP tendons, preserving (as a minimum) the A2 and A4 pulleys if at the zone II level.

Post-operation

Dressing

Light dressings should be applied to the fingers. A dorsal slab is applied with the wrist in neutral and MCPJs are flexed at 45°. The fingers are not bandaged to the slab to allow unresisted accidental flexion in the perioperative period.

Therapy

Physical therapy should start within 3 days of repair. There are a number of different therapy regimens, of which the Belfast regimen is one. The principles are early active and passive motion protected by a dorsal finger and wrist extension block splint. Early motion leads to rapid healing, fewer adhesions and improved excursion.

Complications

Complications can occur with repair of flexor tendon injuries and should be managed as follows:

- Rupture – prompts re-exploration and repair.
- Joint contracture – splintage and physiotherapy.
- Adhesions – if no improvement for several months, consider tenolysis.

Finger-tip injuries

Length preservation is advisable in the thumb but is not always necessary in the fingers.

Digital-tip amputations with skin or pulp loss only

There are two treatment options for digital-tip amputations with skin or pulp loss only:

- Primary closure – if sutures can be placed without much tension.
- Conservative treatment – non-adherent dressing, changed periodically.

Digital-tip amputations with exposed bone

Skeletal shortening and primary closure

Skeletal shortening and primary closure is the preferred treatment for digital-tip amputations with exposed bone. A 'hook nail' should be avoided. The nail bed should not be pulled distally to cover the

Table 6.3. Methods of skin-flap cover for digital-tip amputations.	
Skin-flap method	**Description**
Atasoy-Kleinert volar V-Y flap (5mm advancement)	Better for volar distal-dorsal proximal oblique injuries Cut full-thickness skin only. The base of the triangle is sutured to the cut end of the nail bed, and the rest is closed as a 'Y'
Volar advancement flap (15mm advancement)	The volar skin is advanced on the neurovascular pedicle
Cross-finger pedicle flap	The flap can be based distally, proximally, laterally or medially A full-thickness flap is raised off the extensor tendons It is reflected over and sutured to the palmar defect on three sides. The fourth side is closed in the second stage The donor site is covered with a full-thickness skin graft The pedicle is detached at 2 weeks
Thenar flap	Can be used for the tips of index and long fingers Usually reserved for children; there is a risk of finger stiffness in adults

distal phalanx. Instead, the nail bed is cut back to the level of bone loss so that it does not curve over the end of the bone.

Skin flaps

The use of skin flaps to cover exposed bone is associated with a significant complication rate and is of questionable benefit. Flaps may be considered to preserve length when bone is exposed. A number of skin-flap methods can be used to cover exposed bone in digital-tip amputations (Table 6.3).

Complications

The following complications can occur with repair of finger-tip injuries:

- Hypersensitivity – addressed with a desensitisation program when the wound has healed.
- Stiffness – managed by hand therapy.
- Decreased sensation – advancement flaps and conservatively treated pulp loss often retain good sensation. Full-thickness skin grafting will usually provide only protective sensation.
- Cold intolerance – all finger injuries can develop this. In most patients it resolves after 2-3 years.

Hand infections

Paronychia (infection of the nail fold)

If there is no obvious collection of pus then paronychia can be managed initially with oral antibiotics. A collection on one side of the nail fold is managed by incising along the margin of the nail bed. A collection going across either side of the nail is again managed by incision. If there is also a suspicion of pus under the nail, the nail should be removed.

Felon (infection of the distal phalanx pulp)

The pulp of a digit contains multiple fibrous septa as well as multiple sensory nerve endings. As a result,

even a small amount of pus in a septal compartment (even if not obvious) can cause pressure and significant pain. Increased pressure in the pulp caused by the accumulation of pus can lead to pulp necrosis or osteomyelitis.

Pus is drained either through a lateral incision dorsal to the neurovascular structures (avoiding the sides involved in pinch) or with a volar longitudinal incision. Early infection with mild pain and a soft pulp can initially be treated with antibiotics.

Collar stud abscess

Collar stud abscess is a web-space infection proximal to the superficial transverse metacarpal ligament. The palmar aspect is often the initiating site. Pus can track dorsally to form an abscess above and below the ligament. The palmar aspect of the abscess can spread to the deep palmar space. Drainage is through a dorsal and a palmar longitudinal incision.

Deep fascial space infections

Deep fascial space infections are usually the result of a penetrating injury. The deep palmar space lies deep to the flexor tendons. In the hand it is divided into three spaces separated by septa: the thenar space, the midpalmar space and the hypothenar space. In the forearm, the space is known as Parona's space and lies between the flexor tendons in the distal third of the forearm and the pronator quadratus.

Infections of the deep palmar space present with pain and tenderness over the space involved, swelling (often more noticeable on the dorsum of the hand) and restriction of finger movement.

Drainage of the midpalmar space is through a longitudinal incision in line with the middle finger from the distal palmar crease in a proximal direction. Thenar space infections can be drained through an incision along the proximal side of the thenar crease. Parona's space is drained through an incision on the volar aspect of the forearm ulnar to the midaxial line.

Flexor sheath infection

Flexor sheath infections are usually the result of a penetrating injury. Untreated, they can cause destruction of the gliding mechanism and tendon necrosis.

Diagnosis

Kanavel described four diagnostic signs:

- Flexed position of the finger.
- Symmetric enlargement of the whole finger.
- Excessive tenderness along the course of the sheath.
- Pain on passive extension of finger.

Management

The mainstay of treatment is operative drainage, intravenous antibiotics, rest and splint in the Edinburgh position. Early presentations can be treated with antibiotics alone.

Open drainage is through an oblique palmar incision centred on the DIPJ flexion crease. The synovium is incised between the A4 and A5 pulleys. A counterincision is made in the palm proximal border of the A1 pulley. The tenosynovium is excised, leaving the annular pulleys intact. A small cannula is passed proximally into the sheath, which is irrigated with saline to ensure easy continuous flow. Free drainage should be ensured during irrigation.

A shiny tendon is visualised at both proximal and distal incisions and the finger is allowed to freely flex during irrigation. The flexor sheath of the thumb and small finger may communicate with the bursa of the wrist, in which case the sheath may have to be opened proximal to the wrist flexor crease.

Septic arthritis of the interphalangeal or metacarpophalangeal joints

Infections of the interphalangeal joints and MCPJs are usually the result of direct penetration. Contiguous spread can occur, but is much less common. Infections in the joint can lead to destruction of the articular cartilage and stiffness.

Diagnosis

Movement of the joint is painful and local swelling and tenderness are present. Aspiration of the joint fluid may help in the diagnosis.

Management

Washout of the joint is performed on an urgent basis. Approaches to finger joint washout are as follows:

- MCPJ – access is through a longitudinal split in the extensor digitorum communis tendon. It should not go through the sagittal bands.
- PIPJ – the approach is between the central slip and the lateral band.
- DIPJ – the surgical approach is on either (or both) sides of the terminal extensor tendon.

Carpal tunnel syndrome

Carpal tunnel syndrome is compression neuropathy of the median nerve in the carpal tunnel. In most instances it is idiopathic. Other causes include trauma (distal radius fracture), rheumatoid arthritis, hypothyroidism, pregnancy, diabetes and systemic lupus erythematosus.

Anatomy

The carpal tunnel is bounded dorsally by the arch of carpal bones. The palmar transverse carpal ligament completes the tunnel. The transverse carpal ligament inserts into the hamate and triquetrum on the ulnar side and the scaphoid and trapezium on the radial side.

The contents of the carpal tunnel are the median nerve, the FDS, the FDP and the flexor pollicis longus.

At the distal edge of the retinaculum the median nerve divides into six branches:

- One recurrent motor branch.
- Three proper digital nerves.
- Two common digital nerves.

The palmar cutaneous branch arises from the median nerve, 5cm proximal to the wrist flexion crease from the radiopalmar aspect. It travels along with the nerve for 1.5-2.5cm and then lies between the flexor carpi radialis (FCR) and the palmaris longus (PL). It emerges through the fascia 0.8cm proximal to the wrist flexion crease and divides into ulnar and radial branches. Ulnar branches may be found in superficial tissue when doing a carpal tunnel release.

Variations in the median nerve have been described (Figure 6.3):

- High division separated by a persistent median artery or aberrant muscle.
- The recurrent motor branch passes through or around the distal edge of the flexor retinaculum and can be extraligamentous (50-90%), subligamentous (30%) or transligamentous (25%). It can also arise from the ulnar border of the median nerve and lie on top of the transverse carpal ligament.

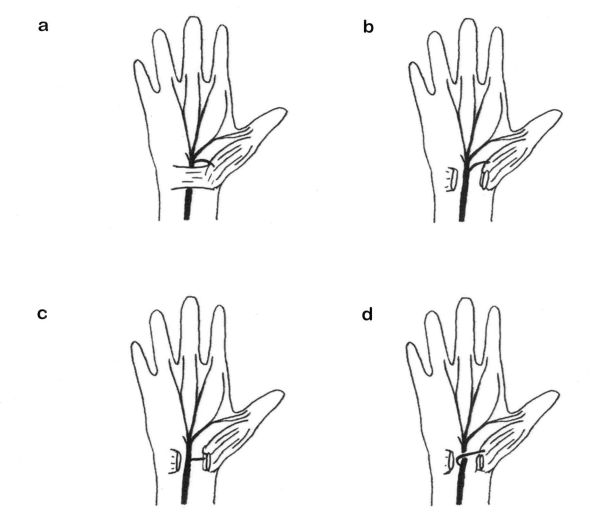

Figure 6.3. Variations in the recurrent motor branch of the median nerve: (a) extraligamentous; (b) subligamentous; (c) transligamentous; and (d) motor branch arising from the ulnar border of the median nerve.

Symptoms

Patients present with pain and paraesthesia in the median nerve distribution in the digits. Symptoms are typically worse at night and may develop with activities involving gripping as the lumbricals are pulled into the tunnel. The palmar cutaneous branch is spared as it travels superficial to the carpal tunnel.

Signs

Phalen's wrist flexion is performed by holding the wrist in flexion for 60 seconds and checking for reproduction of paraesthesia.

Direct compression of the nerve and Tinel's nerve percussion test are also useful tests.

Nerve conduction studies

Carpal tunnel syndrome is a clinical diagnosis and nerve conduction studies are only usually required where the diagnosis is uncertain. A negative result does not exclude carpal tunnel syndrome if the classic symptoms and signs are present.

Abnormal findings:

- Distal motor latencies greater than 4.5ms.
- Distal sensory latencies greater than 3.5ms.
- Asymmetry of conduction between two hands of greater than 1ms for motor and 0.5ms for sensory conduction.

Electromyography of the thenar muscles is useful to look for signs of denervation.

Differential diagnosis

Differential diagnoses are cervical nerve root compression, spinal cord lesions or peripheral nerve disorders.

Non-operative treatment

Night splinting
Where symptoms at night predominate as a result of wrist flexion when sleeping, night splinting can be very effective. The splint prevents wrist flexion.

Steroid injection
A permanent cure is rare following a steroid injection into the carpal tunnel. It is therefore used to confirm a diagnosis in equivocal cases or to provide temporary symptom relief.

Operative treatment

Release of the carpal tunnel can be performed through open surgery or arthroscopically. It is indicated for daytime symptoms and when splinting fails.

With open surgery, there is 96% patient satisfaction and 84% of patients return to their previous job.

With arthroscopic surgery, a general anaesthetic is needed, visualisation is often poor and there is an increased risk of iatrogenic nerve injury.

Note

Ferdinand RD, MacLean JG. Endoscopic versus open carpal tunnel release in bilateral carpal tunnel syndrome. A prospective, randomised, blinded assessment. *J Bone Joint Surg Br* 2002; 84: 375-9. The researchers performed one open and one endoscopic release in 25 patients with bilateral carpal tunnel syndrome. There was no difference in strength, relief or satisfaction between the two hands.

Open release technique
This technique is most commonly performed under local anaesthesia. The incision (approximately 3cm long) is in line with the radial border of the ring finger.

It extends from the distal wrist crease to Kaplan's line. It is not necessary to cross the wrist crease with the skin incision. The transverse carpal ligament extends more proximal to the wrist crease and must be divided.

Kaplan's cardinal line is drawn from the apex of the thumb-index web to the hook of hamate. The deep palmar arch lies under this line. The intersection of the line with the long finger flexed marks the recurrent motor branch. The superficial palmar arch is located between this line and the proximal palmar crease.

If ulnar nerve symptoms are present there is no need to release Guyon's canal, as it enlarges itself following release of the transverse carpal ligament.

Grip strength returns after 3 months and pinch strength returns after 6 weeks following open carpal tunnel decompression.

Bowstringing is not a problem as there is some repair of the flexor retinaculum with time.

Chronic wrist pain

Causes of a chronic painful wrist can be classified according to the site of symptoms (Table 6.4).

Ganglion

Ganglia are the most common benign masses in the hand and wrist. They often arise from the synovial lining of the carpal joints or the tendon sheaths. The dorsal scapholunate ligament is the most common site of origin. The volar ganglia are related to the FCR tendon.

Clinically, ganglia appear as firm, fluctuant swellings, which may be mildly tender on palpation. There is no specific initiating event and these swellings may have been present for a long time before treatment is sought. A sensation of aching or tiredness may sometimes be experienced.

Table 6.4. Causes of chronic wrist pain according to the site of pain.

Site	Causes
Radial-sided pain	De Quervain's tenosynovitis Trapeziometacarpal joint osteoarthritis Scaphoid non-unions and scaphoid non-union advance collapse Scaphotrapeziotrapezoid osteoarthritis Ganglion
Central pain	Scapholunate dissociation and scapholunate advanced collapse Kienbock's disease Intra-osseous ganglion Ganglion
Ulnar pain	Distal radioulnar joint instability, malalignment or osteoarthritis Triangular fibrocartilage tear Pisotriquetral osteoarthritis Hamate hook fracture

Aspiration of the swelling reveals a gelatinous fluid. Aspiration with or without a steroid injection is associated with a high recurrence risk. Surgical excision under general anaesthetic and tourniquet control has the highest cure rate of approximately 95%. Excision involves removal of the stalk of the ganglion as well as a small part of the capsule of the joint from which it arises.

Patients should be warned about the risk of recurrence of the ganglion, which can be up to 30% following excision.

Carpal instability

Carpal instability can be dissociative, non-dissociative or adaptive.

Dissociative carpal instability is instability within a carpal row:

- Scapholunate ligament injury – dorsal intercalated segmental instability, lunate extended, scaphoid flexed.
- Lunotriquetral ligament injury – volar intercalated segmental instability, lunate flexed, scaphoid extended.
- Lunate/perilunate dislocation.

Non-dissociative carpal instability occurs between carpal rows – for instance, midcarpal or radiocarpal instability.

Adaptive carpal instability is carpal malalignment secondary to distal radius malunion.

Management
Scapholunate instability is the most common presentation.

Acute injury is managed with open ligament repair and wire stabilisation.

For chronic injuries (>6 weeks old), ligament reconstruction (modified Brunelli) can be performed if the joint is reducible and there is no arthritis. In the low-demand patient, a dorsal capsulodesis or equivalent procedure is adequate.

Lunotriquetral instability is managed by repair in the acute phase. Lunotriquetral fusion is indicated in the chronic phase.

Acute perilunate dislocation is managed with acute reduction and repair of the ligaments through a dorsal approach.

Kienbock's disease

Kienbock's disease is avascular necrosis and collapse of the lunate. The aetiology is unknown, but it may be related to a single traumatic episode or recurrent microtrauma events.

Management
Treatment is conservative for most patients:

- Radial shortening if ulna-negative.
- Revascularisation procedures.
- Arthrodesis or proximal row carpectomy as salvage procedures.

Congenital anomalies of the hand and upper limb

In 1966, Frantz and O'Rahilly proposed a classification system for congenital upper limb deficiencies that includes four types:

- Type 1 – terminal transverse.
- Type 2 – terminal longitudinal.
- Type 3 – intercalary transverse.
- Type 4 – intercalary longitudinal.

This has been expanded by Swanson, Barsky and Entin to seven categories:

- Type 1 – failure of formation of parts.
- Type 2 – failure of differentiation.
- Type 3 – duplication.
- Type 4 – overgrowth.
- Type 5 – undergrowth.
- Type 6 – congenital constriction-band syndrome.
- Type 7 – generalised skeletal abnormalities.

Note

Swanson AB, Barsky AJ, Entin MA. Classification of limb malformations on the basis of embryological failures. *Surg Clin North Am* 1968; 48(5): 1169-79.

Radial hemimelia

Radial hemimelia is the congenital absence of part or all of a radius and the associated deficiency of radial carpal bones.

Classification is as follows:

- Grade I – absence of the distal radial epiphysis.
- Grade II – complete but short radius.
- Grade III – partial aplasia (absence of the distal radius).
- Grade IV – complete absence of the radius.

Associated conditions include VATER (vertebrae, anal malformations, trachea, oesophagus anomalies and renal) syndrome, cardiovascular anomalies and Fanconi syndrome, and anomalies of the gastrointestinal and genitourinary tracts.

In mild cases, stretching and manipulation may suffice. In more severe cases, the ulna can be centralised and fused to the wrist bones. Pollicisation of the index finger helps to provide opposition, replacing the thumb.

Ulnar hemimelia

Ulnar hemimelia is partial or complete absence of the ulna. Classification is as follows:

- Grade I – hypoplasia of the ulna.
- Grade II – partial aplasia of the ulna.
- Grade III – total aplasia of the ulna.
- Grade IV – radiohumeral synostosis.

Cleft hand

A cleft hand is the central absence of one or more digits and fusion of the other digits. It may be bilateral. The genetic transmission is autosomal dominant.

Syndactyly

Syndactyly is the most common congenital anomaly of the hand. It is partial or complete fusion of two or more digits. Simple syndactyly involves only the skin, while complex syndactyly involves the bones.

Polydactyly

Polydactyly is the presence of supernumerary digits. The accessory digit may be simple soft tissue, or may have a more complex structure with bones and tendons. Rarely, a metacarpal may be present.

Duplication of the thumb

Duplication of the thumb is a common anomaly. It may be associated with cardiac abnormalities or Fanconi syndrome.

The Wassel classification is used:

- Type 1 – bifid distal phalanx.
- Type 2 – duplicated distal phalanx.
- Type 3 – bifid proximal phalanx.
- Type 4 – duplicated proximal phalanx.
- Type 5 – bifid metacarpal.
- Type 6 – duplicated metacarpal.
- Type 7 – triphalangism (similar to type 4, but with an extra phalanx at the end of one distal phalanx).

Hypoplasia of the thumb

Thumb hypoplasia has been classified by Blauth:

- Grade I – short thumb with hypoplastic thenar muscles.
- Grade II – grade I with adducted MCPJ.

- Grade III – deficient metacarpal with abducted thumb.
- Grade IV – floating thumb.
- Grade V – complete absence of the thumb.

Clinodactyly

Clinodactyly is deviation of the little finger laterally. It can be caused by a trapezoidal middle phalanx.

Camptodactyly

Camptodactyly is deviation of the digit in the sagittal plane. Flexion contracture of the little finger is the most common manifestation.

Kirner's deformity is in-curling of the DIPJ of the little finger in prepubertal girls.

Macrodactyly

Macrodactyly is enlargement of one or more digits.

Congenital trigger thumb

The underlying cause of congenital trigger thumb is stenosis of the A1 pulley. A third of cases resolve spontaneously by the age of 1 year. Those that do not resolve are managed by surgical release between the ages of 18 months and 3 years.

Dupuytren's contracture

Dupuytren's contracture was first described by Baron Guillaume Dupuytren (1777-1835).

The palmar fascia is a three-dimensional system of fine ligamentous structures. It forms a framework of guiding channels for the longitudinal structures. It also anchors the skin, allowing the hand to grip and rotate an object without the skin moving. In Dupuytren's contracture this flattened fibrous network thickens to form nodules and then cords. Contraction of these cords results in flexion deformities of the fingers.

Pathology

The proliferation phase is characterised by immature fibroblasts and myofibroblasts in whorl-like patterns. Growth factors, including interleukin-1 and platelet-derived growth factor, are produced by platelets and macrophages.

Once formed, cellular tissue responds to mechanical transduction. Fibroblasts respond to chemical signals and growth factors as well as to mechanical stimuli.

Aetiology

The cause is largely unknown. Dupuytren's contracture is not related to alcohol intake, smoking, trauma or occupation. There is a possible correlation with diabetes or epilepsy medication. There is a genetic element, but only up to 20% of patients have a family history.

Several factors may indicate an increasingly severe disease with a more rapid progression:

- Young age.
- The presence of similar disease process at other sites (e.g., example plantar fibromatosis).
- A positive family history.

Anatomy

The palmar fascia is divided into three layers distally (Table 6.5).

The patterns of cord contraction are as follows:

- Central cord – follows layer 1. Passes distally and attaches to the base of the middle phalanx.
- Lateral cord – runs from the natatory ligament to the lateral digital sheath.
- Spiral cord – formed from the pretendinous band, spiral band, Grayson's ligament and the lateral digital sheet.

The neurovascular bundle is fixed in the midpalm under the palmar fascia and at the base of the middle

Table 6.5. Layers of the palmar fascia.

Layer	Description
1	The superficial layer Inserts into the skin of the palm
2	The spiral band on either side of the flexor tendon – deep to the neurovascular bundle The lateral digital sheet The pretendinous band The natatory ligament Cleland's ligaments – dorsal to the neurovascular bundle Grayson's ligaments – palmar to the neurovascular bundle
3	The deepest layer Passes deep on either side of the metacarpophalangeal joint

phalanx by Grayson's ligament. Between these two points the neurovascular bundle can be displaced.

Clinical features

The presenting features are palpable nodules and cords. There may be pitting of the palmar skin. Finger, thumb and first web-space contractures are present.

Dupuytren's disease may be associated with fibromatoses elsewhere:

- Plantar fibromatosis (Ledderhose disease).
- Garrod's knuckle pads (circumscribed dermal nodules or plaques on the dorsal aspect of the PIPJs or MCPJs).
- Peyronie's disease of the penis.

The underlying cause and associated features are elicited in the history. The degree of flexion contracture of each digit and joint should be recorded. The table-top test of Hueston is performed by placing the palm prone on the table. Flexion of the interphalangeal joints will be evident.

Surgical treatment

Nodules can be painful when they initially form, but the pain decreases as they mature and therefore they rarely need excision. The table-top test of Hueston is a useful test. If the patient cannot place the palm flat on the table because of contractures then surgery is considered.

The aim of treatment is to release contractures by cutting or excising the diseased tissue. Releasing the associated joint contractures is also necessary in severe cases.

MCPJ contracture can be corrected regardless of duration, but PIPJ contracture is more difficult to correct.

Standard limited fasciectomy
All involved fascia are removed by progressive longitudinal dissection. A longitudinal incision is made. The skin deficiency from the contracture is addressed using a Z-plasty, which brings skin from the sides of the finger to the palmar side and lengthens the scar.

Dermofasciectomy
Dermofasciectomy involves the removal of a section of skin and fascia. It is usually reserved for patients with poorly mobile skin and recurrence. A full-thickness skin graft, usually harvested from the antecubital fossa, is used to cover the defect. This helps prevent recurrence as the disease does not reoccur under a graft.

Needle fasciotomy

This is a percutaneous technique performed using a hypodermic needle. It is most suited for well-defined cords causing MCPJ contractures, but the indications have been extended to include cords around the PIPJ.

Segmental fasciectomy

Small, spaced out incisions are made along the cord. A 1cm section of cord is removed through each incision.

Skin defects

Skin defects that remain in the palm after the deformity has been corrected can be left open to heal by secondary intention (open-palm technique) or grafted.

Joint contractures

Residual PIPJ contracture may remain after Dupuytren's cord has been removed. The accessory collateral ligaments are released first, followed by the volar plate if necessary. The more structures that are released, the higher the risk of postoperative stiffness.

Complications

The following complications can occur:

- Injury to digital nerves – rare.
- Injury to the digital artery – may lead to ischaemic flaps and require reconstruction.
- Wound healing – haematoma, infection, ischaemia.
- Reflex sympathetic dystrophy.
- Finger stiffness.

Post-operation rehabilitation

Good therapy is the key to a successful outcome. If it is felt necessary, the hand can be splinted for 2-3 days with the MCPJ flexed and PIPJ extended. If a skin graft is used, a splint is applied for 10 days. A splint is continued in between periods of exercise, and night splintage continues for months. Early movement is encouraged.

Recurrence

There is a reported recurrence rate of 50% within 5-10 years. It is difficult to compare recurrence rates between the different techniques as there are many confounding variables.

Surgery for recurrent disease is made difficult by the presence of scar tissue. Other problems can include an altered anatomy, existing injury to the neurovascular structures, a non-compliant patient and unrealistic patient expectations. If the PIPJ cannot be straightened, consider PIPJ fusion. Amputation is not indicated, unless requested.

Hand osteoarthritis

Before the age of 65 years, osteoarthritis of the hand is more common in men; after 65 years, it is more common in women. The most common joints involved are the DIPJs and PIPJs, and the carpometacarpal joint of the thumb.

Distal interphalangeal joint arthritis

Clinical features

Clinical features include Heberden's nodes and osteophytes. Deformity of the DIPJ may be present in severe arthritis.

Mucous cysts are ganglia arising from the DIPJ, often with an associated underlying osteophyte. These may cause nail deformity secondary to pressure on the germinal matrix. Mucous cysts can be treated by excising the base of the ganglion and the underlying osteophyte.

Management

Arthrodesis using wires or a Herbert screw can be considered for patients with significant malalignment or pain.

Proximal interphalangeal joint arthritis

Clinical features

Patients present with pain, deformity and stiffness due to osteophytes and soft tissue fibrosis.

Management

Treatment is conservative in the majority of cases.

The outcome of surgery is pain relief. It is not usually possible to improve the range of movement.

Arthrodesis is the best way of permanently relieving pain at the cost of losing movement. Tension-band wire techniques, compression screws or plates are all accepted methods.

Arthroplasty is joint replacement surgery. All modern implants have yet to demonstrate good short- to medium-term implant survival. In most cases, range of movement is not improved.

Arthrodesis should be performed on the index and middle fingers. This gives a permanent reliable solution and allows a good stable pinch. Arthroplasty can be performed on the ring and small fingers to maintain range of movement for grip.

Metacarpophalangeal joint arthritis

The symptoms of arthritis in MCPJ are usually well tolerated.

If conservative treatment fails, arthrodesis or excision arthroplasty are poorly tolerated. Joint replacement is a much more reliable option in the MCPJ than in the PIPJ. Unlike in rheumatoid arthritis, the MCPJ in osteoarthritis is stable. Therefore, an unconstrained surface replacement arthroplasty can relieve pain and maintain range of movement and pinch stability.

Trapeziometacarpal joint arthritis

Clinical features
Clinical features of trapeziometacarpal joint (TMCJ) arthritis are pain with use or movement of the thumb, pain on gripping and local deformity. There is tenderness over the capsule of the TMCJ.

There are three main ligamentous stabilisers, of which the beak ligament or the palmar oblique ligament is key for stability. The other two ligaments are the dorsal and lateral ligaments.

Prominence of the subluxed metacarpal base on the radial aspect of the joint is known as the shoulder sign. Pain on axial loading and flexion extension can

be assessed with the crank test, while pain on axial load and rotation can be assessed with the grind test.

Differential diagnosis
- Thumb MCPJ arthritis.
- De Quervain's tenosynovitis.
- Radiocarpal arthritis.

Imaging
Anteroposterior, lateral and oblique X-rays should be obtained. An anteroposterior stress view is achieved by pressing together the tips of the radial aspects of both thumbs. This is useful if testing for laxity.

Staging
The Eaton and Littler system is used to stage TMCJ arthritis:

- Stage 1 – articular contours normal, no subluxation or joint debris.
- Stage 2 – slight narrowing of the thumb TMCJ, contours preserved.
- Stage 3 – TMCJ disruption and sclerotic or cystic changes, osteophytes greater than 2mm in size, subluxation over one-third of the joint.
- Stage 4 – pantrapezial arthritis.

Management
Treatment is based on clinical symptoms and not radiographic findings. Conservative treatment with appropriate splinting should be used first. Steroid injections can help confirm an uncertain diagnosis and offer temporary relief.

Stage 1 TMCJ arthritis is managed by carpometacarpal joint arthroscopy and thermal shrinkage of the palmar beak ligament and capsule. If symptoms return with time, the procedure can be repeated or a more permanent palmar beak ligament reconstruction (with split FCR) performed (Eaton Littler).

Stages 2, 3 and 4 are managed by salvage surgery. A number of options are available (Table 6.6).

Table 6.6. Salvage surgery options for trapeziometacarpal joint arthritis.

Surgery	Description
Trapeziometacarpal arthrodesis (for stages 2 and 3)	Good results, but may lead to wear of the scaphotrapeziotrapezoid joint Suitable for young and high-demand patients
Abduction extension osteotomy	Designed to offload the palmar surface of the joint Can be considered for high-demand young adults with early disease The failure rate is about 20%
Excisional arthroplasty (trapeziectomy)	Good pain relief Weakness in grip and pinch as a result of the operation is rarely noticed by the patient
Excision, ligament reconstruction and interposition – flexor carpi radialis/joint capsule	The additional first metacarpal stabilisation or interposition procedures have yet to be proven superior to excision of the trapezium alone
Trapezial/metacarpal implants	Equivocal/poor results High early failure rate

Table 6.7. Treatment based on location of arthritis.

Location	Treatment
Radiolunate	Radiolunate arthrodesis
Radioscapholunate	Radioscapholunate arthrodesis plus excision of the distal third of the scaphoid (to unlock the midcarpal joint)
Radiolunate and midcarpal	Total wrist fusion Wrist replacement arthroplasty Low-demand patients only

Wrist osteoarthritis

Scaphotrapeziotrapezoid arthritis

Patients present with a painful wrist. Non-operative measures are adopted in early disease. The main surgical treatment is scaphotrapeziotrapezoid fusion.

However, there is progressive TMCJ or radioscaphoid arthritis in 33% of patients. There is also a relatively high non-union rate. Alternatives to scaphotrapeziotrapezoid fusion are trapezium excision or excision of the distal pole of the scaphoid, with or without interposition arthroplasty.

Radiocarpal arthritis

The underlying cause of radiocarpal arthritis may be distal radius fracture, scaphoid fracture, radiocarpal dislocation or scapholunate ligament insufficiency.

Once conservative treatment fails arthrodesis is the treatment of choice (Table 6.7). Partial arthrodesis will preserve some wrist movement.

Scapholunate/scaphoid non-union advanced collapse

Scapholunate advanced collapse and scaphoid non-union advanced collapse can be treated with either of these options:

- Scaphoid excision and four-corner fusion.
- Proximal row carpectomy (remove scaphoid, lunate and triquetrum) with radial styloidectomy.

Rheumatoid hand

Pathology

Rheumatoid arthritis is a chronic, systemic inflammatory disorder that principally attacks the joints. There are several results of this:

- Synovial proliferation and destructive pannus formation.
- Cartilage, ligament and tendon destruction.
- Bone erosion.

Principles of surgery

The following principles should be followed when considering surgery for the rheumatoid hand:

- Maximise medical treatment before considering surgery.
- Assess the timing and the natural course of the disease.

- Surgery should be performed before fixed joint contractures.
- Proximal joints should be operated on before the distal joints.
- Do not combine mobilisation procedures (arthroplasty) with stabilisation procedures (arthrodesis).

Extensor tendons

Patients present with the following:

- Extensor tenosynovitis.
- Tendon rupture due to erosion over the distal ulna – Vaughn-Jackson lesion. There is fraying of tendons, rupture, formation of nodules and pseudotendon.

Causes of inability to extend the fingers:

- Tendon rupture.
- Subluxation of the extensor carpi ulnaris tendon.
- MCPJ dislocation.
- Posterior interosseous nerve palsy.
- Tender nodules.

Management of extensor tendon problems in the rheumatoid hand is shown in Table 6.8.

Flexor tendons

Problems:

- Rupture of the flexor pollicis longus (Mannerfelt syndrome). This tendon ruptures due to erosion or an osteophyte on the scaphoid. It is treated with a tendon bridge graft and a two-stage flexor graft.
- Flexor tenosynovitis – causes pain, triggering and tendon rupture. Steroid injection can be initially attempted, then a tenosynovectomy if the condition fails to respond.

Table 6.8. Management of extensor tendon problems in the rheumatoid hand.

Problem	Treatment
Rupture of little finger	Little finger to ring finger extensor transfer
Rupture of ring and little fingers	Combine little and ring extensors and transfer extensor indicis proprius to both
Rupture of small, ring and middle fingers	Combine little and ring extensors and transfer extensor indicis proprius to both Suture middle finger extensor to index finger
Rupture of all four extensor digitorum tendons	Tendon graft or ring finger flexor digitorum superficialis transfer
Rupture of extensor pollicis longus	Extensor indicis to extensor pollicis longus transfer

Wrist

Problems:

- Carpal supination – rupture of the dorsal radiocarpal ligaments leads to the ulna head becoming prominent.
- Carpal ulnar subluxation – the carpus migrates down the radial slope secondary to erosive changes.
- Synovitis – involves the distal radioulnar and radiocarpal joints. A synovectomy can be considered for pain.
- Joint destruction and pain – consider wrist arthrodesis or replacement.
- Distal radioulnar joint pain – consider synovectomy with or without ulnar head excision. A Sauvé-Kapandji procedure is an option in young patients with a preserved ulnar head. This allows the ulna head to support the carpus.

Metacarpophalangeal joint

Problems:

- Palmar dislocation of the proximal phalanges and ulnar deviation. Causes:

  - synovitis predominantly on the radial side, weakening the radial collateral ligament;
  - weakening of the radial sagittal band;
  - ulna subluxation of the extensor tendons;
  - normal pinch forces against the radial side of the fingers.
- Synovitis – managed by synovectomy with or without extensor realignment.
- Joint destruction and pain – managed by implant arthroplasty with a silicone implant such as Swanson's, together with extensor tendon realignment.

Interphalangeal joint

Swan-neck deformity

Swan-neck deformity is predominantly caused by PIPJ synovitis with attenuation of the volar plate and collateral ligaments, allowing hyperextension. In addition, patients may have intrinsic tightness.

A DIPJ mallet can be the initiating problem, with the PIPJ being susceptible to hyperextension because of an attenuated volar plate.

Treatment varies depending on the type of deformity (Table 6.9).

Table 6.9. Treatment of swan-neck deformity.

Type	Description	Treatment
I	Good passive motion at the PIPJ and no pain	A figure of eight splint to prevent hyperextension. Tendon procedures (e.g., lateral band transfer) should be used to statically prevent extension
II	A positive result for the intrinsic test. MCPJ extension limits PIPJ flexion	As for type I, plus intrinsic release
III	Loss of PIPJ motion without PIPJ destruction on X-ray	PIPJ manipulation with a temporary wire, with or without intrinsic release. Once mobile, treatment is as for type I
IV	Limited PIPJ motion and joint destruction	Arthrodesis for the index and middle fingers. Implant arthroplasty for the little and ring fingers

MCPJ = metacarpophalangeal joint; PIPJ = proximal interphalangeal joint

Boutonnière deformity

Boutonnière deformity is caused by synovitis at the PIPJ. This attenuates the extensor mechanism and elongates the central slip. The lateral bands then start to migrate towards the volar aspect.

Again, treatment varies depending on the stage of deformity (Table 6.10).

Table 6.10. Treatment of Boutonnière deformity.

Stage	Description	Treatment
I	Pre-Boutonnière deformity. Normal PIPJ movement, but may have decreased DIPJ movement	Splint or synovectomy
II	Passively correctable PIPJ flexion of 30°	Synovectomy and central slip repair or reconstruction using lateral bands
III	Fixed PIPJ contracture	Arthrodesis or arthroplasty
IV	Contracture >70°	Arthrodesis

DIPJ = distal interphalangeal joint; PIPJ = proximal interphalangeal joint

Table 6.11. Treatment of problems of the rheumatoid thumb.

Problem	Description	Treatment
Swan-neck deformity	Proximal interphalangeal joint flexed, MCPJ extended, carpometacarpal joint flexed/adducted	If originating from carpometacarpal joint degeneration and adducted first metacarpal – trapeziectomy If originating from the MCPJ – MCPJ arthrodesis
Boutonnière deformity	PIPJ extended, MCPJ flexed, carpometacarpal joint extended or normal	If comfortable and mobile – divide the extensor pollicis longus distally and transfer to the proximal phalanx
MCPJ pain	-	Arthrodesis

MCPJ = metacarpophalangeal joint; PIPJ = proximal interphalangeal joint

Thumb

Problems associated with the thumb include swan-neck and Boutonnière deformities, as well as MCPJ pain (Table 6.11).

Tendon transfers for peripheral nerve dysfunction

Before tendon transfers can take place, certain prerequisites must be met (Table 6.12).

There are many different types of tendon transfers. Those below mention some of the accepted transfers for the conditions described.

Low median nerve palsy

Problem

Loss of thumb abduction and opposition. Thumb abduction and opposition are frequently retained after an isolated median nerve injury because of innervation by the ulnar nerve. Even with marked thenar muscle wasting, adequate abduction and opposition is possible.

Table 6.12. Prerequisites for tendon transfers.

Category	Prerequisites
Joints	Good preoperative range of motion
Donor muscle/tendon	Good power Sufficient excursion for satisfactory function Preferably synergistic Preferably has a straight line of pull Under voluntary control with independent action Expendable
Patient	Motivation and mental capacity to re-train

Management

Treatment depends on the presence of the PL. If the PL is present, a Camitz transfer is performed. This transfer restores palmar abduction. When abducted, the flexor pollicis longus can then oppose the thumb.

A strip of palmar fascia is dissected in continuity with the PL tendon. This effectively extends the length of the tendon. This is passed subcutaneously and attached to the abductor pollicis brevis insertion. Release of the carpal tunnel is performed.

Donor tendons are used if the PL is absent:

- Extensor indices proprius.
- FDS to ring or long fingers.
- Abductor digiti minimi (Huber transfer).

High median nerve palsy

Problem

Restoration of thumb flexion, opposition and index finger flexion can be achieved by transferring:

- Forearm pronation.
- Wrist flexion.
- Index finger, middle finger and thumb flexion.
- Thumb opposition.

Management

Restoration of thumb flexion, opposition and index finger flexion can be achieved by transferring:

- Brachioradialis to flexor pollicis longus.
- Extensor indicis proprius to restore opposition.
- Extensor carpi radialis longus to the index finger FDP.

Low ulnar nerve palsy

Problem

- Loss of intrinsic muscles.
- Loss of thumb to index finger pinch.

Management

- Static clawing – MCPJ volar plate advancement.
- Dynamic clawing – the FDS of the long finger tendon transfer is split to attach A2 pulleys to all fingers.
- Thumb adduction – the extensor carpi radialis brevis, brachioradialis or ring finger FDS can be used to provide motor function.
- Index finger abduction – accessory slip of the abductor pollicis longus transfer.

High ulnar nerve palsy

Problem

Loss of flexor carpi ulnaris and FDP to ring and little fingers.

Management

Treatment is similar to that for low ulna nerve palsy, with suturing of the FDP tendon of the little and ring fingers to that of the middle finger.

Radial nerve palsy

For low radial nerve palsy, the extensor carpi radialis longus, extensor carpi radialis brevis and brachioradialis are spared. The available muscles are the wrist flexors: flexor carpi ulnaris, FCR, FDS, PL and pronator teres (Table 6.13).

Table 6.13. Tendon transfers for low radial nerve palsy.

Function needed	Common method
Wrist extension (extensor carpi radialis brevis)	Pronator teres
Finger extension	Flexor carpi ulnaris
Thumb extension	Palmaris longus
Thumb abduction	Palmaris longus

Procedures for the paralytic hand

Trying to improve hand function for patients who have cerebral palsy or suffered a stroke is complex. The surgical options depend on the following and are assessed on an individual patient basis:

- Extent of motor involvement.
- Degree of spasticity.
- Extent of contracture.
- Voluntary control of the muscles.
- Mental capacity to maximise function following surgery.

In principle, the following treatment options can be used:

- Muscles with high resting tone or spasticity can be lengthened to weaken them.
- Tendons can be transferred if there is a degree of motor control.
- An improved functional position of the hand can be achieved with arthrodesis.

In most cases the condition is too severe for a useful tendon transfer. Most often, a mixture of tendon lengthening/division, joint releases and arthrodesis can improve function and personal care.

Replantation

Indications

The factors that influence the decision for replantation are shown in Table 6.14.

Table 6.14. Factors influencing replantation.	
Factor	**Implications for replantation**
Level of injury	Replantation is considered for: • Amputation of the thumb • Multiple-digit amputations • Amputation through the palm, wrist and distal forearm Single-digit amputation is a controversial indication (unless in a child) Results are variable with amputation through the proximal forearm, elbow and arm
Age	Outcomes worsen with age
General medical condition	Cardiac disease and diabetes reduce the success rate
Ischaemic time	Cold ischaemia of 12 hours and warm ischaemia of 6 hours are the upper limit for proximal amputations These limits can be doubled for digit amputations
Injury mechanism	Avulsion and crush are negative factors

Reattachment

The order of reattachment is flexible, but in general:

- Obtain skeletal stability.
- Arteries.
- Veins.
- Tendons.
- Nerves.

Post-transplantation

Patients with successful digit replantations commonly complain of stiffness, cold intolerance and poor sensibility. As a result, the patient often excludes the digit from use following a single finger replantation.

Hand transplants

Eighteen hand transplant operations were performed from 1998 to early 2004. Two of the transplanted hands had to be re-amputated and several patients experienced osteomyelitis or skin necrosis. Most patients had protective sensation, but poor localisation.

Most patients were hospitalised for several months. Prolonged immunosuppression is required.

Chapter 7 Bone and soft tissue tumours

Assessment of tumours

Assessment of patients with any potential bone or soft tissue tumour should include a full history (particularly including previous malignancies and family history), a detailed clinical examination including the breasts or prostate and appropriate imaging.

After local and systemic staging (Table 7.1), a biopsy should be undertaken either in or following discussion with the regional sarcoma unit.

Biopsy and staging of tumours

Biopsy for bone tumours should be performed by or in conjunction with the surgeon who will be definitively resecting the tumour and who is therefore familiar with the surgical approach that will be required for that resection.

Indications for biopsy

The following features are indications for biopsy:

- Lesions that are large, deep to fascia, painful and growing.
- When an accurate diagnosis cannot be made on imaging or when the lesion appears aggressive on imaging.

Biopsy is not needed for the following:

- Non-ossifying fibromas.
- Unicameral bone cysts.
- Osteochondroma.

Table 7.1. Plan for evaluating bone and soft tissue tumours.

Staging	Primary bone tumour	Soft tissue sarcoma	Skeletal metastasis
Local	Plain radiograph Whole bone MRI	Plain radiograph Lesion MRI	Plain radiograph
Systemic	Chest X-ray Chest CT Isotope bone scan ?PET-CT	Chest X-ray Chest ± abdomen CT ?PET-CT	Chest and abdomen CT* Isotope bone scan*

* = where appropriate; CT = computed tomography; MRI = magnetic resonance imaging; PET-CT = positron emission tomography-CT

Table 7.2. Advantages and disadvantages of core needle biopsy compared with open biopsy.

Advantages	Disadvantages
Less contamination	Small sample size – insufficient/unrepresentative tissue
Less invasive	Diagnostic accuracy is 85% (better at tumour centres)
Local anaesthetic (may need image guidance)	Needle track has to be excised *en bloc* with main mass
Useful in spine and pelvis	

- Enchondromas.
- Soft tissue ganglion.
- Fatty tumours that completely suppress on magnetic resonance imaging (MRI) (e.g., lipoma, atypical lipomatous tumours, low-grade liposarcomas) – these should be marginally excised.

Types of biopsy

Closed/core needle biopsy
Core needle biopsy (CNB) is used by most sarcoma services worldwide. Typically a Tru-Cut needle type should be used for soft tissue lesions and a Jamshidi or Harlow-Wood type for bone lesions.

CNBs are used for bone lesions with large soft tissue extensions and soft tissue tumours. The advantages and disadvantages of CNB are shown in Table 7.2.

Open biopsy
The advantages and disadvantages of open biopsy are shown in Table 7.3.

There are a number of types of open biopsy: incisional, excisional and primary wide excision (where the entire lesion is excised with a cuff of normal tissue).

In incisional biopsy, all tissue touched or manipulated, including sutures and drain sites at definitive resection, is considered contaminated and is excised *en bloc*.

Incisional biopsy is indicated for several types of lesions:

- Larger than 3-4cm.
- Distal to the elbow and ankles, even for small lesions.
- Close to major vessels and nerves.

Table 7.3. Advantages and disadvantages of open biopsy compared with core needle biopsy.

Advantages	Disadvantages
Large sample size	More time and expense – needs an operating theatre
Diagnostic accuracy is 96%	Risk of pathological fracture, infection or haematoma
	Biopsy tract must be excised with definitive surgery
	Higher risk of contamination

Table 7.4. Advantages and disadvantages of excisional and primary wide excision biopsy.

Type of biopsy	Advantages	Disadvantages
Excisional	Large sample size Serves as treatment	Extensive contamination if the tumour proves aggressive and a wide margin is not achieved Nerve or vascular contamination can result in need for amputation
Primary wide excision	Single operation	Lesion may not be malignant Negates role of neoadjuvant chemotherapy

It can also be useful for lesions in the axilla, groin, antecubital and popliteal fossae, hand and foot.

The advantages and disadvantages of excisional and primary wide excision methods are shown in Table 7.4.

Surgical technique for open biopsy

Incision
- A tourniquet can be used, with elevation rather than exsanguination and deflation prior to closure.
- A longitudinal incision is used with short oblique segments when crossing joint creases.
- The planned definitive resection incision for limb salvage should be marked and utilised in part.
- The most direct approach is used, going directly through the compartment, not in between compartments.
- Flaps should not be raised.
- Dissection should not be in between muscle planes.
- To prevent contamination, vessels, nerves or tendons should not be exposed.

Biopsy
- Obtain a peripheral soft tissue mass.
- Do not biopsy Codman's triangle, as periosteal new bone can be misdiagnosed as tumour.
- A round window (3.5mm drill bit) is made in the bone if necessary – a biopsy can then be taken through this hole.

- A frozen section is helpful to confirm the tissue is representative.
- Obtain a culture sample before administering antibiotics – biopsies are always sent for histology and microbiology.

A frozen section should ideally be utilised for all patients being biopsied under general anaesthetic. The accuracy of frozen section for diagnosis is approximately 80%, but is less reliable for cartilage and fat lesions. The real role of the frozen section is to ensure representative tissue has been obtained.

Closure
- Meticulous haemostasis is mandatory.
- If a drain is necessary, it should exit through the same compartment in line with the longitudinal incision.
- Tight closure is performed in layers.
- A light pressure dressing is applied.

Note

Mankin HJ, Lange TA, Spanier SS. *The hazards of biopsy in patients with malignant primary bone and soft-tissue tumours. J Bone Joint Surg Am* 1982; 64: 1121-7. **Open biopsy had a 20% inaccuracy rate when performed in a referring centre. The complication rate was higher when biopsy was performed by non-tumour surgeons.**

Note

Mankin HJ, Mankin CJ, Simon MA. The hazards of the biopsy, revisited. Members of the Musculoskeletal Tumor Society. *J Bone Joint Surg Am* 1996; 78: 656-63. **The authors found no improvement from the 1982 study.**

Note

Pollock RC, Stalley PD. Biopsy of musculoskeletal tumours – beware. *ANZ J Surg* 2004; 74: 516-9. **Definitive treatment was hindered by a badly performed open biopsy in 38% of patients biopsied by the referring surgeon. In 25%, treatment had to be changed either to a more radical procedure than would originally have been necessary or to palliative rather than curative intent.**

Note

Ashford RU, McCarthy SW, Scolyer RA, *et al*. Surgical biopsy with intra-operative frozen section. An accurate and cost-effective method for diagnosis of musculoskeletal sarcomas. *J Bone Joint Surg Br* 2006; 88: 1207-11. **Accuracy was 99% and there were no inadequate biopsies. Surgical biopsy with intra-operative frozen section was 38% more expensive than CT-guided biopsy.**

Staging of malignant bone tumours

Staging is based on three factors:

- Grade of tumour – low grade (G1) or high grade (G2).
- Anatomic site – intracompartmental (T1) or extracompartmental (T2).
- Metastasis – no distant metastasis (M0) or presence of distant metastasis (M1).

These three factors determine the staging (Table 7.5).

Table 7.5. Staging of malignant bone tumours.

Stage	Grade	Site	Metastasis
IA	G1	T1	M0
IB	G1	T2	M0
IIA	G2	T1	M0
IIB	G2	T2	M0
III	Any grade	Any site	M1

Table 7.6. Classification of benign bone tumours.

Type	Characteristics	Tumour type
Latent	Well-defined margin Grows slowly then stops Remains static/heals	Non-ossifying fibroma Chondroma Eosinophilic granuloma Osteoid osteoma
Active	Progressive growth Limited by natural barriers Recurs	Aneurysmal bone cyst Osteoblastoma Chondroblastoma
Aggressive	Aggressive growth, not limited by natural barriers Grows from bone to soft tissues	Giant cell tumour

Classification of benign tumours

Benign bone tumours are classified into latent, active and aggressive, based on Enneking's classification (Table 7.6).

Note

Enneking WF. A staging system of musculoskeletal neoplasms. *Clin Orthop Relat Res* 1986; 204: 9-24.

Benign cartilaginous tumours

Benign cartilaginous tumours include osteochondroma, chondroma, chondroblastoma and chondromyxoid fibromas (CMFs).

Osteochondroma

Osteochondroma is the most common benign bone tumour. It is a cartilage-capped projection on the external surface of bones. Lesions can be solitary or multiple. Solitary osteochondroma is a different pathological entity to multiple osteochondroma (multiple hereditary exostoses [MHE]).

Aetiology

The aetiology of osteochondroma is linked to the *EXT* gene. The underlying process is abnormal growth of cartilage.

MHE is associated with bone deformities and bone growth abnormalities and occurs with an incidence of 1:50,000. It is autosomal dominant in 70% of patients and sporadic in 30%.

Clinical features

Patients most commonly present with osteochondroma in the second decade of life, and the male to female ratio is 2:1. The actual incidence of osteochondroma in the general population is unknown because osteochondromas are often asymptomatic.

Osteochondromas are seen as bony prominences at the metaphyseal ends of long bones – usually around the knee, although the pelvis and scapula are also commonly involved. They can occur in any bone.

MHE can interfere with joint movements and lead to flexion deformities. Clinical features include abnormal bone growth, leg-length inequalities, forearm bowing and valgus knees and ankles.

The risk of malignant transformation is about 1% in solitary osteochondromas and increases to 10% in MHE. Malignant transformation never occurs before skeletal maturity. Increasing size, onset of pain and an increase of more than 1cm in the thickness of the cartilage cap indicate possible malignant transformation. Malignant transformation is usually to a low-grade chondrosarcoma with a local recurrence rate of less than 2%.

> **Note**
>
> Staals EL, Bacchini P, Mercuri M, Bertoni F. Dedifferentiated chondrosarcomas arising in preexisting osteochondromas. *J Bone Joint Surg Am* 2007; 89: 987-93. **Dedifferentiated chondrosarcomas from osteochondroma were extremely rare, but were associated with a poor prognosis.**

Imaging

On radiographs, the osteochondroma can be a pedunculated or sessile outgrowth from the metaphyseal region. The direction of growth of the pedunculated lesion is away from the adjoining joint. The cortex of the osteochondroma is always contiguous with the normal cortex.

There is a hyaline cartilage cap on the bony prominence, the thickness of which decreases with skeletal maturity. This is easily demonstrated on ultrasound. An increase in the thickness of the cartilage cap indicates possible malignant transformation.

> **Note**
>
> Malghem J, Vande Berg B, Noël H, Maldague B. Benign osteochondromas and exostotic chondrosarcomas: evaluation of cartilage cap thickness by ultrasound. *Skeletal Radiol* 1992; 21: 33-7. **Ultrasound is accurate for assessing cartilage cap thickness.**

Management

The removal of a benign osteochondroma may be indicated by functional limitation of the adjoining joint, formation of painful bursa overlying the growth, neurological or vascular pressure symptoms, fracture or cosmetic concern.

Osteochondromas should be investigated for pain or growth after skeletal maturity. Recurrence after excision raises suspicions of malignancy. The risk of malignancy is 5-25%.

> **Note**
>
> Porter DE, Lonie L, Fraser M, *et al.* Severity of disease and risk of malignant change in hereditary multiple exostoses. A genotype-phenotype study. *J Bone Joint Surg Br* 2004; 86: 1041-6. **The presence of an *EXT1* mutation indicated significantly worse disease. The lifetime sarcoma risk was 3%.**

Chondromas

Chondromas are common cartilaginous tumours, second only to osteochondromas in prevalence. Broadly, chondromas can be divided into two groups: enchondromas, which occur within the bone; and periosteal chondromas, which occur on the bone surface.

Enchondroma

Patients usually present with enchondroma in the second decade of life. Enchondroma commonly involve the small bones of the hand; other sites include the long bones, pelvis and scapula. Long bone lesions are located in the metaphysis and diaphysis.

The tumour is usually asymptomatic, although local swelling due to bone expansion is sometimes evident. Pain is commonly due to a pathological fracture, which can draw attention to the presence of an enchondroma. If the lesion is painful without pathological fracture, consider chondrosarcoma.

Histologically, the tumour is composed of well-differentiated mature hyaline cartilage cells. It can be extremely difficult to distinguish between enchondroma and low-grade chondrosarcoma.

Imaging shows an intraosseous radiolucent lesion with a varying amount of mineralisation and calcification. The edges are rounded and well defined. The cortex is well preserved in long bones, while in small bones there can be cortical thinning and expansion. There is a high MRI signal on T2 and a low MRI signal on T1.

Periosteal chondroma

Periosteal chondroma is an often painful tumour on the bone surface. It is rare and usually occurs in adolescents or young adults.

The pathological appearance is similar to that of enchondroma. The tumour is usually smaller than 5cm in diameter. A mass lies on the bone surface, with scalloping of the underlying cortex and a dense sclerotic rim.

Multiple chondromas

Conditions resulting in multiple chondromas are much rarer than MHE:

- Ollier's disease – caused by an error in osseous development. It is characterised by multiple intraosseous and subperiosteal cartilage tumours. The development of bone destruction or soft tissue masses suggests malignant transformation. The risk of secondary malignancy is 10-25% and the lifetime risk of malignancy is 25%.
- Maffucci's syndrome – a congenital condition characterised by the same skeletal lesions as Ollier's disease, plus soft tissue haemangiomas. Calcified phleboliths are a feature on radiographs. The risk of secondary malignancy is 15-56% and the lifetime risk of malignancy is 100%.

Management of chondromas

Benign asymptomatic chondromas can be simply followed up with regular radiographs. In the presence of a pathologic fracture, the fracture is

allowed to heal with non-operative measures and the lesion is subsequently managed by curettage and bone grafting. Alternatively, the fracture can be stabilised internally along with bone grafting of the lesion.

Chondroblastoma

Chondroblastomas are small cartilaginous tumours in the epiphysis of long bones, appearing as well-demarcated lytic lesions. They account for less than 1% of all primary bone tumours.

Clinical features

Patients usually present with chondroblastoma in the second decade of life, and the male to female ratio is 3:2. The knee is a common site, while other sites include the upper end of the femur and the upper end of the humerus. Patients present with local pain and restricted movement. Pain has often been present for many months.

Pathology

The tumour is composed of round or polyhedral cells with large nuclei. Mitotic figures can be present but are never atypical. Multinucleated giant cells may be present. Pericellular chicken-wire-like calcifications are pathognomonic of chondroblastoma and stain positively for S100. The histological appearance of the pulmonary nodules is similar to that of bone lesions.

Imaging

The neoplasm appears as a lytic lesion in the centre of the epiphysis. Aggressive tumours may sometimes extend to the metaphysis or the soft tissues. Mineralisation is present in approximately 50% of lesions. MRI scans demonstrate 'vigorous' oedema surrounding the lesion.

Management

Management of the vast majority of chondroblastomas is with curettage and bone grafting. Local recurrence occurs in up to 15% of patients. Recurrent chondroblastoma is likely to be malignant and is best managed by *en bloc* resection.

Chondromyxoid fibroma

Clinical features

CMF is the least common benign bone tumour of chondrogenic origin. The male to female ratio is 2:1. CMF shows a predilection for the tibia, the small bones of the feet and the ilium. There are two peaks of incidence: one in the first and second decades of life, and a second at ages 50-70 years.

Pathology

Histologically, the lesion is lobulated and well demarcated from the surrounding bone. The lesion is hypocellular centrally and hypercellular peripherally. Spindle cells are present in an abundant myxoid matrix.

Imaging

The main features are well-circumscribed, round or oval osteolytic lesions with an eccentric metaphyseal location. The cortex is frequently eroded. With MRI scanning, there is a low signal on T1 sequences of the lesion and a high signal on T2.

Management

Management of CMF is by curettage (consider adjuvants) with bone grafting if necessary. Local recurrence is less than 5%. *En bloc* resection with appropriate reconstruction may be necessary for extensive lesions.

> **Note**
>
> Rahimi A, Beabout JW, Ivins JC, Dahlin DC. Chondromyxoid fibroma: a clinicopathologic study of 76 cases. *Cancer* 1972; 30: 726-36. **CMF was aggressive locally and distinguishable from chondrosarcoma on imaging. It will recur if not treated properly.**

Benign osteoblastic tumours

Osteoid osteoma

Osteoid osteoma is a benign bone neoplasm.

Clinical features

The common age of presentation is 5-35 years and the male to female ratio is 2:1. The main presenting symptom is pain. The pain can be severe, is often worse at night and is relieved by non-steroidal anti-inflammatory drugs (NSAIDs). The common sites of osteoid osteoma are the diaphysis and metaphysis in the long bones.

Lesions in the spine involve the posterior elements and the resulting pain leads to a non-structural, painful, concave scoliosis on the side of the lesion.

Pathology

The pain in osteoid osteoma is related to a high level of local prostaglandins, and hence is effectively alleviated by NSAIDs.

The nidus is composed of immature osteoid trabeculae and mineralised matrix, with blood vessels and a fibrovascular stroma. The nidus is surrounded by dense sclerotic bone.

Imaging

The radiographic appearance is of a small lytic lesion with surrounding cortical sclerosis. A fine-cut computed tomography (CT) scan is the best imaging modality to use to demonstrate the nidus and plan management.

Management

The management options for osteoid osteoma include the following:

- Intralesional resection with a burr.
- Intralesional resection and the use of phenol or hydrogen peroxide.
- Wide resection of the nidus.
- CT-guided radiofrequency/laser ablation.

Surgery is the preferred option for easily accessible lesions as it provides tissue for histological diagnosis and is associated with a low rate of recurrence (5-10%).

The radiofrequency/laser ablation method is useful for lesions that are difficult to access surgically. It is minimally invasive, but the procedure often has to be performed under general anaesthetic. There is a risk of injury to nearby nerves and soft tissues, and histological diagnosis can be difficult due to the limited amount of tissue obtained. This method cannot be used in spinal lesions due to the risk of nerve damage. Furthermore, the recurrence rate (10-15%) is higher than with surgical excision.

Note

Hoffmann RT, Jakobs TF, Kubisch CH, *et al*. Radiofrequency ablation in the treatment of osteoid osteoma – 5-year experience. *Eur J Radiol* 2010; 73: 374-9. **Biopsy was possible in 50% of patients. Thirty-eight of 39 patients were successfully treated. One patient developed an infection and there was one broken needle.**

Osteoblastoma

Osteoblastoma is a benign neoplasm. It is also known as giant osteoid osteoma.

Clinical features
Patients usually present with osteoblastoma in the second and third decades of life. Men are more commonly affected than women.

The posterior element of the spine is the most common site of osteoblastoma, although any bone can be involved. The metaphysis is the preferred location in long bones.

Neurological symptoms may arise from pressure or pathologic fracture. Osteoblastoma in the spine can cause painful scoliosis.

Pathology
Osteoblastomas are predominantly lytic with a fibrovascular stroma. There is less surrounding sclerosis than in osteoid osteomas. Immature osteoid trabeculae and giant cells are seen.

Imaging
The lesions are either mixed lytic and blastic or predominantly lytic.

A CT scan is the ideal imaging method to assess the size and location of the neoplasm. The presence of mineralisation within the lesion helps to differentiate it from an aneurysmal bone cyst (ABC).

An MRI scan may reveal oedema in the surrounding tissues and bone, known as 'flare phenomenon'. This can give the impression of malignancy.

Management
Wide surgical excision is the treatment of choice to achieve the lowest recurrence rate. If the location of the tumour precludes wide excision then curettage and treatment with adjuvants (e.g., phenol) or cryosurgery is an option. Bone grafting is often required and prophylactic fixation should be considered for larger lesions.

Benign cystic lesions

Unicameral (simple) bone cyst

Clinical features
Patients present with unicameral bone cysts (UBC) in the first two decades of life. The male to female ratio is 2:1.

The majority of UBCs are asymptomatic, although some patients can present with pain and pathological fractures or swelling.

UBCs are usually located in the metaepiphyseal areas and most frequently involve the proximal humerus (60-70%), proximal femur (15%), and proximal tibia (5%).

Pathology
The pathological features are of a unilocular cyst with clear fluid, a thin fibrous wall, dilated vessels and scattered lymphocytes.

Imaging
On imaging there is a central lucency within the medullary cavity, with a narrow zone of transition. A fallen fragment sign may be seen in pathological fractures. With MRI, the lesion is very bright on T2 sequences and there is a low signal on T1.

Management

Management is usually observation. If a pathological fracture occurs then it should be allowed to heal. In the event of recurrence, curettage and adjuvants can be considered. Injections of steroid, bone marrow or calcitonin have been tried to stimulate healing, with variable results.

If there is an expanding lesion in weight-bearing bone, curettage and bone grafting is the treatment of choice.

Aneurysmal bone cyst

Clinical features

ABCs are benign cystic lesions of bone that expand the cortex. They can be primary (arising *de novo*) or secondary (as a result of cystic change in a giant cell tumour [GCT] or chondroblastoma); approximately 50% are secondary. The male to female ratio is 1:1.

The symptoms are usually pain and swelling. Occasionally a pathological fracture is the presenting feature.

Pathology

At surgery the feature is typically a 'hole containing blood'. Histologically ABCs are cavernous spaces with walls that lack any endothelial cell lining.

Imaging

ABCs are typically expansile, lytic lesions, eccentrically located in the medullary cavity of long bones. They can arise in the cortex or periosteum and can cross joints.

MRI of fluid levels often reveals multiple and markedly expansile ABCs.

Differential diagnosis

The differential diagnosis of ABC includes the following:

- GCT.
- Giant cell reparative granuloma.
- Telangiectatic osteosarcoma.

Management

The management of ABC depends on the location. Most lesions are treated with intralesional curettage, with or without bone grafting or cementation. Recurrence occurs in 10-20% of patients and is reduced by adjuvants. Expendable bones can be excised. Embolisation should be considered for large and pelvic lesions.

> **Note**
>
> Marcove RC, Sheth DS, Takemoto S, Healey JH. The treatment of aneurysmal bone cyst. *Clin Orthop Relat Res* 1995; 311: 157-63. **With curettage alone, the authors reported 59% recurrence. Curettage plus cryosurgery resulted in an 82% rate of cure, rising to 96% with a second treatment.**

Benign, locally aggressive tumours

Giant cell tumour (osteoclastoma)

A GCT is a mesenchymal tumour. The cell of origin is a mononuclear stromal cell that produces type I and II collagen. Most GCTs are benign (80%) and the risk of local recurrence is 20-50%. Malignant transformation occurs in 10% of GCTs at recurrence. A small percentage of apparently benign lesions (1-4%) have pulmonary metastasis.

Clinical features

Almost half of GCTs occur around the knee. Other common sites are the distal radius, proximal humerus and pelvis. GCTs are typically epiphyseal and have an eccentric location in the bone. Patients usually present in the second to fourth decade of life, and the male to female ratio is 1.5:1.

Clinically, GCT presents with local swelling, warmth and pain unrelated to weight bearing. Pathologic fracture occurs in up to 15% of cases.

Pathology

GCTs arise from undifferentiated mesenchymal cells in the bone marrow. The giant cells are derived from fusion of mononuclear stromal cells or nuclear division. They are approximately 60 microns in size and the nuclei are arranged centrally. The giant cells stain positively for tartrate-resistant acid phosphatase (TRAP) and have receptors for calcitonin.

Mononuclear stromal cells have two cell lines:

- Round cells – non-neoplastic and express TRAP.
- Spindle-shaped neoplastic cells – produce type I and II collagen and alkaline phosphatase, and have receptors for parathyroid hormone. These cells are genetically unstable and have high expression of *p53*. They secrete macrophage colony-stimulating factor, interferon-γ, and tumour necrosis factor-α.

Round cells and giant cells are the reactive components of the tumour, while spindle cells represent the neoplastic component.

Histology

Confirmatory needle biopsy should usually be obtained prior to definitive management.

Immunohistochemical staining can be used to assess the relationship between the rate of proliferation and recurrence. Overexpression of the *p53* and *MYC* oncogenes is seen in tumours metastasising to the lung.

Imaging

With CT, the density is 20 to 70 HU. CT is useful for evaluating the intraosseous extent of the tumour. With MRI, GCTs are typified by a high signal in T2-weighted images. They demonstrate high contrast enhancement. MRI is useful to detect extension of the tumour into the bone marrow. Secondary ABC formation can occur.

Differential diagnosis

Differential diagnosis of GCT includes the following:

- ABC.
- Brown tumour of hyperparathyroidism.
- Giant cell reparative granuloma.
- Non-ossifying fibroma.
- Giant-cell-rich osteosarcoma.

Grading

GCTs are graded using the Enneking and Campanacci staging system (Table 7.7).

> **Note**
>
> Campanacci M, Baldini N, Boriani S, Sudanese A. Giant-cell tumor of bone. *J Bone Joint Surg Am* 1987; 69: 106-14.

Table 7.7. Giant cell tumour grading with the Enneking and Campanacci staging system.

Grade	Nature	Description
1	Benign, latent	Minimal cortical involvement with a static pattern of growth
2	Benign, active	Extensive cortical thinning and bulging Often clinically symptomatic
3	Aggressive	Cortical breach and a soft tissue component Symptomatic and rapidly growing Often cause a pathological fracture

GCTs can be polyostotic, which can either be simultaneous or metachronous with an interval of many years. Malignancy can occur and can either be primary and sarcomatous from the onset (1-3%) or secondary due to malignant transformation of a recurrent tumour (5-10%).

Rarely, GCTs can occur in a benign metastasising form, with nodules in the lung (1-3%). This is believed to be due to embolisation. Lung metastases may be present at the first presentation of the tumour or a few years later.

Management

Benign GCT

For benign tumours, wide local excision (*en bloc* resection) is associated with a recurrence rate of 0-5%. This usually requires resection of the articular surface and reconstruction with an endoprosthetic replacement or allograft.

The indications for *en bloc* resection are as follows:

- Extensive grade 3 tumour with no remaining mechanically supportive bone.
- Repeated recurrences.
- Displaced intra-articular fracture.
- Distal radial site.
- Articular collapse after previous curettage.
- Involvement of 50% of the distal femur (a relative indication).

The distal radius is the third most common site for GCT and reconstruction is challenging. Options include ulnocarpal arthrodesis or replacing the bone defect with a vascularised or non-vascularised fibular graft.

Simple curettage can have a recurrence rate of 20-50%. This is decreased with the use of adjuvants and when performed in a specialist centre.

Radiotherapy is utilised for GCT in the pelvis, vertebra or technically inoperable sites. The form is 40-60 Gy using a linear accelerator and supervoltage therapy. Local control is achieved in 85-90% of patients. The risk of radiation-induced sarcoma is 0-8%.

> **Note**
>
> Feigenberg SJ, Marcus RB Jr, Zlotecki RA, *et al*. Radiation therapy for giant cell tumours of bone. *Clin Orthop Relat Res* 2003; 411: 207-16. **From 26 tumours, 20 were controlled locally. One patient developed a radiation-induced sarcoma.**

Recurrent GCT

Several factors influence recurrence:

- Original tumour stage – stage 1, recurrence rate of 7%; stage 2, 20%; stage 3, 41%.
- Surgical margin.
- Aggressiveness of curettage.
- Adjuvant agents.
- Tumour behaviour.

Pathologic fracture does not increase the risk of recurrence. Recurrent GCT can be managed with wide excision or repeat curettage with adjuvants.

Adjuvants help to reduce recurrence. These include high-speed burr, liquid nitrogen, polymethyl methacrylate (PMMA), phenol, hydrogen peroxide and alcohol. Bone cement (PMMA) is useful because it is cheap and helps detect recurrence. Liquid nitrogen is also very effective and has been associated with a 7.9% recurrence rate. The use of a dental burr to remove tumour tissue has been found to reduce recurrence rates to 12%.

> **Note**
>
> Malawer MM, Bickels J, Meller I, *et al*. Cryosurgery in the treatment of giant cell tumor. A long-term follow-up study. *Clin Orthop Relat Res* 1999; 359: 176-88.

> **Note**
>
> Blackley HR, Wunder JS, Davis AM, *et al*. Treatment of giant-cell tumors of long bones with curettage and bone-grafting. *J Bone Joint Surg Am* 1999; 81: 811-20.

Malignant GCT

Malignant GCT has a mortality rate of 15-20%. Lung lesions should be excised or treated with whole-lung radiotherapy.

> **Note**
>
> Campanacci M, Baldini N, Boriani S, Sudanese A. Giant-cell tumor of bone. *J Bone Joint Surg Am* 1987; 69: 106-14. **Of nearly 300 patients, 74% had grade 2 GCT and 22% grade 3. Nine percent presented with a pathological fracture. The local recurrence rates were 27% for intralesional procedures, 8% for marginal procedures and 0% for wide excision.**

> **Note**
>
> Zhen W, Yaotian H, Songjian L, *et al.* Giant-cell tumour of bone. The long-term results of treatment by curettage and bone graft. *J Bone Joint Surg Br* 2004; 86: 212-6. **This study looked at 92 patients with a 5- to 11-year follow-up. The patients were treated with 50% zinc chloride for 5 minutes and auto- or allograft bone grafting. The recurrence rate was 13%, and 93% achieved at least good function. Patients underwent wide excision of soft tissues if the lesion perforated through the cortex.**

> **Note**
>
> Prosser GH, Baloch KG, Tillman RM, *et al.* Does curettage without adjuvant therapy provide low recurrence rates in giant-cell tumors of bone? *Clin Orthop Relat Res* 2005; 435: 211-8. **The local recurrence rate of GCTs confined to bone (Campanacci grades 1 and 2) was only 7%, compared with 29% in tumours with extraosseous extension (Campanacci grade 3).**

Malignant primary bone tumours

Osteosarcoma

Osteosarcoma is a malignant bone tumour characterised by spindle cells and the production of osteoid matrix. It is the most common primary malignant bone tumour (excluding multiple myeloma).

Epidemiology

Osteosarcoma has a bimodal distribution. It is most common in the second decade of life and in men (male to female ratio, 2:1). Adults in the fifth to sixth decades of life may develop osteosarcoma in association with Paget's disease (with a 1% incidence of malignant transformation). Ionising radiation predisposes to osteosarcoma.

Hereditary retinoblastoma and Li-Fraumeni syndrome are linked to the development of osteosarcoma. *c-MYC* and *c-FOS* proto-oncogenes are overexpressed in the disease.

Clinical features

Osteosarcoma tumours are usually metaphyseal and the symptoms are related to fast bone growth. The most common sites are the distal femur, proximal tibia and proximal humerus. Half of osteosarcomas occur around the knee, as this area has the most active bone growth.

The most common presenting symptoms are pain (85%) and a tender swelling. Pain at rest and at night indicates the diagnosis. Occasionally, a patient will have a pathologic fracture.

In up to one in five patients, the disease has metastasised to the lungs at the time of presentation. Less common sites of metastasis include bone, kidneys, lymph nodes, brain and pleura. The presence of metastasis at initial presentation is a poor prognostic sign.

Note

Widhe B, Widhe T. Initial symptoms and clinical features in osteosarcoma and Ewing sarcoma. *J Bone Joint Surg Am* 2000; 82: 667-74. **Strain-related pain was reported in 85% of patients with osteosarcoma and 64% of those with Ewing's sarcoma. Night pain was experienced by 21% and 19%, respectively, and 39% and 34% had a mass. Symptoms developed at 9 weeks with osteosarcoma and at 19 weeks with Ewing's sarcoma.**

Pathology

Osteoblasts are the malignant cells that produce the osteoid matrix. Pleomorphism and anaplasia are seen.

Laboratory studies

Alkaline phosphatase levels are usually raised. Lactate dehydrogenase (LDH) elevation carries a poor prognosis.

Imaging

Radiographs show a metaphyseal lesion with bone destruction. Soft tissue calcification may be visible and is described as having a 'star-burst' appearance. The periosteum is elevated at the periphery of the lesion due to rapid growth, and laying down of bone under the elevated periosteum is known as Codman's triangle. There is little endosteal bone formation and the transition zone is wide.

A chest X-ray and CT scan of the chest are used to look for metastasis. A Tc-99m bone scan is used to identify other lesions or bone metastasis, as well as the extent of the lesion in the affected bone.

MRI of the whole bone is undertaken to evaluate the extent of the tumour and skip lesions – both in the soft tissues and the medullary canal. The relationship of the tumour to the neurovascular structures is of particular importance.

Types of osteosarcomas

- Classic high-grade central osteosarcoma (about 90% patients).
- Parosteal osteosarcoma (4% of osteosarcomas) – a low-grade tumour commonly arising from the cortex of the posterior surface of the distal femur. It is seen in older patients (the third and fourth decades of life) than classic osteosarcoma. It is densely mineralised. Surgical resection gives a high cure rate.
- Periosteal osteosarcoma (1.5% of osteosarcomas) – a moderate-grade lesion commonly occurring on the proximal tibia. It presents in the second decade of life. It is intermediate in malignancy between parosteal and classic osteosarcoma. Surgery and chemotherapy are recommended.
- Juxtacortical osteosarcoma – a rare, high-grade osteosarcoma occurring on the surface of the bone rather than arising in the metaphysis like classic osteosarcoma.
- Secondary osteosarcoma – a tumour developing in Paget's disease or following exposure to radiation. It carries a poor prognosis.
- Multifocal osteosarcoma – a tumour developing at more than one site, either simultaneously or after a period of time. Tumours developing at an alternative location after a time gap are known as metachronous lesions.
- Telangiectatic osteosarcoma (3.6% of osteosarcomas) – a high-grade, vascular lesion with little osteoid formation. The radiographic differential diagnosis is ABC. Management is similar to that of classic osteosarcoma and the response to chemotherapy is usually good.

Management

Surgery and chemotherapy are the mainstays of management.

Surgery

Surgical resection should have a negative margin (wide excision), and this is an important factor determining local recurrence. The inability to achieve wide margins at resection is a contraindication to limb salvage. Other relative contraindications include very young patients, distal tumours and pathologic fracture, although recent studies have found pathologic fractures to be salvageable as long as the fracture haematoma is resected *en bloc* with the primary tumour.

Following resection, typical reconstruction options include allograft, metal prosthesis or allograft-prosthesis composites (Table 7.8). Novel reconstructions such as extracorporeal irradiation and reimplantation supplemented by vascularised fibular grafting, rotationplasties, lengthening and bone transport procedures are sometimes used.

> **Note**
>
> Jeys LM, Kulkarni A, Grimer RJ, *et al.* Endoprosthetic reconstruction for the treatment of musculoskeletal tumors of the appendicular skeleton and pelvis. *J Bone Joint Surg Am* 2008; 90: 1265-71. **At 10 years, implant survival was 75% with mechanical failure as the endpoint and 58% with failure from any cause as the endpoint. The limb salvage rate was 84% at 20 years.**

> **Note**
>
> Sewell MD, Spiegelberg BG, Hanna SA, *et al.* Total femoral endoprosthetic replacement following excision of bone tumours. *J Bone Joint Surg Br* 2009; 91: 1513-20. **This study looked at 33 patients with a mean age of 31 years. Total femoral endoprosthetic replacement resulted in no cases of aseptic loosening and no recurrence.**

Resection options for the upper extremities include intra- and extra-articular resection. Excision of the entire scapula is known as Tikhoff-Linberg resection.

Resection of tumours around the knee follows similar principles and a range of reconstruction prostheses are available. A consideration in young people is to use an expandable prosthesis that makes up for growth of the limb. Repeated procedures may be required to lengthen the prosthesis, or an implant that is expandable without surgical intervention may be used.

Table 7.8. Relative advantages and disadvantages of endoprosthesis and allograft reconstruction.

Reconstruction	Advantages	Disadvantages
Allograft	Reattachment of soft tissues Maintains joint anatomy with restoration of tendons and ligaments	High infection rate Graft failure and fracture are possible Chemotherapy and radiotherapy interfere with host-graft union Resorption of graft
Metal endoprosthesis	Durable Easily available Stable (immediately) Immediate mobilisation	Soft tissue reconstruction is required and may be difficult or unsatisfactory Loosening* Mechanical failure*

* Loosening and mechanical failure are late disadvantages and better survival is seen with improved technology, including the use of rotating-hinge knee prostheses and hydroxyapatite coating of collars.

Rotationplasty is a procedure in which a knee tumour is excised and reconstructed with the tibial segment arthrodesed to the distal femur and the ankle rotated 180° to function as the knee joint. Extensive patient counselling and information is imperative prior to planning this procedure. Good function is achievable, but the procedure is still unacceptable to many patients (and parents), who will often choose endoprosthetic replacement ahead of rotationplasty.

Chemotherapy

The development of effective chemotherapy regimens has improved the survival of patients with osteogenic sarcoma. Chemotherapy is often part of a multinational trial – for this tumour type, the main group currently recruiting patients for trials is the European and American Osteosarcoma Study Group (EURAMOS).

Induction (preoperative) chemotherapy is used to improve chances of limb salvage and reduce tumour size, although there is a lack of evidence for this practice. The main role is to eradicate the disease from distant sites.

In the EURAMOS trial, induction chemotherapy is with the combination of cisplatin, doxorubicin and methotrexate (CDM). This has shown to produce a survival benefit and locally control the disease. After surgery, patients are randomised based on their response rate to induction chemotherapy. Good responders (>90% tumour kill) are randomised to CDM with or without interferon-α. Poor responders (>10% viable tumour) receive CDM with or without ifosfamide and etoposide.

Drug resistance is the failure of tumour cells to respond to chemotherapy. P-glycoprotein is a membrane pump that pumps doxorubicin out of the cells. The *MDR1* (multidrug resistance) gene encodes P-glycoprotein and the presence of *MDR1* significantly reduces patient survival. Chemotherapeutic agents have been tested for their ability to block the action of P-glycoprotein, but toxicity limits their regular use.

Note

Grimer RJ, Taminiau AM, Cannon SR; Surgical Subcommittee of the European Osteosarcoma Intergroup. Surgical outcomes in osteosarcoma. *J Bone Joint Surg Br* 2002; 84: 395-400. **In this study of 202 patients following surgery, the survival rates were 57% at 5 years and 54% at 10 years. The local recurrence rate was 8%, and all local occurrences were in patients undergoing limb salvage surgery using endoprosthetic replacements (there were no local recurrences in amputations). Local recurrences did not occur when the necrosis rate was over 90%.**

Note

McDonald DJ, Capanna R, Gherlinzoni F, *et al.* Influence of chemotherapy on perioperative complications in limb salvage surgery for bone tumours. *Cancer* 1990; 65: 1509-16. **In this study of 304 patients, the incidence of complications was 25.2% (29/115) for no chemotherapy, 32.8% (20/61) for adjuvant chemotherapy and 55.4% (71/128) for neoadjuvant chemotherapy.**

Prognostic indicators

The following factors are indicators of poor prognosis:

- Metastases at initial presentation.
- Skip lesions – separate foci within the same bone.
- Tumours of the axial skeleton and more proximally located tumours.
- Elevated LDH levels.
- Poor response to chemotherapy (<95% necrosis).
- Pathological fracture.

Ewing's sarcoma

Ewing's sarcoma is the second most common bone tumour in childhood and the second most common bone malignancy. It belongs to a family of tumours known as primitive neuroectodermal tumours, as the cell of origin of this tumour is considered to be neuronal. The incidence is 0.6 per 1 million and the male to female ratio is 1.6:1.

Aetiology

The gene associated with the development of Ewing's sarcoma is *EWS*, which is responsible for triggering changes in fibroblasts. The translocation t(11;22) is present in 85% of patients with Ewing's sarcoma.

Clinical features

The bones commonly involved in Ewing's sarcoma are the femur, tibia, humerus, fibula, pelvis, ribs, scapula, clavicle and spine. The location within the bone is usually diaphyseal.

The common presenting features are pain (90%) and swelling (70%) in the involved extremity. There may be a history of incidental trauma. Tumours involving the spine may present with neurological disturbance. Pathological fractures are the presenting feature in 5-10% of patients.

Systemic signs may be present, including fever, weight loss and malaise.

Laboratory studies

Typically there is an elevated white blood cell count and erythrocyte sedimentation rate and normochromic normocytic anaemia.

LDH and alkaline phosphatase levels may be elevated. The rise and fall in LDH levels correlate with tumour progression or response to chemotherapy, respectively. A raised LDH level indicates a poor prognosis.

Imaging

The lesion is usually diaphyseal and may extend to the metaphysis. In plain radiographs, the pattern of bone destruction is permeative and is accompanied by cortical changes. The appearance is described as 'onion skin' due to the lamellated appearance and Codman's triangle may be seen due to rapid growth of the lesion.

MRI is used to show the soft tissue component, intramedullary extent and presence of skip lesions.

Metastasis is commonly to the lungs, but also to other sites in the skeleton. This can be detected early on the bone scan.

Histology

Sheets of closely packed small, round, blue cells with large nuclei are evident on microscopy. The presence of glycogen makes them stain positive with periodic acid-Schiff staining.

Management

Chemotherapy is the first line of treatment for Ewing's sarcoma. Systemic control is usually achieved by induction chemotherapy, which is generally part of a clinical trial. The Euro-EWINGS clinical trial investigated the role of adjuvant therapy in patients with Ewing's sarcoma. Every patient received vincristine, ifosfamide, doxorubicin and etoposide as induction therapy. Subsequently, there were two randomisation groups. The first compared vincristine, actinomycin-D and ifosfamide (VAI) with vincristine, actinomycin-D and cyclophosphamide. The second randomisation was split between local and pulmonary disease. For local disease, the second randomisation was to VAI or busulphan and melphalan. For pulmonary disease, the randomisation was to VAI plus lung irradiation or busulphan and melphalan. The trial showed patients with primary disseminated multifocal Ewing's sarcoma have better survival with mutimodal therapy.

Radiation is effective for local control but the disadvantages are substantial. The recurrence rate is 10% and there is a 20% risk of development of secondary neoplasm. Radiation can also cause growth arrest in the immature skeleton, avascular necrosis in the femoral head, joint contracture, muscle atrophy and pathological fracture.

Surgery is used after induction chemotherapy to achieve local control of the disease and is followed by adjuvant chemotherapy. If adequate margins can be achieved, local recurrence is reduced. Surgery has the advantages of preserving function and avoiding the complications of radiation therapy. Radiation may be needed after surgery if there is a possibility of residual tumour tissue.

Prognostic indicators

The following factors are indicators of poor prognosis in Ewing's sarcoma:

- Metastatic disease at presentation.
- Large tumours.
- Pelvic tumours.
- Older age at presentation.
- Increased LDH levels.
- Poor response to chemotherapy.

Chondrosarcoma

Chondrosarcoma is the third most common primary bone tumour and has varying malignant potential. Even within the same tumour mass, different areas may have different malignant potentials.

Two-thirds of chondrosarcomas occur in the trunk, proximal humerus or femur. The genetic translocation t(9;22) is present in 25% of tumours.

Several factors are associated with a higher rate of malignancy:

- Larger tumour.
- Older patient.
- Persistent or night pain.
- Multiple lesions (Maffucci's syndrome, Ollier's disease or hereditary multiple exostoses).
- Lesions within the bone.
- Centrally placed tumours.
- Increased uptake on bone scan.
- Local recurrence.

Clinical features

Most chondrosarcomas present as a slowly growing mass. Pain may indicate possible malignant growth. Pathologic fractures can be present with enostotic lesions.

Imaging

The soft tissue calcification seen in chondrosarcoma is typically described as having a 'popcorn-ball' appearance. There is a thick cap of cartilage and the presence of a soft tissue mass indicates malignancy. Bone destruction is often evident.

Classification

Chondrosarcoma is classified using the following categories:

- Grade:
  - ½ – atypical enchondroma;
  - 1 – low;
  - 2 – medium/intermediate;
  - 3 – high.
- Primary or secondary.
- Central or peripheral.
- Histological subtype:
  - clear cell;
  - mesenchymal;
  - chondrosarcoma of soft parts;
  - dedifferentiated.

Management

For grade 1 lesions, curettage plus cementation is usually appropriate – careful histological examination is necessary to ensure the tumour is not more aggressive.

The mainstay of management of grade 2 and 3 lesions is wide surgical excision. The adequacy of the margin can be planned depending on the site of the lesion. Reconstruction options after surgery range from allografts to endoprostheses and allograft-prosthesis composites.

There is a lack of standard guidelines regarding use of chemotherapy and radiotherapy, but these modalities are employed where there is a dedifferentiated tumour, which has a poor prognosis.

Patients should be followed up regularly for the development of local recurrence and metastasis in the chest. If a lesion is detected, surgical excision is planned.

Note

Daly PJ, Sim FH, Wold LE. Dedifferentiated chondrosarcoma of bone. *Orthopedics* 1989; 12: 763-7. **Patients had a 5-year survival rate of 10%.**

Note

Barnes R, Catto M. Chondrosarcoma of bone. *J Bone Joint Surg Br* 1966; 48: 729-64.

Note

Dahlin DC, Beabout JW. Dedifferentiation of low-grade chondrosarcomas. *Cancer* 1971; 28: 461-6. **Ten percent of low-grade chondrosarcomas had areas of dedifferentiation. These patients rapidly deteriorated.**

Note

Giuffrida AY, Burgueno JE, Koniaris LG, et al. Chondrosarcoma in the United States (1973 to 2003): an analysis of 2890 cases from the SEER database. *J Bone Joint Surg Am* 2009; 91: 1063-72. **Current treatment protocols have not improved the survival of chondrosarcoma patients over the last 30 years.**

Soft tissue sarcomas

Incidence

The incidence of soft tissue sarcomas is 20-30 per 1 million of the population. There are approximately 1,500 cases per year in the UK, and 46% of these occur in the lower extremities.

Clinical features

Concerning features are a size larger than 5cm, the lesion located in the deep fascia or a painful and growing lesion. Approximately 20% of lesions are small and superficial.

Pathology

There are many subtypes of soft tissue sarcomas based on tissue of origin.

The common subtypes are:

- Liposarcoma:
  - myxoid liposarcoma;
  - pleomorphic liposarcoma.
- Leiomyosarcoma.
- Rhabdomyosarcoma:
  - embryonal (two-thirds of patients) – ages 10-20 years (alveolar, botyroid or spindle-cell);
  - pleomorphic (one-third) – ages 50-70 years.
- Synovial sarcoma.
- Malignant peripheral nerve sheath tumour.

Pathogenesis

Several different factors contribute to the pathogenesis of soft tissue sarcomas:

- Environmental factors:
  - trauma (anecdotal) or implants (surgical);
  - chemicals (asbestos, phenoxyacetic acid herbicides, vinyl chloride);
  - radiation.
- Oncogenic viruses:
  - Epstein-Barr virus in smooth muscle tumours of patients positive for HIV;
  - human herpes virus 8 in Kaposi's sarcoma.
- Immunologic factors:
  - immunodeficiency/therapeutic immuno-suppression associated with leiomyosarcomas;
  - acquired regional immunodeficiency associated with angiosarcomas in lymphoedema.

- Genetic factors:
  - bilateral retinoblastoma is associated with secondary sarcoma (germline deletion of *RB1* locus on chromosome 13);
  - Li-Fraumeni syndrome (germline deletion of *p53* locus) results in familial rhabdomyosarcoma.

The genetic factors associated with soft tissue sarcomas are shown in Table 7.9.

Post-radiation sarcoma

The criteria for post-radiation sarcoma were first defined by Cahan and later modified by Arlen:

- The sarcoma developed in an irradiated field.
- Histological confirmation.

- Latency of 3 years or more.
- The region bearing the tumour was normal prior to irradiation.

Note

Cahan WG, Woodard HQ, *et al.* Sarcoma arising in irradiated bone; report of 11 cases. *Cancer* 1948; 1: 3-29.

Note

Arlen M, Higinbotham NL, Huvos AG, *et al.* Radiation-induced sarcoma of bone. *Cancer* 1971; 28: 1087-99.

Table 7.9. Genetic factors associated with soft tissue sarcomas.

Genetic factor	Sarcoma	Gene	Chromosome
Neurofibromin type 1	Malignant peripheral nerve sheath tumour	*NF-1*	17q11.2
Retinoblastoma	Soft tissue sarcoma or osteosarcoma	*RB1*	13q14
Li-Fraumeni	Soft tissue sarcoma or osteosarcoma	*TP53*	17p13
Gardner	Fibrosarcoma or desmoid	*APC*	5q21
Werner	Soft tissue sarcoma	*WRN*	8p12
Gorlin	Fibrosarcoma or rhabdomyosarcoma	*PTC*	9q22.3
Tuberous sclerosis	Rhabdomyosarcoma	*TSC1, TSC2*	9q34 16p13.3

APC = adenomatous polyposis coli; *NF-1* = neurofibromin 1; *PTC* = patched; *RB1* = retinoblastoma 1; *TSC* = tuberous sclerosis; *TP53* = tumour protein p53; *WRN* = Werner syndrome

Management

Surgical excision with wide margins (>2cm) is the treatment of choice for local control of soft tissue sarcomas. Planned marginal resection is sometimes used (e.g., in elderly patients when major nerve resection would otherwise be needed).

Adjuvant radiotherapy is used for large (>5cm), deep and high-grade tumours or where margins are suboptimal.

Chemotherapy is reserved for second-line treatment where the disease is metastatic, and typically comprises doxorubicin and ifosfamide.

> **Note**
>
> Tunn PU, Kettelhack C, Dürr HR. Standardized approach to the treatment of adult soft tissue sarcoma of the extremities. *Recent Results Cancer Res* 2009; 179: 211-28.

> **Note**
>
> Khatri VP, Goodnight JE Jr. Extremity soft tissue sarcoma: controversial management issues. *Surg Oncol* 2005; 14: 1-9.

Skeletal metastases

Skeletal metastases are much more common than primary bone tumours. In the USA alone, 1.2 million new cases of skeletal metastases are diagnosed each year compared with 2,700 primary bone tumours. The skeleton is the third most common site for metastasis, after the lungs and liver.

Metastasis sites

The common sites for skeletal metastasis are the spine, sacrum, pelvis, ribs, femur and humerus. Metastasis distal to the elbow and knee is uncommon.

Lung cancer may sometimes cause metastasis in the distal part of the extremities (acrometastases).

Cortical metastases are less common, but can be detected early on plain films. The appearance is of punched-out lesions known as 'cookie-cutter' metastasis. These lesions are generally from the lung and the most common site is the femur.

Tumours metastasising to bone

Any tumour can metastasise to bone. The breast, prostate, lung, kidney and thyroid directly drain to the vertebral venous system. Less common causes include gastric and colon carcinoma, melanoma and neurogenic tumours. Neuroblastoma and leukaemia can cause bone metastases in children.

Evaluation of a patient presenting with an unknown primary tumour should focus on identifying the primary tumour sites. Lung and prostate tumours can often spread to bone and present as a metastasis with an unknown primary lesion. Melanoma and colon cancer are less common. In lymphoma and leukaemias, bone metastasis may be the first presentation.

A detailed investigation of patients presenting with skeletal metastases from cancer of an unknown primary origin is probably unnecessary. A CT scan of the chest, abdomen and pelvis, an isotope bone scan and a biopsy of the most accessible lesion will usually give sufficient information on most tumours.

Pathology

Bone destruction is most often through activation of osteoclasts by the tumour cells. The pathological steps are shown in Figure 7.1.

Several mechanisms are involved in osteoclast-mediated bone resorption:

- Increased osteoclasts binding to bone.
- Stimulation of osteoclastic bone resorption.
- Increased osteoclast formation from precursors and increased osteoclast survival.

Type I collagen is a chemotactic factor for tumour cells in bone.

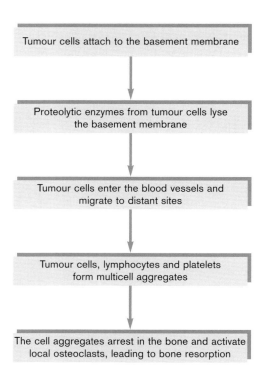

Figure 7.1. The pathological process of osteoclast activation in skeletal metastasis.

Lesion	Differential diagnosis
Table 7.10. Differential diagnosis of lytic lesions in patients aged over 40 years.	
Benign	Paget's disease
	Hyperparathyroidism
Malignant	Haematological malignancy – myeloma, lymphoma
	Chondrosarcoma
	Malignant fibrous histiocytoma
	Secondary osteosarcoma
	Metastasis

Clinical features

Skeletal metastases may be incidentally identified on radiographs, although this is relatively uncommon. Usually a radiograph will have been performed for pain, which may have been misinterpreted as pain from osteoarthritis. The features of skeletal metastases are typically as follows:

- Pain – typically at night. The pain may be localised to the lytic area. Pain on mobilisation with femoral or tibial metastases often indicates an imminent pathological fracture. Activity-related pain with upper limb metastasis may also indicate an impending fracture.
- Swelling – this is generally a late sign and tumours are often identified before they get to this stage. Swelling signifies soft tissue extension or a pathological fracture with haematoma.
- Neurological dysfunction – sometimes seen with vertebral tumours.

In a solitary lesion, the diagnosis should be confirmed before treatment is undertaken. Patients aged over 40 years may have primary bone tumours and the management of these is fundamentally different to that of metastases (Table 7.10).

Evaluation

Radiographs (whole bone and chest)

Radiographs of the lesion and the whole bone are taken in the anteroposterior and lateral views. Approximately 30-50% of the mineral content of the bone has to be lost before the lesions are apparent on radiographs.

Lytic lesions are common in renal cell and thyroid metastasis. Other tumours may produce varied appearances. Prostate cancer is typically sclerotic, while breast cancer is usually lytic or mixed. Lung cancer produces a lytic or permeative, moth-eaten appearance. Myeloma produces punched-out lesions with no surrounding sclerosis.

The risk of pathologic fracture is usually determined by plain radiographs (although there is increasing

evidence for the role of CT). It is necessary to visualise the whole bone for further metastases prior to planning stabilisation.

A chest radiograph is taken to check for lung metastases, which are a poor prognostic indicator.

Radiographs help to assess response to treatment, as evidenced by increased sclerosis, reduced size or lesion disappearance.

Computed tomography of the chest, abdomen and pelvis

A CT scan is useful for spinal and pelvic lesions where plain radiographs may not provide sufficient information. CT scans are also necessary for staging the primary disease and planning appropriate surgery.

A Tc-99m isotope bone scan indicates 'hot' areas with increased blood flow and increased bone turnover. It is useful for determining singularity versus multiplicity of a lesion. A bone scan may be positive before the lesion is evident on radiographs. It also helps to assess response to treatment.

In myeloma, a Tc-99m bone scan is often negative because of low bone turnover. Renal cell carcinoma may give a false-negative bone scan because of its highly aggressive nature, with little or no reactive bone.

Diffuse metastasis can lead to a high level of diffuse uptake in the skeleton while inhibiting uptake in the kidneys and bladder, which are normally visible on the bone scan. The appearance of the entire skeleton as 'hot' is known as a superscan.

Plain radiographs should be obtained of any areas with increased uptake.

Magnetic resonance imaging

MRI is extremely sensitive for the detection of bony metastatic disease. Because of a high water content in metastases, they usually appear dark on T1 and bright on T2 imaging.

T1 imaging is more sensitive for detection and the low-signal (dark) metastases show up well against the background of high-signal (bright) marrow fat. Short tau inversion recovery (STIR) sequences are useful to detect metastases on T2 as the fat signal is suppressed. Sclerotic metastases are dark on T1 and T2. Ideally, T1 should be combined with T2 or STIR sequences to detect metastases.

For spinal metastases, MRI can detect cord compression and soft tissue extension. MRI is less sensitive for differentiating acute fractures from metastases, but is able to differentiate old fractures from metastases.

MRI is a good modality for detecting and staging primary breast tumours, which may be undetected by clinical examination and mammography (positron emission tomography is also a good investigation here).

MRI is not a good screening tool because of its cost and because only a part of the skeleton can be assessed at any one time. Whole-body scans are expensive and time consuming, although scanners are improving in quality and scans are becoming cheaper. A Tc-99m bone scan is currently a better screening tool for metastases.

Blood tests

A full blood count and electrolyte levels should be taken for all patients. Positive findings often include anaemia or a low platelet count.

Serum electrophoresis often demonstrates features consistent with myeloma and there is usually an elevated sedimentation rate (>100mm/hour).

Serum calcium, phosphate and liver function tests should be performed. Alkaline phosphatase can be elevated and is a poor prognostic indicator.

Carcinoembryonic antigen levels are often elevated in gastrointestinal or hepatocellular carcinoma. These are helpful in monitoring response to treatment, but are not a good diagnostic test.

The prostate-specific antigen (PSA) level is useful in screening for prostate cancer. This should be evaluated in light of PSA density (the rise in the PSA level in relation to the size of the gland on ultrasound) and PSA velocity (the rate of rise of PSA over a period of time).

Positron emission tomography

Positron emission tomography (PET)-CT uses the 18F-fluorodeoxyglucose tracer and helps to detect occult primary tumours (particularly in the head and neck area) and differentiate scar tissue from recurrent disease. There may be a role for this imaging modality in cancers of unknown primary origin and surveillance for sarcoma recurrence.

Note

Yanagawa T, Shinozaki T, Iizuka Y, *et al.* Role of 2-deoxy-2-[F-18] fluoro-D-glucose positron emission tomography in the management of bone and soft-tissue metastases. *J Bone Joint Surg Br* 2010; 92: 419-23. **In this study, PET scanning was not helpful in evaluating occult primary lesions in patients with bone metastasis.**

Needle biopsy (image guided)

Multiple specimens should be obtained and checked for adequacy by frozen section. Biopsies are ideally obtained from areas of bone destruction. Reactive bone, which may not have tumour cells, and the centre of the lesion, which may be largely necrotic tissue, should be avoided.

Indications for biopsy

There are several indications for taking a biopsy of a lesion suspected of being a bone malignancy:

- A patient with a known primary malignancy but no known metastases who develops a first bony lesion.
- A patient with a history of long stable malignancy (e.g., breast, renal, prostate cancer) who was considered cured, but develops a new bony lesion.
- A patient with a known malignancy who presents with a pathological fracture.
- A previously healthy patient who presents with new multiple bony lesions indicative of disseminated metastatic disease, as yet of unknown origin.

- A healthy patient who presents with a pathological fracture suspected of being metastatic in origin.

Preparation for surgery

Surgery for skeletal metastases is rarely an emergency (excluding spinal cord compression). Patients should be medically optimised and ideally operated on from a planned list within normal hours. A number of measures should be undertaken prior to performing surgery:

- Check cervical spine radiographs – metastases can lead to instability.
- Correct hypercalcaemia (rehydration and bisphosphonates).
- Consider preoperative embolisation, especially for renal or thyroid tumours and multiple myeloma. Surgery should be undertaken soon after embolisation (within 24 hours) to avoid the formation of a collateral circulation.
- Check the white blood cell count and avoid surgery when the count is low after chemotherapy or radiotherapy.
- Correct anaemia and thrombocytopenia and any other haematological or biochemical abnormalities.

Prediction of fracture possibility

The prediction of pathologic fractures in skeletal metastasis is based on Mirels' scoring system (Table 7.11).

> **Note**
>
> Mirels H. Metastatic disease in long bones: a proposed scoring system for diagnosing impending pathologic fractures. *Clin Orthop Relat Res* 1989; 249: 256-64. Patients with a score of 8 had a 15% risk of fracture, while those with a score of 9 had a 33% risk. Hence, impending fracture is indicated by a score of 9 or more.

> **Note**
>
> Capanna R, Campanacci DA. The treatment of metastases in the appendicular skeleton. *J Bone Joint Surg Br* 2001; 83: 471-81. Patients with fracture had a mean score of 10, while those without fracture had a mean score of 7.

Table 7.11. Mirels' scoring system for pathologic fractures.

	Score		
	1	2	3
Site	Upper limb	Lower limb	Peritrochanteric
Pain	Mild	Moderate	On weight bearing
Lesion type	Blastic	Mixed	Lytic
Relation to bone diameter	<1/3	1/3-2/3	>2/3

Mirels' scoring system is a guide and the decision to prophylactically stabilise a possible fracture should be based on the characteristics of the individual lesion and the patient.

A CT scan and rigidity analysis are research tools that may help in predicting the risk of an impending fracture.

Prognosis

The prognosis is worse with the following:

- Site:
  - extraosseous/visceral metastasis;
  - metastasis below the lumbosacral junction.
- Duration:
  - a short interval from the diagnosis of the primary tumour to metastasis;
  - metastasis at presentation.

- Pathology:
  - non-small-cell lung cancer;
  - cancer of unknown primary origin.
- Laboratory results and imaging:
  - hypercalcaemia, elevated alkaline phosphatase levels;
  - lytic lesions.

Survival following skeletal metastases is variable and generally ranges from 6 months to 4 or more years. Patients with breast and prostate skeletal metastasis often survive for 2-3 years.

Clinical evaluation of the unknown primary tumour

A clinical evaluation should be performed to identify the unknown primary tumour (Table 7.12).

Table 7.12. Clinical features of primary tumours.

Primary tumour	Clinical features
Lung	History of smoking or exposure to asbestos Cough, haemoptysis Bronchial breathing, consolidation, pulmonary effusion Clubbing
Breast	Breast lumps, enlarged axillary lymph nodes (mammography, magnetic resonance imaging)
Prostate	Symptoms of prostate enlargement – hesitancy, frequency, dysuria Rectal examination for enlargement or mass
Renal	Haematuria Palpable mass, flank pain
Thyroid	Swelling or enlargement of the thyroid gland
Colorectal	Altered bowel habits, blood with faeces
Melanoma	History of pigmented or non-pigmented lesions with a recent increase in size, asymmetric shape, change in colour, itching or bleeding

Non-surgical management of bone metastasis

Non-surgical management aims to achieve local or systemic control of the tumour, or both. It usually has two aims:

- Control of the primary tumour by anticancer measures.
- Reducing the effect of the tumour on the bone.

Anticancer measures

Radiotherapy
Once the bone has been surgically stabilised, postoperative radiotherapy is essential to control tumour growth. Radiotherapy can be given once the surgical incision is well healed, usually 2-4 weeks after surgery. In the event of an intramedullary nailing, the whole bone should be irradiated (the nail will disseminate the tumour).

A short course of radiotherapy over 1-2 weeks is preferred, usually with a total dose of 20-30 Gy. A palliative single dose may be appropriate in some circumstances.

Cytotoxic chemotherapy
The indications for cytotoxic chemotherapy include the following:

- Breast cancer that is hormone-receptor-negative and patients with aggressive visceral disease.
- Lung cancer – chemotherapy is usually palliative.

Endocrine therapy
Endocrine therapy is the treatment of choice for hormone-receptor-positive breast cancer. Cancer cells that express oestrogen and progesterone receptors are more susceptible to endocrine therapy. Luteinising hormone-releasing hormone (LHRH) agonists are frequently prescribed to premenopausal women and tamoxifen is prescribed to postmenopausal women.

Prostate cancers can respond to endocrine therapy in the form of LHRH agonists and antiandrogens.

Radioisotopes
The increased uptake of radioisotopes by tumour cells allows the use of radioisotopes to control metastases. Commonly used isotopes include ^{131}I for metastatic thyroid carcinoma, ^{131}I MIBG (mono-iodo benzylguanidine) for neuroblastoma and ^{89}Sr for blastic prostate and breast metastasis.

Reducing the effect of the tumour

Management of bone pain
The causes of bone pain in metastasis have been postulated to include the following:

- Increased intraosseous pressure.
- Periosteal stretching.
- Local inflammation and release of mediators that activate pain receptors.

The management of bone pain is based on the analgesic ladder. Patients with mild to moderate pain are managed with NSAIDs. Weak opioids can be added to NSAIDs in a fixed-dose combination if pain is not controlled. Severe pain requires opioid analgesia. The dosage of opioid analgesia is determined by the response to the drug and the susceptibility to adverse effects.

Fentanyl patches can be considered where pain is not controlled by oral analgesia. Bisphosphonates can also be useful for metastatic bone pain.

Management of hypercalcaemia
Hypercalcaemia causes nausea, vomiting, dehydration, polyuria, polydipsia, confusion and, in severe cases, coma.

Several mechanisms contribute to hypercalcaemia:

- Paraneoplastic production of parathyroid hormone-related peptide.
- Local osteolytic hypercalcaemia due to bone resorption.
- Reduced renal elimination.

Initial management of hypercalcaemia is by saline rehydration to restore intravascular volume, followed by intravenous bisphosphonate therapy. It can take 3-5 days to restore calcium ion levels to normal. Long-term management is normally aimed at controlling the neoplastic process.

Surgical management of bone metastasis

The prerequisites for surgery to treat skeletal metastases are as follows:

- A single operation can be performed with a reconstruction that will not fail in the patient's lifetime.
- The whole bone can be stabilised.
- The operation will enable immediate weight bearing.
- The recovery time from surgery is not longer than the probable life expectancy.

With improved survival rates, more aggressive management strategies (e.g., endoprosthetic replacement) are becoming necessary to restore quality of life.

> **Note**
>
> Katagiri H, Takahashi M, Wakai K, *et al*. Prognostic factors and a scoring system for patients with skeletal metastasis. *J Bone Joint Surg Br* 2005; 87: 698-703. **This study identified five significant prognostic factors for survival: the site of the primary lesion, performance status, the presence of visceral or cerebral metastases, previous chemotherapy and multiple skeletal metastases. The prognostic score was calculated by totalling the scores for individual factors. Patients with a prognostic score of six or more had a survival rate of 31% at 6 months and 11% at 1 year. By contrast, patients with a prognostic score of two or less had survival rates of 98% and 89%, respectively.**

Pelvic metastasis

A thorough preoperative evaluation is performed to assess the extent of the lesions and integrity of the remaining bone. Percutaneous options such as cementoplasty may be appropriate and should be considered. The surgical options include reconstruction using cemented hip replacement with augmentation of the acetabular bone defects using cage reconstruction. Extensive disease that cannot be treated with acetabular replacement requires either a saddle prosthesis or resection (Girdlestone) arthroplasty.

Harrington described a reconstruction technique of the pelvis using threaded pins inserted into the intact hemipelvis to transfer load. This requires an extensile exposure and is technically demanding. Tillman described a modified version through a percutaneous approach augmented by a cemented hip arthroplasty.

> **Note**
>
> Harrington KD. The management of acetabular insufficiency secondary to metastatic malignant disease. *J Bone Joint Surg Am* 1981; 63: 653-64.

> **Note**
>
> Tillman RM, Myers GJ, Abudu AT, *et al*. The three-pin modified 'Harrington' procedure for advanced metastatic destruction of the acetabulum. *J Bone Joint Surg Br* 2008; 90: 84-7. **In this study of 19 patients, there were no deep infections, dislocations or nerve or major vessel injuries.**

Femoral neck pathologic fracture

Plain radiographs of the entire femur and acetabulum are necessary to identify occult lesions. A Tc-99m isotope bone scan or MRI scan is also undertaken to detect any radiologically occult lesions. Preoperative embolisation is employed for renal metastasis unless the metastasis is being excised *en bloc*.

Arthroplasty is the treatment of choice for femoral neck fractures due to the high risk of failure of fixation implants.

Long-stem cemented implants should be used and the tip of the stem should bypass the most distal lesion by twice the bone diameter. Long stems are preferable even if there are no identifiable lesions distally because of the possibility of later lesion development.

Acetabular involvement requires appropriate reconstruction. If possible a cemented acetabulum is preferable, as a cementless socket can have impaired bone ingrowth if radiation is required following surgery.

Intertrochanteric fractures

The recovery time from surgery should not be longer than the life expectancy. Patients are more likely to mobilise early following internal fixation than with extensive joint replacement surgery.

The treatment method chosen should be expected to function beyond the life expectancy of the patient.

A dynamic hip screw is inappropriate for the management of intertrochanteric metastatic fractures because of the following:

- There is a high risk of failure because of the nature of the device.
- A dynamic hip screw does not address any distal defects.
- Non-union and cut-out are major problems.
- Postoperative irradiation can lead to a stress riser at the distal end of the implant.
- Disease progression will result in failure of the reconstruction.

Cephalomedullary nails

Cephalomedullary nails (reconstruction nails or long intramedullary hip screw/Gamma nails) can be used. These should be long and should stabilise the entire femur to avoid the risk of fracture at the tip of the nail, which is a problem with the short version of the nail locked in the diaphysis.

Arthroplasty

Total hip replacement can use a conventional cemented design or a calcar replacement design that supports the deficient medial wall. The greater trochanter and abductor attachments are important for hip stability and should be preserved if possible. If the greater trochanter is involved, conversion to a proximal femoral replacement may be needed. Arthroplasty for metastatic disease is palliative; therefore, even if the greater trochanter is involved, it can be preserved and residual disease irradiated.

Cemented stems are preferred to achieve primary stability in bone. Ingrowth is unreliable due to pathologic bone and the radiation requirement. The exothermic reaction by which bone cement cures will also kill tumour cells.

The arthroplasty can be technically difficult and has a higher risk of infection and dislocation than primary hip arthroplasty. Consideration should be given to larger-diameter heads to reduce the dislocation rate.

Postoperative radiotherapy

Postoperative radiotherapy is routinely used to control disease progression. The efficacy is well proven.

Subtrochanteric fractures

Mechanisms for internal fixation include an intramedullary implant and proximal femoral replacement.

Intramedullary implant

Intramedullary fixation is the preferred treatment, if possible. It avoids the risk of implant failure associated with extramedullary implants (there is no place for sliding hip screws because of the risk of disease progression or implant failure) and the risk of instability associated with proximal femoral replacement endoprostheses.

Second-generation (reconstruction-type) nails provide secure fixation proximally in the femoral head using two screws and distal interlocking.

The mode of failure is generally by screw cut-out from the femoral head. This can be caused by involvement of the head in the disease process or inappropriate positioning of the implant (technical error).

Third-generation nails (long intramedullary hip screw/Gamma nails) have a single large proximal-locking screw as well as distal locking. Failure is less frequent.

Proximal femoral replacement

Proximal femoral replacement is useful in the event of intramedullary fixation failure, disease progression or extensive disease involving the entire proximal femur. The surgery is more extensive than with internal fixation, with greater blood loss and an increased risk of infection. Stability can be a concern and reattachment of the abductors to the prosthesis or vastus lateralis may provide some support. Because this is a palliative procedure, preserving the greater trochanter and its soft tissue attachment will improve stability, as will the use of unipolar heads (hemiarthroplasty), bipolar heads, constrained liners and large-diameter metal-on-metal resurfacing-type heads.

> **Note**
>
> Chandrasekar CR, Grimer RJ, Carter SR, et al. Modular endoprosthetic replacement for tumours of the proximal femur. *J Bone Joint Surg Br* 2009; 91: 108-12.

Proximal humerus metastasis

Involvement of the head and neck requires hemiarthroplasty. A long stem may be needed to achieve distal fixation. The tuberosities (if salvageable) or the rotator cuff can be reattached to the prosthesis.

Using an allograft-prosthesis composite can help the reattachment of the host rotator cuff to the soft tissue on the allograft.

Humerus diaphysis

Options for reconstruction include an intramedullary nail with or without cement augmentation, or prosthetic intercalary spacers. The latter allow excision of the tumour. They also provide good axial and rotational stability, but reduced function.

> **Note**
>
> Spencer SJ, Holt G, Clarke JV, *et al.* Locked intramedullary nailing of symptomatic metastases in the humerus. *J Bone Joint Surg Br* 2010; 92: 142-5. **Thirty-five patients had a mean postoperative survival of 7.1 months. There were no failures of fixation and no reoperations.**

Distal humerus metastasis

There are two surgical reconstructive options:

- Double plating with cement augmentation. The plates are placed in different planes for maximum mechanical advantage and the defect is curetted and filled with cement.
- Excision of the lesion and endoprosthetic distal humeral replacement.

Spinal metastasis

The aim of management of spinal metastases is to alleviate pain, restore stability and prevent the compression of neural elements.

Diagnostic surgical procedures include open or percutaneous biopsy to establish a tissue diagnosis. Percutaneous biopsy can be performed under fluoroscopy, CT or MRI guidance.

Radiotherapy

Malignant spinal cord compression is often best treated with radiotherapy, but surgical management is more appropriate in some cases. Based on the British Orthopaedic Association guidelines, the following are indications for radiotherapy:

- No spinal instability.
- Radiosensitive tumour.
- Stable or slowly progressive neurology.
- Multilevel disease.
- Surgery is precluded by the general condition.
- Poor prognosis.
- Postoperative adjuvant treatment.

It is possible to deliver radiotherapy to the posterior vertebral body. Supplemental dexamethasone should be administered and the course of radiotherapy should be short (24 Gy in 6 fractions or 30 Gy in 10 fractions).

Surgery

The indications for surgical management of malignant spinal cord compression are as follows:

- Spinal instability evidenced by pathological fracture, progressive deformity and/or neurological deficit.
- Clinically significant neurological compression, especially by bone.
- The tumour is insensitive to radiotherapy, chemotherapy or hormonal manipulation.

Surgical stabilisation is indicated where there is impending instability. The Denis three-column concept has been extended to include a left and right division in each column, making a total of six columns. Involvement of three or four columns out of six is an indication for stabilisation. Those with involvement of five or six columns will often require anterior and posterior stabilisation.

For the dorsal and lumbar spine, the anterior approach is preferred as the disease commonly involves the body of the vertebrae. The posterior approach can be used for isolated posterior disease (which is quite rare) or in conjunction with the anterior approach when the disease extends to more than two vertebral levels.

The anterior approach is also best for lower cervical spine disease. The upper cervical spine may require posterior stabilisation with or without anterior reconstruction.

> **Note**
>
> Fürstenberg CH, Wiedenhöfer B, Gerner HJ, Putz C. *The effect of early surgical treatment on recovery in patients with metastatic compression of the spinal cord. J Bone Joint Surg Br 2009; 91: 240-4.* **In 35 patients with incomplete cord compression, those who underwent decompression within 48 hours had better neurologic outcomes than those with compression delayed for more than 48 hours.**

Chapter 8 Infections

Acute osteomyelitis

Incidence

The incidence of acute osteomyelitis varies, but has been reported as 1 in 5,000 per year in children, peaking in late summer. Boys are three times more prone to infection than girls. It generally involves rapidly growing bones, hence the predominance in children.

Pathogenesis

The common infective organisms in acute osteomyelitis are *Staphylococcus aureus*, group A *Streptococcus*, *Strep. pneumoniae* and group B beta-haemolytic *Streptococcus*.

Staph. aureus and group B *Streptococcus* are common in neonates. In children, *Staph. aureus*, group A *Streptococcus* and coliform bacteria are more commonly seen. *Staph. aureus* continues to be the most common organism in adults with acute osteomyelitis. Salmonella is the characteristic infective organism in patients with sickle-cell anaemia.

The infection is commonly haematogenous. Several features of the metaphysis make it a common site of infection:

- The blood flow is slow, allowing bacteria to migrate through fenestrations in the capillary wall.
- Endothelial cells are unable to phagocytose particles in the metaphysis.
- Medullary vessels become thrombosed and white cells cannot reach the bacteria.

Figure 8.1 shows the arrangement of blood vessels in the metaphysis.

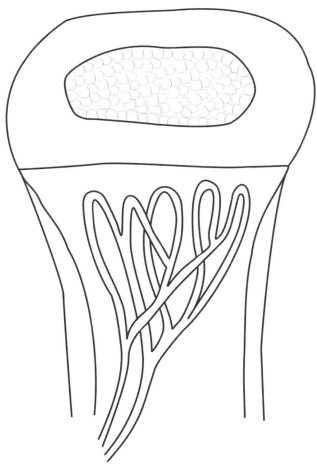

Figure 8.1. Arrangement of blood vessels in the metaphysis.

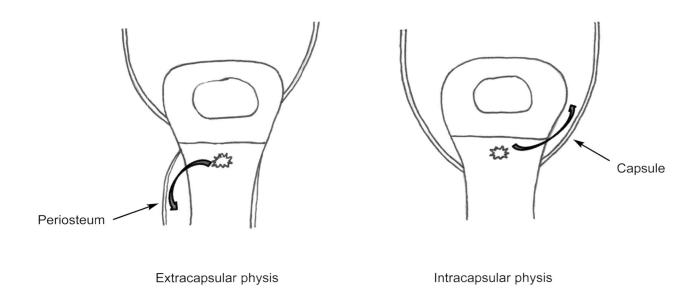

Periosteum

Capsule

Extracapsular physis

Intracapsular physis

Figure 8.2. Intra-articular spread of infection from the metaphysis.

The initial phase is inflammatory with rising intraosseous pressure causing intense pain. Pus formation follows. In long bones, pus exits laterally and forms a subperiosteal abscess. Because of pressure the blood supply to the cortex is cut off, which can lead to the formation of a sequestrum.

Intra-articular metaphysis is found in the proximal femur, proximal humerus, distal tibia and the radial neck. At these sites, the joint can become infected by contiguous spread from the metaphysis (Figure 8.2).

In the later phase, after about 2 weeks, new bone formation takes place under the elevated periosteum. This new bone over sequestrum is called involucrum.

Clinical features

Patients commonly present with pseudoparalysis, pain, a limp and refusal to walk. Sympathetic effusion may be present in the adjoining joint. Acute infection is often associated with systemic signs.

Investigation

Blood tests

The white cell count (WCC) is normal in 75% of patients. The erythrocyte sedimentation rate (ESR) is elevated in 90%, but can be normal in people with sickle-cell disease, those undergoing steroid therapy and neonates. The ESR rises 3-5 days after the onset of infection and starts declining in 1-2 weeks.

The C-reactive protein level peaks in 2 days, and starts declining within 6 hours of appropriate therapy. This is the most sensitive indicator of the course of infection and response to treatment.

Blood cultures are positive in 30-50% of patients.

Imaging

Radiographs within 3 days may show displacement of the muscle planes. In 7 days, the muscle planes are typically obliterated. Bone changes appear after 1-2 weeks.

A Tc-99m bone scan has a high false-negative rate. It should be performed within 48 hours of aspiration, otherwise false-positivity is high. Patients with cold bone scans may have more aggressive infection.

Other radioisotope scans with increasing sensitivity and specificity are available. These include gallium 67, indium-111-labelled white blood cells, indium-111-labelled immunoglobulin and Tc-99m ciprofloxacin scans.

A computed tomography (CT) scan will show bone changes. This can help to differentiate osteomyelitis from chondroblastoma and osteoid osteoma.

Magnetic resonance imaging (MRI) can detect changes caused by bone oedema within 3-5 days. Gadolinium enhancement helps define areas of necrosis. MRI is a sensitive and commonly used investigation.

An ultrasound scan can be performed to detect subperiosteal abscesses ('sandwich appearance of periosteum'). Elevation of the periosteum by 2mm is suggestive of an underlying infection.

Positron emission tomography scanning has nearly 99% sensitivity for the detection of bone infections.

Bone marrow aspiration

Bone marrow aspiration is performed to obtain material for Gram stain and culture.

If the patient has underlying chronic diseases then the aspirate should be tested for anaerobes, acid-fast bacilli and fungi.

Polymerase chain reaction can detect bacteria and help in determining the causative organism.

Management

Empiric therapy can be started once samples have been obtained for bacteriological diagnosis. Commonly used antibiotics are oxacillin, cefazolin, clindamycin and vancomycin. Once the infecting organism has been identified, the choice of antibiotic therapy depends on sensitivity.

Bacteraemia may interfere with the absorption of oral agents. Hence, antibiotics are given intravenously for 3 weeks and then orally for a further 3 weeks.

Indications for surgery include a subperiosteal abscess, intramedullary pus, sequestrum and secondary septic arthritis.

Long-term sequelae include limb-length discrepancy, recurrent infection, joint deformity and gait abnormalities.

Brodie's abscess

Brodie's abscess is subacute osteomyelitis in the metaphysis of long bones. It appears as a lytic area surrounded by sclerotic bone.

Chronic osteomyelitis

Chronic osteomyelitis can be the result of persistent infection following acute osteomyelitis or local/haematogenous spread. Open fractures and post-surgery infection can lead to chronic osteomyelitis. Immune deficiency predisposes to chronic infection.

Three types of patients are identified on the basis on immune resistance:

- Type A – normal immune response, non-smoker.
- Type B – mild systemic disorders or smoker.
- Type C – major nutritional or systemic disorder.

Anatomically, chronic osteomyelitis can be of four types:

- Superficial.
- Medullary.
- Localised.
- Diffuse.

Chronic osteomyelitis may or may not be associated with a sinus tract.

Note

Cierny G 3rd, Mader JT. Approach to adult osteomyelitis. *Orthop Rev* 1987; 16: 259-70.

Investigation

In addition to blood tests and radiographs, MRI will help determine soft tissue involvement, the presence of marrow oedema and areas of pus collection.

Culture from the sinus tract is not helpful because it is colonised by a variety of bacteria. Deep cultures are more representative of the causative organism.

The radioisotope scans mentioned in the section on acute osteomyelitis (above) and polymerase chain reaction techniques can aid diagnosis.

Management

Management is based on thorough debridement of all dead and infected tissue, appropriate antibiotics, obliteration of dead space and soft tissue cover. In the localised form of chronic osteomyelitis, local debridement may involve excising dead bone; the diffuse form is managed by *en bloc* resection of a segment of bone, with the defect filled by distraction histogenesis.

A flap cover is very useful to cover soft tissue defects and bring a greater blood supply to the local area. Open cancellous grafting (Papineau technique) is rarely used.

McNally described a technique that was performed in two stages. The first stage was radical debridement with the use of gentamicin beads. The second stage, performed 3-6 weeks later, involved further debridement and bone grafting. The reported success rate was 92%.

Note

McNally MA, Small JO, Tofighi HG, Mollan RA. Two stage management of chronic osteomyelitis of the long bones. The Belfast technique. *J Bone Joint Surg Br* 1993; 75: 375-80.

Another technique (from Oswestry) describes excision of sinus tracts, removal of internal fixation devices and double-ended reaming. An endoscope is passed into the canal to ensure bleeding bone surfaces. A closed suction irrigation tube is inserted and removed at the end of treatment. Only one operation is planned, although some patients may require repeat debridement.

Note

Caesar BC, Morgan-Jones RL, Warren RE, *et al*. Closed double-lumen suction irrigation in the management of chronic diaphyseal osteomyelitis: long-term follow-up. *J Bone Joint Surg Br* 2009; 91: 1243-8. **Oswestry technique. Thirty-five patients were managed by reaming, arthroscopic debridement of the medullary canal and closed double-lumen suction irrigation. Infection was cleared in 85%.**

Vascularised bone grafts are indicated for long defects (>6cm) and require close coordination between plastic and orthopaedic surgeons.

The Ilizarov method of corticotomy, bone transport and distraction histogenesis is helpful when a bone segment must be excised. Docking of the two ends can be performed acutely and then length regained by distraction, or the length can be maintained and a segment transported to fill the gap.

Septic arthritis

Septic arthritis is acute bacterial infection of a joint. The most common route of spread is via the blood. Local spread, trauma or surgery may be responsible in some instances.

Clinical features

Septic arthritis can present in any age group, but is most common in boys younger than 2 years. There may be a history of upper respiratory tract infection or local infection.

Common presenting symptoms include fever, local pain, swelling, tenderness and inability to bear weight.

Blood parameters

An ESR of more than 40mm/hour and a WCC of greater than 12,000/mm^3 are suggestive of septic arthritis.

If three out of these four characteristics – fever, inability to bear weight, raised ESR and raised WCC

– are present, there is a 93% chance of septic arthritis. If all four characteristics are present, the odds rise to 99.6%.

Imaging

X-ray features include joint-space widening, obliteration of normal fat planes and soft tissue swelling. Later, bone destruction is sometimes evident.

A Tc-99m bone scan is useful in detecting multifocal lesions. In addition, clinical and radiological signs may not be readily evident in certain areas such as the foot, pelvis, hip, spine and scapula. These can be evaluated with a Tc-99m or single-photon emission CT scan.

CT and MRI cannot differentiate infection from non-septic inflammation. Ultrasound is non-specific and operator-dependent.

Aspiration

Joint aspiration can provide a definitive diagnosis. Table 8.1 shows the tests performed on the fluid and indicators of infection.

Table 8.1. Tests performed on the joint aspiration fluid and indicators of infection.

Test	Indicator of infection
Gram stain	Positive
Culture – aerobic, anaerobic	Positive Cultures are positive in 50-60% of patients
WCC count	WCC >50,000/mm^3 with >90% polymorphonuclear neutrophils
Synovial glucose test	Ratio of synovial fluid glucose to blood glucose of <0.5
Mucin clot test	Acetic acid is added to the fluid, and an appearance like curdled milk indicates infection In rheumatic fever, a mucin clot forms a rope-like appearance

Management

Septic arthritis is an emergency. The immediate management is resuscitation of the patient, ensuring adequate analgesia and hydration. Blood should be sent for culture, and it is worth taking a sample for microbiology analysis prior to starting antibiotics. Open irrigation and debridement is undertaken and the joint closed over drains. In gonococcal arthritis, aspiration only may be sufficient.

Intravenous antibiotics, usually cephalosporins, are started pending culture results. Oxacillin and ceftriaxone are used in immunocompromised patients. The duration of antibiotic therapy is a debated issue, but in most cases it should continue for 6 weeks.

With early diagnosis and adequate treatment, a 90% cure rate can be expected. Ongoing infection and damage to the physis account for most of the disability following septic arthritis. A damaged physis leads to deformity, shortening or sometimes compensatory overgrowth. A pathological fracture can occur through the infection site.

Osteoarticular tuberculosis

Tuberculosis of the skeletal system is caused by *Mycobacterium tuberculosis* and *M. bovis*. It is common in the developing world. In developed countries, it is predominantly seen in those with compromised immune systems.

Primary tuberculosis presents as a pulmonary infection in children and often resolves. The primary lesion is subpleural and is known as a Ghon focus. Reactivation of the primary tuberculosis, often related to a drop in immune resistance, leads to a more severe infection. Haematogenous spread of the infection leads to involvement of the bones and joints.

Clinical features

The features of post-primary tuberculosis include cough, haemoptysis, weight loss, night sweats and lymphadenopathy. The systemic signs depend on the system involved.

Investigation

Microscopic identification of *Mycobacteria* is performed using Ziehl-Neelsen staining. Culture is on Lowenstein-Jensen medium for 6 weeks. The histology is characterised by a delayed-type hypersensitivity picture, with granulomas, giant cells, central caseating necrosis, abundant lymphocytes and macrophages.

Management

The management of osteoarticular tuberculosis is mainly medical and is based on combination therapy with rifampicin, isoniazid and ethambutol. These are continued for 6 months. Resistant or recurrent tuberculosis requires second-line drugs.

Involvement of the hip or knee joint leads to joint destruction and arthroplasty is an option. Adequate debridement must be performed and the implant can be inserted as a single- or two-stage procedure. Antitubercular medication should be given both pre- and postoperatively to minimise the risk of recurrent infection.

Prevention of surgical site infections

Surgical site infections account for substantial morbidity in the postoperative period. A range of practices have been proposed to minimise surgical site infection, and include patient-dependant aspects as well as factors related to the operation room environment and perioperative management:

- An adequate nutrition status and control of concurrent infections is essential before elective procedures.
- An impaired immunological response is associated with a higher risk of infection.
- Local hair removal, if needed, should be performed using clippers and not razors. It should be performed just before the operation, preferably in the anaesthetic room.
- The use of clean-air operation theatres with vertical laminar flow significantly reduces the risk of infection.

- Chlorhexidine is more effective and longer-lasting than iodine-based antiseptics. Iodine antiseptics should be allowed to dry for maximal efficacy.
- High-pressure pulse lavage can increase damage to soft tissues and increase the penetration of bacteria.
- The use of drains has not been shown to make a difference to the infection rate or wound breakdown following elective surgery. Drains may increase the transfusion rate, but this can be offset by the use of reinfusion drains. Reinfusion drains are contraindicated where the operation is performed for infection.
- Sutures are considered to be better than skin clips for wound closure.
- The maintenance of normal glucose levels, normothermia and oxygenation reduces the risk of infection.
- Occlusive dressing allows a hypoxic and acidic environment, which retards the growth of skin pathogens and improves healing.

Prophylactic antibiotics

Prophylactic antibiotics should be given prior to starting an operation. For closed fractures and elective orthopaedic procedures, cefuroxime or cefazolin is considered to be effective against the common infective organisms (*Staph. aureus* and *Staph. epidermidis*). In some hospitals, the emergence of resistance has led to the use of co-amoxiclav, vancomycin or teicoplanin as the prophylactic antibiotics of choice.

Antibiotics are given for a maximum of 24 hours postoperatively. A longer period of therapy does not reduce infection risk and may increase the risk of resistant organisms and systemic infections.

Chapter 9 Non-union

Non-union, in general, is defined as cessation of the normal biological healing process at the fracture site, with no progression of healing for at least 3 months. Non-unions require intervention for union to be achieved.

Delayed union is a delay in the healing of a fracture. There is some progression, but the rate of healing is less than expected for that site.

In view of the various factors that influence fracture healing, it is difficult to provide a standard fixed timescale to define non-union.

The rate of delayed and non-union varies with the site and type of injury. In tibial fractures, for instance, the non-union rate is around 2.5% and the delayed union rate is about 5%. The actual risk in an individual patient depends on a variety of injury and treatment-related factors.

Causes

The causes of non-union can be related to the patient, the injury or surgery.

Patient factors

- Smoking.
- Malnutrition – a serum albumin level of less than 3.4g/dL and a lymphocyte count of less than 1,500/mm^3 is suggestive of a reduced nutrition level.

Injury-related factors

- Initial displacement of fragments.
- Degree of comminution.
- Degree of periosteal stripping.
- Bone loss.
- Local infection.
- Disruption of blood supply.

Surgical factors

- Inadequate stabilisation.
- Ongoing sepsis.
- Distraction at fracture site.
- Lack of contact between the fragments.

Types

Radiologically, non-union can be of three types:

- Hypertrophic – there is abundant callus and an adequate blood supply at the fracture fragments, but insufficient stability to allow healing.
- Oligotrophic – the blood supply to the fragments is adequate, but there is a lack of callus formation. Oligotrophic non-unions result from a lack of reduction or lack of contact of the fracture fragments.
- Atrophic – the blood supply is lacking and there is no callus formation. The biologic process is deficient.

Table 9.1. Mora and Paley classification of non-unions.

Type A non-unions (<1cm bone loss)	Type B non-unions (>1cm bone loss)
A1: lax non-unions	B1: non-union with bone loss but no shortening
A2: stiff non-unions	B2: non-union with shortening but no bone defect
A2-1: stiff non-unions without deformity	B3: non-union with shortening and bone defect
A2-2: stiff non-unions with deformity	

The distinction between these types is based on the vascularity of the bone ends. This can be determined with strontium-85 scanning.

Mora and Paley have classified non-unions into type A (<1cm bone loss) and type B (>1cm bone loss) (Table 9.1). They can be further classified based on deformity and shortening.

Note

Mora R, Paley D. *Nonunion of the Long Bones: Diagnosis and Treatment with Compression-Distraction Techniques.* Springer, 2006.

Diagnosis

Plain radiographs are the basis for the diagnosis of non-union. Tomography (plain film) or computed tomography (CT) scans may be used for detecting a gap between the fragments if it is not obvious on plain films. CT scans are more commonly available than tomography in most radiology departments.

Ultrasound examination can reveal a discontinuity in the cortex, implying incomplete healing.

General management

Evaluation for the cause of non-union is an integral part of management. Bone loss, sepsis, malalignment and previous operations can affect planning of the treatment modality.

The principles of management are as follows:

- Radical debridement to minimise the risk of sepsis.
- Adequate stability and contact between bone ends.
- Preservation of blood supply.
- Adequate soft tissue cover.
- Bone grafting.
- Use of supplementary treatments (e.g., bone morphogenetic protein [BMP]) to encourage healing.

Management of tibial delayed union and non-union

The commonest long bone non-union which is a major cause of morbidity involves the tibia. The options available to deal with this are outlined below.

Nailing

An intramedullary nail is commonly used to treat tibial fractures. In the absence of sepsis, it is an effective method of treatment. In the presence of sepsis the use of nails is debatable, with some studies showing a higher risk of persistent infection with the use of nails in infected non-unions.

Reaming stimulates healing by generating an autogenous graft. In fractures managed with external fixation, removal of the fixator and insertion of a nail is an option, but carries a high risk of infection.

Dynamisation of the nail involves removal of the locking screws, which allows the fracture fragments to impact together. The value of dynamisation has been questioned by Court-Brown.

> ### Note
>
> Court-Brown CM, Christie J, McQueen MM. Closed intramedullary tibial nailing. Its use in closed and type I open fractures. *J Bone Joint Surg Br* 1990; 72: 605-11. **In this study involving 125 patients, all healed with closed intramedullary tibial nailing and no use of dynamisation. Forty-one percent of patients experienced knee pain and 26% had the nail removed.**

Exchange nailing involves removing the existing nail and replacing with a larger-diameter nail. It is an effective treatment for delayed union in the tibia.

> ### Note
>
> Templeman D, Thomas M, Varecka T, Kyle R. Exchange reamed intramedullary nailing for delayed union and nonunion of the tibia. *Clin Orthop Relat Res* 1995; 315: 169-75. **In this study involving 28 patients, 93% healed after exchange nailing and the rest healed after a second exchange nailing. The infection rate was 11%.**

In view of the high risk of infection reported with exchange nailing, the reaming should be cultured and antibiotics given for 6 weeks if positive. Fibular osteotomy is not required in exchange nailing and the nails can be left unlocked if adequate stability has been achieved.

Bone grafting

A variety of bone grafts and substitutes have been used in the management of non-unions. The ideal graft is an autogenous cancellous graft, usually obtained from the iliac crest.

Grafts can be onlay or inlay grafts. The recommended approach for the tibia is posterolateral, which is through less traumatised tissue compared with the anterolateral approach. The incision is medial to the fibular border and the dissection plane is along the interosseous membrane, lifting the deep posterior compartment from the tibia.

Compression plate

Hypertrophic non-union can be managed with compression plating, which provides enough stability to allow healing. Atrophic non-union will require supplementary bone grafting. The disadvantages of using a compression plate include soft tissue damage, infection and the inability to bear weight until satisfactory union.

External fixator

External fixators are commonly used for the management of open tibial fractures. Uniplanar fixation can be converted to an intramedullary nail within 1-2 weeks. Applying fixators for more than 2 weeks carries the risk of pin-site infection, which can lead to intramedullary infection when the fixator is exchanged for a nail.

In the presence of bone loss, circular fixators provide stability and allow bone regeneration through distraction histogenesis. Advantages are minimal trauma to the soft tissues, the ability to correct deformities and the ability to compress and regenerate bone. In addition, the patient can immediately bear weight. Disadvantages are pin-site infection, a prolonged period in a fixator, joint stiffness and the risk of damage to neurovascular structures.

Corticotomy along with circular fixators improves vascularity and encourages union.

Note

Paley D. Treatment of tibial nonunion and bone loss with the Ilizarov technique. *Instr Course Lect* 1990; 39: 185-97.

Electrical stimulation

Electrical stimulation has been shown to enhance fracture healing. Stimulation can be delivered by implantable devices, percutaneously or non-invasively.

In most studies, the reported healing rate for these methods is 75-90%. The implantable device allows weight bearing, while the other two methods involve a period of non-weight bearing. Implantable devices require surgery for implantation and removal.

The clinical efficacy of electrical stimulation in randomised controlled studies is debatable.

Note

Sharrard WJ. A double-blind trial of pulsed electromagnetic fields for delayed union tibial fractures. *J Bone Joint Surg Br* 1990; 72: 347-55. **Out of 45 patients with tibial shaft non-unions, 20 had electrical stimulation and 25 a dummy device. Significantly better healing was observed in patients with the functioning electrical stimulation device.**

Note

Goldstein C, Sprague S, Petrisor BA. Electrical stimulation for fracture healing: current evidence. *J Orthop Trauma* 2010; 24 (Suppl. 1): S62-5. **This review identified four meta-analyses on the use of electrical stimulation in fracture healing. The authors concluded that the evidence in support of electrical stimulation in non-union is debatable.**

Ultrasound

Ultrasound has been used to help healing in tibial fractures. Hypertrophic non-unions respond better to ultrasound than atrophic non-unions.

Bone morphogenetic protein

Recombinant human (rh)BMP-7 has been shown to be as effective as an autogenous graft in the management of tibial non-unions.

The rhBMP is applied to an absorbable collagen sponge placed over the fracture site.

Note

Friedlaender GE, Perry CR, Cole JD, *et al.* Osteogenic protein-1 (bone morphogenetic protein-7) in the treatment of tibial nonunions. *J Bone Joint Surg Am* 2001; 83-A (Suppl. 1): S151-8. **A total of 122 patients with established tibial non-unions were treated with a nail with rhBMP7 or a nail with autogenous graft. At 9 months, 81% of patients with BMP and 85% of patients with an autogenous graft showed healing.**

Note

Govender S, Csimma C, Genant HK, *et al.* Recombinant human bone morphogenetic protein-2 for treatment of open tibial fractures: a prospective, controlled, randomized study of four hundred and fifty patients. *J Bone Joint Surg Am* 2002; 84-A: 2123-34. **Patients were divided into three groups: nail only; nail plus 0.75mg/ml rhBMP2; and nail plus 1.5mg/ml rhBMP2. The group with 1.5mg/ml rhBMP2 underwent significantly fewer secondary interventions.**

Chapter 10 Inflammatory joint disorders

Rheumatoid arthritis

Rheumatoid arthritis is the most common inflammatory joint disease, with a prevalence of 0.9%. It is more common in females than males (ratio 3:1) and can present at any age, with a peak between 30 and 50 years. It is polygenic, with 30% identical twin and 5% non-identical twin concordance.

The joints are involved in the following order of frequency (most frequent first):

- Hands – metacarpophalangeal and proximal interphalangeal joints.
- Wrists.
- Feet.
- Knees.
- Elbows.
- Ankles.
- Shoulders.
- Cervical spine.
- Temporomandibular joints.
- Cricoarytenoid joints (causing hoarseness).
- Stapedius (causing deafness).

Pathology

The underlying process is characterised by synovitis, nodules and vasculitis. Synovitis occurs in all patients. Histopathology of the involved synovium reveals an increase in the synovial lining layer, increased vascularity and an abundance of T- and B-lymphocytes, macrophages and activated cells of all types, with increased production of cytokines and their receptors.

Diagnosis

Rheumatoid arthritis presents in the following ways:

- Insidious onset – low-grade persistent inflammation.
- Palindromic onset – bursts of severe inflammation that may settle after a few days.
- Polymyalgic onset – limb-girdle pain and stiffness, which may progress to involve joint synovitis.
- Systemic onset – presenting with fever and general malaise.
- Acute polyarthritis – a sudden onset of inflammation in multiple joints. Consider infection as a trigger (e.g., parvovirus, streptococcal infection).

Based on the 1987 American College of Rheumatology criteria for rheumatoid arthritis, four out of seven of the following characteristics should be positive to establish a diagnosis:

- Morning stiffness of longer than 1 hour, for more than 6 weeks.
- Arthritis of at least three areas – soft issue swelling of exudation lasting for more than 6 weeks.
- Arthritis of hand joints – wrist, metacarpophalangeal or proximal interphalangeal joint lasting for more than 6 weeks.
- Symmetrical arthritis – at least one area, lasting for 6 weeks or longer.
- Rheumatoid nodules – as observed by a physician.

- Serum rheumatoid factor – by a method positive in less than 5% of controls.
- Radiographic changes – on anteroposterior films of hands and wrists.

Prior to these criteria being met, a patient may be considered to have early synovitis with a strong suspicion of rheumatoid arthritis. Treatment is initiated as for rheumatoid arthritis.

> **Note**
>
> Arnett F, Edworthy S, Bloch D, *et al*. The American Rheumatism Association 1987 revised criteria for the classification of rheumatoid arthritis. *Arthritis Rheum* 1988; 31: 315-24.

Although widely used, these criteria have been criticised for a lack of sensitivity in early disease. To address this, in 2010 the American College of Rheumatology and the European League against Rheumatism (EULAR) proposed joint criteria for the diagnosis of rheumatoid arthritis. The diagnosis is based on four areas:

- Joint involvement.
- Serology.
- Acute-phase reactants.
- Duration of symptoms.

A score of 6 or more from the system outlined in Table 10.1 is suggestive of a diagnosis of rheumatoid arthritis.

> **Note**
>
> Aletaha D, Neogi T, Silman AJ, *et al*. 2010 Rheumatoid arthritis classification criteria: an American College of Rheumatology/ European League Against Rheumatism collaborative initiative. *Arthritis Rheum* 2010; 62: 2569-81.

Investigation

The following investigations should be performed:

- Full blood count.
- Erythrocyte sedimentation rate, C-reactive protein level or plasma viscosity (dependent on availability).
- Serum electrolytes.
- Liver function tests.
- Bone profile – serum calcium and alkaline phosphatase levels.
- Autoantibody tests.
- Rheumatoid factor and anti-citrullinated protein antibody.
- Antinuclear antibodies – if positive, test extractable nuclear antigens and anti-double-stranded DNA to exclude connective tissue diseases and overlap syndromes.
- Radiology – hands and feet, other involved joints and chest X-ray.
- ~~Rheumatoid factor.~~ *duplated* ?

Antibodies can be immunoglobulin (Ig)M/G or IgA. Agglutination tests (Latex/SCAT) detect IgM rheumatoid factor and are specific for seropositive disease. Radioimmunoassays and ELISAs detect IgG rheumatoid factor, and may detect seronegative disease with low-titre borderline-positive results.

To be valid, a laboratory test must be positive in less than 4% of the population. Therefore, up to 4% of the population may be positive for rheumatoid factor with no evidence of rheumatoid arthritis. Conversely, up to 30% may have rheumatoid arthritis by diagnostic criteria, but no rheumatoid factor.

Rheumatoid factor may be positive in the presence of chronic infections (e.g., syphilis, pulmonary tuberculosis), other rheumatological conditions (e.g., connective tissue diseases) or sarcoidosis. Its prevalence tends to increase with increasing age.

Radiology

Early plain radiological changes include soft tissue swelling and juxta-articular osteoporosis. Joint-space

Table 10.1. American College of Rheumatology – European League against Rheumatism 2010 criteria for the diagnosis of rheumatoid arthritis.

Criteria	Score
Joint involvement	
One large joint	0
Two to 10 large joints	1
One to three small joints, with or without large-joint involvement	2
Four to 10 small joints, with or without large-joint involvement	3
More than 10 joints, with involvement of at least one small joint	5
Serology	
Negative RF and negative ACPA	0
Low positive RF or low positive ACPA	2
High positive RF or high positive ACPA	3
Acute-phase reactants	
Normal C-reactive protein level and normal erythrocyte sedimentation rate	0
Abnormal C-reactive protein level or abnormal erythrocyte sedimentation rate	1
Duration of symptoms	
Less than 6 weeks	0
6 weeks or more	1

ACPA = anti-citrullinated protein antibody; RF = rheumatoid factor

narrowing and erosions follow, progressing to bone and joint destruction and joint subluxation.

Diagnostic ultrasound and magnetic resonance imaging (MRI) may be helpful in the diagnosis of early synovitis, as these techniques demonstrate early bony change before they are apparent on plain X-ray.

Extra-articular features

Rheumatoid arthritis is a systemic disease, variably affecting many other systems and causing extra-articular disease as follows:

- Systemic – malaise, fever, weight loss, myalgia, elevation of acute-phase reactants (inflammatory markers), serositis causing pericarditis or pleurisy.

- Haematological – anaemia caused by impaired iron utilisation related to disease activity or medication (especially non-steroidal anti-inflammatory drugs [NSAIDs]), bone marrow suppression related to disease-modifying anti-rheumatic drugs, haemolysis, Felty's syndrome.
- Skin – cutaneous vasculitis, rheumatoid nodules, drug rashes, palmar erythema, skin atrophy.
- Eyes – keratoconjunctivitis sicca, scleritis and episcleritis, scleromalacia perforans.
- Lungs – nodules (granulomas), pleurisy and pleural effusions, interstitial fibrosis, recurrent infections, bronchiectasis, obliterative bronchiolitis, Caplan's syndrome (severe nodules of coal and silica in miners).
- Heart – pericarditis, cardiomyopathy, nodules causing conduction or valvular defects, accelerated coronary artery disease.
- Nervous system – entrapment peripheral neuropathy, mononeuritis multiplex, autonomic neuropathy, cervical myelopathy due to atlantoaxial subluxation, cervical nerve root syndromes.
- Kidney – amyloid, analgesic nephropathy and other drug-related renal effects, glomerulonephritis (rarely).

Note

Aviña-Zubieta JA, Choi HK, Sadatsafavi M, et al. Risk of cardiovascular mortality in patients with rheumatoid arthritis: a meta-analysis of observational studies. *Arthritis Rheum* 2008; 59: 1690-7.

Note

Gupta A, Fomberstein B. Evaluating cardiovascular risk in rheumatoid arthritis. *J Musculoskelet Med* 2009; 26: 481-94.

Management

The medical management of rheumatoid arthritis has improved dramatically in recent years, with the aggressive use of disease-modifying agents and the development of biologic agents. Early diagnosis is vital.

Medication

Simple analgesia, NSAIDs and corticosteroids must be considered in all patients.

Treatment is started early, using guidelines such as those published by the British Society for Rheumatology or EULAR. The general principle of early management is to use combinations of disease-modifying agents (of which the most commonly used is methotrexate), followed by biologic therapies. Disease-modifying agents include:

- Weekly low-dose (7.5-25mg/week) methotrexate.
- Sulphasalazine (2-3g/day).
- Leflunomide (10-20mg/day).
- Hydroxychloroquine.

All these drugs are subject to monitoring protocols.

Evidence-based triple therapy consists of methotrexate, sulphasalazine and hydroxychloroquine; methotrexate can be used with leflunomide with careful liver function monitoring. Other agents are occasionally used, including intramuscular gold, cyclosporine, azathioprine and rarely penicillamine, although these have largely been superseded.

Biologic therapy

Biologic therapies have revolutionised the management of severe aggressive rheumatoid arthritis. In the UK, the use of biologic therapies is determined by guidance from the National Institute for Heath and Clinical Excellence (NICE). Some other developed countries (e.g., Scandinavia) have less stringent criteria, but these drugs are often unavailable in developing countries because of high costs.

Tumour necrosis factor α (TNFα) is a proinflammatory cytokine secreted by macrophages. It has a pivotal role in proinflammatory processes. The anti-TNFα agents etanercept, adalimumab, infliximab and certolizumab pegol are all approved by NICE. Other drugs that are also licensed, but not approved for use on the National Health Service, include abatacept and the anti-interleukin-6 agent tocilizumab.

Biologic therapies are delivered according to specific guidance that requires two other drugs to have been used first, one of which must be methotrexate. The anti-B-cell agent rituximab is used in combination with methotrexate in patients who have failed anti-TNFα therapy. The criteria for use are under constant review and differ between countries.

Surgery

The improvements in medical therapy have reduced the need for joint replacement surgery in patients with rheumatoid arthritis. Nevertheless, surgery is often needed at some point to correct deformities and replace damaged joints.

Note

The National Collaborating Centre for Chronic Conditions. Rheumatoid Arthritis: National Clinical Guideline for Management and Treatment in Adults. Royal College of Physicians, 2009.

Note

Saag KG, Teng GC, Patkar NM, *et al*. American College of Rheumatology 2008 recommendations for the use of nonbiologic and biologic disease-modifying antirheumatic drugs in rheumatoid arthritis. *Arthritis Rheum* 2008; 59: 762-84.

Spondyloarthropathies

The spondyloarthropathies (SpAs) are a group of disorders characterised by sacroiliitis, peripheral arthritis (mainly lower limb, large joint and asymmetric), absence of rheumatoid factor, enthesitis and an association with human leukocyte antigen (HLA)-B27.

EULAR defines five broad types of SpA:

- Ankylosing spondylitis (AS).
- Psoriatic SpA.
- Inflammatory bowel disease-associated SpA.
- Reactive SpA.
- Undifferentiated SpA.

Epidemiology

The overall prevalence of the SpAs is 0.5% (one in 200), with some ethnic variation (Table 10.2).

Table 10.2. Prevalence of the spondyloarthropathies in various countries.

Ethnicity	Prevalence	HLA-B27 positivity (%)
Norway	1.1-1.4	16
UK	0.2	8
Japan	0.04	<1
Haida Indians	6	50

The incidence is approximately seven people per 100,000 per year.

The gender ratio is 3:1 (men to women) and the peak age of onset is 20-40 years. The mean age at diagnosis is 33 years and there is a mean diagnostic delay of 7 years.

For a diagnosis of 'inflammatory' back pain, four out of the five following criteria have to be positive.

- Onset at age <40 years.
- Symptoms >3 months.
- Insidious onset.
- Early morning stiffness lasting for >60 minutes.
- Improvement of pain with exercise.

Clinical features

Enthesitis (inflammation at the bone tendon junction) is a cardinal feature of SpA and may be the initiating event in this inflammatory arthritis.

Sites of enthesopathy include the sacroiliac joints, spinal ligaments, manubriosternal joint, symphysis pubis, iliac crests, trochanters, patellae, clavicles and calcanei. Synovitis also occurs and the peripheral arthritis is usually an asymmetric, large-joint oligoarthritis (30% of patients). Joints commonly involved include the hips, shoulders and sternoclavicular, temporomandibular and cricoarytenoid joints. Dactylitis (sausage fingers or toes) may be present.

Ankylosing spondylitis

The British Society for Rheumatology recommends using the modified New York criteria for diagnosis of AS. For a definitive diagnosis, radiological change with at least one clinical criterion is required. For a probable diagnosis, either radiological change must be identified or all three clinical criteria met.

Clinical criteria:

- Low back pain for >3 months, improved by exercise but not relieved by rest.

- Limitation of lumbar spine movement in both the sagittal and frontal planes.
- Limitation of chest expansion relative to normal for sex and age.

Radiological criterion:

- Sacroiliitis on X-ray.

Investigation

Haematological investigations at onset are similar to those for rheumatoid arthritis. Patients may have normocytic or normochromic anaemia. Inflammatory markers (erythrocyte sedimentation rate, C-reactive protein or viscosity) are normal in a third of patients. Radiology includes sacroiliac and lumbar spine views, with thoracic and cervical spinal films if symptomatic (Ferguson oblique views are necessary). MRI scanning with short tau inversion recovery sequences may be required for the sacroiliac joints if plain X-ray is not diagnostic.

HLA-B27 is also checked. It has a prevalence of 10% in the white UK population and 90% of patients with AS are HLA-B27 positive. An HLA-B27-positive individual has a 50-100 times increased relative risk of developing AS, and HLA-B27-negative AS patients may have a more benign disease course. The presence of HLA-B27 is associated with extra-articular manifestations of AS such as ocular involvement (Table 10.3).

People with AS have an increased prevalence of fractures and osteoporosis occurs in 10-20% of patients with a relative risk of 6-8. Osteoporosis mostly involves the thoracic spine, with contributing factors of inflammation and reduced mobility. Bone mineral densitometry should be performed in all patients.

Prognosis

Maximal deterioration occurs during the first 10 years of disease and the severity correlates with peripheral arthritis and spinal radiographic change. Untreated there is significant disability, and 80% of patients have daily pain and stiffness after 20 years of disease.

Table 10.3. Extra-articular manifestations of ankylosing spondylitis.

	Manifestations
A	Aortic regurgitation, ascending aortitis, conduction defects, diastolic dysfunction and pericarditis (10% of patients)
N	Neurological: atlantoaxial subluxation and cauda equina syndrome
K	Kidney: secondary amyloidosis and chronic prostatitis
S	Spine: cervical fracture, spinal stenosis, significant spinal osteoporosis
P	Pulmonary: upper-lobe fibrosis, restrictive defect
O	Ocular: anterior uveitis (25-30% of patients)
N	Nephropathy (immunoglobulin A)
D	Discitis

Note

Barlow JH, Wright CC, Williams B, Keat A. Work disability among patients with ankylosing spondylitis. *Arthritis Rheum* 2001; 45: 424-9. **This study found that 31% of those with AS were unable to work.**

The standardised mortality ratio is 1.5. The causes of death are amyloidosis, spinal fracture, cardiovascular disease, gastrointestinal bleeding, renal involvement or pulmonary disease.

Note

Lehtinen K. Mortality and causes of death in 398 patients admitted to hospital with ankylosing spondylitis. *Ann Rheum* 1993; 52: 174-6.

Management

It is important for the patient to have the support of a multidisciplinary team, delivering physiotherapy, hydrotherapy, orthotics (footwear), occupational therapy and psychological support.

The NSAIDs, both conventional (e.g., naproxen, diclofenac) and cyclo-oxygenase-2 selective (e.g., etoricoxib), provide some symptom control and may have a disease-modifying role if used continuously. The disease-modifying antirheumatic drugs (methotrexate, sulphasalazine, leflunomide) are effective for peripheral disease only; corticosteroid injections are given to peripheral joints and trigger points.

The anti-TNFα agents have revolutionised the management of AS. To be prescribed anti-TNF agents in the UK, patients must meet the AS modified New York criteria, have active disease defined by a visual analogue scale and have had a trial of NSAID therapy. Patients respond better if they have early disease and high inflammatory markers. Etanercept and infliximab increase bone mineral density in AS patients, and infliximab and adalimumab are effective for iritis.

Surgical management includes hip replacement surgery and neck surgery in advanced AS.

Note

Boonen A, Brinkhuizen T, Landewe R, *et al.* Impact of ankylosing spondylitis on sick leave, presenteeism and unpaid productivity, and estimation of the societal cost. *Ann Rheum Dis* 2010; 69: 1123-8.

Note

Wang CY, Chiang PY, Lee HS, Wei JC. The effectiveness of exercise therapy for ankylosing spondylitis: a review. *Int J Rheum Dis* 2009; 12: 207-10.

Note

Thomas GP, Brown MA. Genetics and genomics of ankylosing spondylitis. *Immunol Rev* 2010; 233: 162-80.

Psoriatic arthritis

Psoriatic arthritis is considered with the SpAs even though the pathogenic pathway between psoriasis and arthritis is unknown, and the condition is heterogeneous with some overlapping features with rheumatoid arthritis.

Psoriatic arthritis occurs in approximately 10% of patients with psoriasis. There is a link to the severity of skin disease and the presence of nail disease, but only a weak temporal relationship between severity of disease affecting the joints and skin. Furthermore, patients may have a disease typical of psoriatic arthritis without any apparent skin disease.

Patterns of disease

The following patterns of disease may appear in psoriatic arthritis – they are not mutually exclusive and may evolve with time:

- Oligoarticular.
- Polyarticular (rheumatoid-like).
- Spondylitis – more asymmetrical than in AS; there may also be more florid paraspinal ossification and new bone formation further away from the vertebrae (paramarginal syndesmophytes).
- Mutilating arthritis – a very severe destructive disease with both axial and peripheral involvement.
- Predominant distal interphalangeal joint disease.

Radiological features

There is greater asymmetry in the peripheral joints than in rheumatoid arthritis. Osteolysis (i.e., complete resorption of bone) may occur, causing 'pencil-in-cup' deformity and fluffy periosteal new bone around involved joints. Joint fusion may be seen.

Management

The disease-modifying agents sulphasalazine, methotrexate and leflunomide are most commonly used in management. The anti-TNF-α agents, etanercept and adalimumab, are licensed and approved for this indication by NICE in the UK.

Note

Pipitone N, Kingsley GH, Manzo A, *et al.* Current concepts and new developments in the treatment of psoriatic arthritis. *Rheumatology* (Oxford) 2003; 42: 1138-48.

Note

Sterry W, Ortonne JP, Kirkham B, *et al.* Comparison of two etanercept regimes for treatment of psoriasis and psoriatic arthritis: PRESTA randomised double blind multicentre trial. *BMJ* 2010; 340: c147.

Inflammatory bowel disease-associated spondyloarthritis

Up to 60% of patients with AS have inflammation on ileocolonoscopy and up to 25% of patients with Crohn's disease have inflammatory arthritis. The arthritis may occur either in association with flares of inflammatory bowel disease (enteropathic arthritis) or as an independently active seronegative arthropathy.

The biologic agents infliximab and adalimumab may be effective for treating both inflammatory bowel disease and SpA.

Reactive arthritis

Reactive arthritis is triggered by a bacterial or viral infection. Gut infections (e.g., *Salmonella*) and sexually acquired infections (e.g., *Chlamydia*) are common triggers. *Streptococcus* or parvovirus may also trigger arthritis. The joint inflammation may be accompanied by inflammation of the eye (conjunctivitis), rash, urethritis, diarrhoea and mouth ulcers. The triad of joint inflammation, urethritis and eye inflammation is termed Reiter's syndrome. The skin may also be involved, with scaly patches on the genitalia or the sole of the foot (keratoderma blennorrhagica).

The joints involved are usually the lower limbs (knees, ankles or toes), but upper limb joints and the spine may also be involved. As in other seronegative arthropathies, the tendons (e.g., Achilles) may be involved. Tendon involvement in the fingers and toes causes swelling, leading to the appearance known as 'sausage digits'.

Management
- Antibiotics to treat the initial triggering infection, if persistent.
- Symptom control (e.g., NSAIDs, analgesia).
- Disease-modifying agents for persistent arthropathy (e.g., steroids locally or systemically and sulphasalazine).

In 85% of patients the condition is self-limiting, lasting for up to 6 months. More persistent disease may occur, however, particularly if the patient is positive for HLA-B27.

Undifferentiated spondyloarthropathy

Undifferentiated SpA is when the symptoms and signs do not match a specific disease pattern. Some of these patients may develop a classic pattern in due course, but in others a specific diagnosis may not be achieved. Management is largely directed at symptom control.

Juvenile idiopathic arthritis

Juvenile idiopathic arthritis (JIA) occurs in children younger than 16 years. Symptoms may be non-specific initially, including lethargy, flu-like symptoms, reduced physical activity and poor appetite. Limping may occur.

The knees, ankles, wrists and small joints of the hands and feet are most commonly involved. Swelling may be difficult to detect clinically, especially for joints such as those of the spine, sacroiliac joints, shoulder, hip and jaw, where imaging techniques such as ultrasound or MRI are very useful.

Pain and morning stiffness occur, but young children may have difficulty in communicating this. The late effects of arthritis include joint contracture and joint damage.

The three major types of JIA are oligoarticular, polyarticular and systemic.

Oligoarticular (pauciarticular) JIA

Oligoarticular JIA accounts for about 50% of JIA cases. It affects four or fewer joints in the first 6 months of illness. Antinuclear antibody positivity is more likely than in other types of JIA.

It usually involves the knees, ankles and elbows, but smaller joints such as those of the fingers and toes may also be affected. The hip is not affected. The condition is usually asymmetrical.

Chronic iridocyclitis or uveitis is a feature that often goes unnoticed. These children should be closely monitored by an ophthalmologist or optometrist.

Polyarticular JIA

Polyarticular JIA accounts for about 40% of JIA cases. It affects five or more joints in the first 6 months of disease. The smaller joints are usually affected, such as those of the fingers and hands, although weight-bearing joints such as the knees, hips, ankles, neck and jaw may also be affected. The joints affected are usually symmetrical.

Polyarticular JIA is more common in girls than boys. Chronic iridocyclitis or uveitis may occur and rheumatoid factor may be positive.

Systemic JIA

Systemic JIA accounts for about 10% of JIA cases. It is characterised by arthritis, fever and a salmon-pink rash. Unlike the other two subtypes of JIA, it affects girls and boys equally.

Systemic JIA may have internal organ involvement and lead to serositis (e.g., pericarditis). It is closely related to adult-onset Still's disease.

Extra-articular features and complications

JIA is a chronic disorder that if neglected can lead to serious complications.

Joint deformities
Children who delay treatment or do not participate in physical therapy often develop joint deformities of the hand and fingers. Over time, hand function is lost and is almost impossible to recover.

Eye disease
Iridocyclitis affects about one child in five with JIA and can lead to permanent eye damage, including blindness. This complication may be asymptomatic and requires regular screening by an ophthalmologist using a slit lamp. It is most common in girls.

Growth disturbance
Children with JIA may have a reduced overall rate of growth, especially if the disease involves many joints or other body systems. Individually affected large joints (e.g., the knee) may grow faster due to an inflammation-induced increased blood supply to the bone growth plates situated near the joints. Corticosteroids may affect overall growth.

Management

The multidisciplinary team approach is particularly important. The major emphasis of management is to help the child regain normal levels of physical and social activities. This is accomplished with the use of physical therapy, pain management strategies and social support.

Most children are treated with NSAIDs and intra-articular corticosteroid injections. Methotrexate is the most effective disease-modifying drug and anti-TNFα blockers, particularly etanercept, are increasingly being used.

Surgery is only used to treat the most severe cases of JIA.

Note

Weiss JE, Ilowite NT. Juvenile idiopathic arthritis. *Rheum Dis Clin North Am* 2007; 33: 441-70.

Note

Lovell DJ, Reiff A, Ilowite NT, *et al.* Safety and efficacy of up to eight years of continuous etanercept therapy in patients with juvenile rheumatoid arthritis. *Arthritis Rheum* 2008; 58: 1496-504.

Connective tissue diseases

These conditions are rarely the primary reason for orthopaedic intervention, although they may cause considerable musculoskeletal pain (polyarthralgia).

Sjögren's syndrome

Described in 1933 by the Swedish ophthalmologist, Henrik Sjögren, Sjögren's syndrome is probably the most common of the connective tissue diseases. It may occur as a primary disorder or secondary to other rheumatic diseases, especially rheumatoid arthritis. It is characterised by dry eyes and mouth, caused by inflammation and damage to tear and salivary glands (sicca symptoms), as well as polyarthralgia, muscular aching and fatigue. The salivary glands may become visibly swollen.

It occurs most mostly in women between the ages of 40 and 60 years, with a 10:1 female to male ratio. Viruses (e.g., Epstein-Barr virus, retroviruses) may trigger the syndrome in genetically susceptible people.

The antinuclear antibodies anti-Ro and anti-La are present in some patients. These may be linked to complete heart block in the babies of women with the syndrome.

Rare sequelae include peripheral neuropathy and lung fibrosis. The risk of non-Hodgkin's B-cell lymphoma is increased in patients with the syndrome.

Management may require a multidisciplinary team, including a rheumatologist, ophthalmologist and dentist. Topical lubricants can be used for the sicca symptoms, and hydroxychloroquine and occasionally prednisolone for the polyarthralgia.

Note

Voulgarelis M, Skopouli FN. Clinical, immunologic, and molecular factors predicting lymphoma development in Sjögren's syndrome patients. *Clin Rev Allergy Immunol* 2007; 32: 265-74.

Systemic lupus erythematosus

Systemic lupus erythematosus (SLE) is a diverse condition, varying in organ involvement and severity. It mainly affects young women (age range 10-50 years), particularly black (one in 250-500), followed by South Asians and then white (one in 4,000) women. The main symptoms of lupus include a facial rash, joint pain, Raynaud's phenomenon (impaired circulation in fingers and toes on exposure to cold) and abnormal sensitivity to sunlight on exposed skin. Patients may also experience fever, weight loss, lymphadenopathy, mouth ulceration and hair thinning.

Approximately one in three people develop glomerulonephritis. Inflammation of the pleura or pericardium may occur, causing pleurisy or pericarditis. The condition may also affect the bone marrow, depressing haemoglobin, white cell or platelet counts. Patients are at a significantly increased risk of vascular disease and thrombosis may occur, particularly if anti-phospholipid antibodies are present.

Approximately 95% of patients with SLE are positive for the antinuclear antibody, although healthy people can also have this antibody. Double-stranded DNA is more specific to SLE and its level may correlate with disease activity. Anti-Ro-positivity may occur and overlapping features with Sjögren's syndrome are more likely in these patients. A low complement level (C3 or C4) correlates with SLE activity.

Patients with SLE are treated with hydroxychloroquine for the joint manifestations and rash, with corticosteroids and immunosuppressive medications (including azathioprine, methotrexate, mycophenolate mofetil, cyclophosphamide and rituximab) for more serious organ involvement.

Note

Rahman A, Isenberg DA. Systemic lupus erythematosus. *N Engl J Med* 2008; 358: 929-39.

Scleroderma

The term 'scleroderma' means hard skin, but the condition may affect the connective tissues surrounding the joints, blood vessels and internal organs. It is uncommon, affects women more often than men (4:1) and usually begins between the ages of 25 and 50 years. It may be localised (termed 'morphoea'), just affecting an area of skin, or systemic, affecting the blood vessels, joints, any part of the gut and occasionally the lungs, heart, kidneys and muscles.

Scleroderma is a variable, gradual and long-term disorder. It may start slowly, with the patient gradually deteriorating and then stabilising. Raynaud's phenomenon can be very severe, resulting in digital ischaemia. Patients may experience synovitis and digestive problems due to weakness of the oesophagus or involvement of both the small and large bowel. Other symptoms are pulmonary fibrosis, pulmonary hypertension, accelerated atherosclerosis and renal disease.

Antinuclear antibodies may be positive, with various specificities linked to disease patterns. Blood pressure monitoring and annual pulmonary function tests and echocardiography are routinely used to monitor the condition.

Frequent reviews and multidisciplinary involvement specific to the needs of the patient are particularly important. Individual manifestations are treated with specific therapies (e.g., angiotensin-converting enzyme inhibitors in hypertension). Evidence for agents with an overall benefit in modifying the disease remains poor, although specific aspects of scleroderma are being treated more effectively. Mycophenolate mofetil may have a role in modifying skin disease. Cyclophosphamide is used for active pulmonary fibrosis; vasodilators for severe Raynaud's disease (iloprost, sildenafil); and endothelin antagonists and vasodilators for pulmonary hypertension.

Note

Gabrielli A, Avvedimento EV, Krieg T. Scleroderma. *N Engl J Med* 2009; 360: 1989-2003.

Crystal arthropathies

The crystal arthropathies can cause joint damage and accelerate the need for joint replacement surgery.

Gout

Gout is the most common crystal arthropathy, affecting around 1-2% of the Western population. It presents with an intensely painful arthritis, which usually begins overnight. Men are most often affected and gout is rare in women before the menopause. Gout has increased in frequency in recent decades, related to risk factors in the population such as the metabolic syndrome, longer life expectancy and changes in diet. With time the attacks become more frequent, involve greater numbers of joints and may cause joint damage.

The metatarsophalangeal joint at the base of the big toe is the most commonly affected joint (being involved in around half of all cases), but gout may involve the ankles, knees, finger joints and wrists. It may be accompanied by a fever, and infection should be excluded.

Gout is caused by elevated levels of urate in the blood. These crystallise and are deposited in the joints, tendons and surrounding tissues. Renal underexcretion occurs in about 90% of patients, with overproduction of urate in less than 10%. Longstanding hyperuricemia may result in tophi. Elevated levels of urate may also lead to crystals precipitating in the kidneys, resulting in stone formation and a urate nephropathy.

Diagnosis is confirmed clinically by the visualisation of the crystals in joint fluid. Plasma urate may be suppressed during an acute attack of gout.

Management
Gout can be prevented and effectively cured in the majority of patients.

NSAIDs, steroids or colchicine improve the symptoms. Modification of other medications, (e.g., diuretics) may help.

Lifestyle changes are recommended, including weight loss and a reduced intake of alcohol, fructose-sweetened drinks, meat and seafood.

Drugs to lower urate levels

The xanthine-oxidase inhibitor, allopurinol, is the mainstay of treatment. The uricosuric agents, probenecid and sulphinpyrazone, provide long-term prevention in some patients. Benzbromarone with liver function monitoring is used in some countries. Febuxostat has recently been approved by NICE in the UK, but its use is cautioned in those with cardiovascular disease pending further data.

Rapid changes in urate may precipitate an attack of gout. Patient education, NSAIDs, colchicine or steroids for symptom relief are vital when initiating treatment.

> **Note**
>
> Chen LX, Schumacher HR. Gout: an evidence-based review. *J Clin Rheumatol* 2008; 14(Suppl.): S55-62.

> **Note**
>
> Schlesinger N. Diagnosing and treating gout: a review to aid primary care physicians. *Postgrad Med* 2010; 122: 157-61.

> **Note**
>
> Terkeltaub R. Update on gout: new therapeutic strategies and options. *Nat Rev Rheumatol* 2010; 6: 30-8.

Pseudogout and calcium crystal diseases

Calcium pyrophosphate dihydrate disease is caused by the accumulation of calcium pyrophosphate dihydrate crystals in the connective tissues. 'Pseudogout' refers to the acute symptoms of synovitis resembling acute gout.

Chondrocalcinosis refers to the radiographic evidence of calcification in hyaline or fibrocartilage. Pyrophosphate arthropathy is a term that refers to pseudogout.

The knees, wrists, and hips are the most commonly affected areas in crystal diseases and women are more often affected than men (1.4:1). Often no trigger is identified, but an injury or intercurrent illness may trigger an attack.

Hyperparathyroidism, haemochromatosis, hypophosphataemia, renal osteodystrophy and Wilson's disease may be associated with chondrocalcinosis.

Diagnosis of pseudogout is by evaluating joint fluid, which shows rhombus-shaped, positively birefringent crystals. Plain X-rays show chondrocalcinosis.

Intra-articular corticosteroid injection, systemic corticosteroids, NSAIDs or colchicine may be used in treatment.

Chapter 11 Arthrodesis and amputation

Arthrodesis

Hip

Hip arthrodesis (fusion) has been carried out for over 100 years for infection, arthritis and hip dysplasia. Hip arthrodesis can be achieved by intra-articular or extra-articular techniques, or a combination of the two. Internal fixation to achieve union was first proposed by Watson-Jones and Charnley.

> **Note**
>
> Morris JB. Charnley compression arthrodesis of the hip. *J Bone Joint Surg Br* 1966; 48: 260-79.

In modern practice hip arthrodesis is a rare operation, although it may be indicated in young people with advanced arthritis who are involved in heavy labour. A normal lumbar spine, contralateral hip and ipsilateral knee are prerequisites. Active sepsis is a contraindication.

The recommended position for hip arthrodesis is 30° of flexion, 0-5° of adduction and 0-15° of external rotation. Abduction and internal rotation should be avoided.

Various techniques have been described for hip arthrodesis:

- Debridement of the joint and fixation with transacetabular cancellous screws. A subtrochanteric osteotomy can be performed at the same time.
- Application of a cobra plate to the lateral aspect of the femur, fixed to the outer surface of the ilium. A greater trochanter osteotomy is performed to elevate the abductors to preserve abductor function. After plate fixation the greater trochanter is reattached to the femur over the plate. The distal end of the plate may act as a stress riser.
- Fixation after arthrodesis is performed with a dynamic compression screw and supplemented by cancellous screws.

Conversion of hip arthrodesis to total hip arthroplasty is associated with a high risk of complications, including infection and poor mobility. Total knee arthroplasty for knee pain after hip arthrodesis should be performed after conversion of the arthrodesis to arthroplasty. Knee replacement below a hip arthrodesis has a poor outcome.

Knee

With the reliability and success of knee arthroplasty, knee arthrodesis is an increasingly rare operation. Historically, the indications included gross instability, tuberculosis of the knee, pyogenic infection and neuropathic joints. They were also sometimes performed in young patients with arthritic knees who were involved in heavy manual work.

Most of these situations are now managed by knee arthroplasty. Failed knee arthroplasty with extensive bone loss or recurrent infection is now the most common indication for knee arthrodesis. Other indications include a grossly unstable knee in a young patient or a neuropathic joint.

A successful knee arthrodesis alleviates pain, but imposes significant limitations in mobility and the ability to perform activities of daily living. A preoperative trial using a long leg cast for 2-3 weeks is sometimes recommended to emphasise the limitations following knee arthrodesis.

A relatively normal contralateral limb is essential to allow optimum mobility after knee arthrodesis. Contralateral knee disease and ipsilateral hip or ankle disease are contraindications to this procedure.

The recommended position for knee arthrodesis is 10-15° of flexion and physiological valgus (3-5°).

Several techniques have been proposed to achieve arthrodesis:

- External fixator.
- Compression plate.
- Intramedullary nail.

External fixators

In the early days of the technique, external fixators were effectively used by Sir John Charnley, achieving 98.5% union using a pin above and below the knee connected to clamps on either side. Problems included pin-site infections and difficulty mobilising.

More recently, ring fixators have been used to stabilise fusions. Extensive bone loss results in shortening, and compressing with a fixator accentuates the problem. However, ring fixators can be used in conjunction with debridement in patients with ongoing sepsis. It is possible to adjust the alignment postoperatively with external fixators.

Note

Charnley J, Lowe HG. A study of the end-results of compression arthrodesis of the knee. *J Bone Joint Surg Br* 1958; 40: 633-5.

Compression plates

Compression plates can be used when the knee is opened for debridement, using the same exposure for stabilising the arthrodesis with one or two plates. Two plates at right angles or a medial and lateral plate can be used. The plates should be staggered to avoid a stress riser at the end of the plate. Wound closure can be difficult due to the added bulk of the plates. Weight bearing is restricted until the fusion is solid.

Intramedullary rods

Intramedullary rods provide reliable fixation without the problems associated with external fixation. They allow debridement and nail insertion, with early weight bearing.

The nails can be a long intramedullary nail or comprise a separate femoral and tibial nail connected at the level of the knee joint. Long intramedullary nails can be locked proximally and distally for added stability, but have the same diameter throughout, which means a relatively narrow nail in the femoral segment. Using separate femoral and tibial nails has the advantage of using different diameters for the two segments, but the disadvantage of difficult removal if required. Removal in this situation requires opening a window in the bone at the arthrodesis site and cutting the nail with a metal burr.

Ankle

The common indications for ankle arthrodesis include post-traumatic arthritis, rheumatoid arthritis, chronic infections, neuromuscular conditions, tumours around the ankle and failed ankle replacement. Restriction of hind foot movement after ankle arthrodesis makes walking on uneven surfaces difficult.

The recommended position for ankle arthrodesis is 0° of flexion, 0-5° of valgus and 5-10° of external rotation.

The surgical technique should allow thick skin flaps, a large cancellous surface for contact, rigid internal fixation and optimum alignment. The approach can be anterior through the sheath of tibialis anterior, transmalleolar, transfibular or posterior. The joint surfaces are denuded and fixation can be with an external fixator, cancellous screws or intramedullary rod.

Arthroscopic ankle arthrodesis is increasingly popular as it creates minimal soft tissue disruption and better cosmesis. The technique is useful in patients with minimal deformity. Success rates of 80% have been reported in most series.

In patients with severe deformity an open technique is the gold standard, but success has been reported with arthroscopic techniques.

Note

Smith R, Wood PL. Arthrodesis of the ankle in the presence of a large deformity in the coronal plane. *J Bone Joint Surg Br* 2007; 89: 615-9. **The researchers performed open fusion using compression screws in a consecutive series of 23 patients (25 ankles). Primary union was achieved in 24 ankles.**

Note

Gougoulias NE, Agathangelidis FG, Parsons SW. Arthroscopic ankle arthrodesis. *Foot Ankle Int* 2007; 28: 695-706. **Arthroscopic ankle arthrodesis was performed in 30 ankles with more than 15° deformity. A good outcome was reported in 80% of the ankles.**

Shoulder

Shoulder arthrodesis has been used for over 100 years for the management of chronic shoulder infections. Extra-articular arthrodesis was initially proposed to reduce the risk of infection, and Charnley devised an external fixator with pins in the proximal humerus and the acromion to achieve compression.

The success of shoulder arthroplasty and stabilisation procedures has led to a reduction in arthrodesis procedures. The current indications for arthrodesis are paralytic disorders, brachial plexus injury, massive cuff tears, tumours around the shoulder and failed shoulder arthroplasty. Chronic infections in the shoulder can also be managed with arthrodesis. The optimum position for arthrodesis is 25-40° of abduction, 20-30° of flexion and 25-30° of internal rotation.

A contoured plate along the spine of the scapula, acromion and proximal humerus provides stable support following arthrodesis.

Elbow

Elbow arthrodesis is indicated in patients with chronic infections or post-traumatic arthritis, and in severely comminuted fractures in young patients. Elbow arthroplasty provides good function, but limited long-term survival of the implant makes arthrodesis a viable option in younger patients.

The optimum position for arthrodesis is individualised to the needs of the patient and varies from 70° to 90° of flexion.

Arthrodesis is performed by debridement of the joint and bone grafting. Cancellous screws or plates and external fixators can be used to stabilise the arthrodesis until bone healing.

Wrist

Wrist arthrodesis is indicated for post-traumatic arthritis in young patients, chronic infection, tumours, paralytic disorders and failed wrist arthroplasty. It is contraindicated in patients with an open physis (i.e., aged <17 years).

The optimum position for wrist arthrodesis is 10-20° of extension, with the long axis of the third metacarpal lined up with the long axis of the radius in the sagittal plane. Dorsiflexion improves grip strength.

The preferred method of arthrodesis is iliac crest bone grafting along with internal fixation with a plate.

Amputation

The aim of amputation is to remove diseased or non-functional parts of an extremity to reduce morbidity and mortality, and enable restoration of function.

Indications for amputations are as follows:

- Peripheral vascular disease – irreversible ischaemia in a limb is an absolute indication for amputation.
- Trauma with an insensate limb.
- Uncontrolled infection.
- Thermal injury – burns or frostbite.
- Tumour.
- Congenital anomalies.

Peripheral vascular disease is the most common indication for amputation. Revascularisation techniques may avoid the need for amputation and an assessment must be made for this possibility. Infection should be treated and the nutritional status optimised prior to amputation.

Table 11.1. The Mangled Extremity Severity Score (MESS). A score >7 indicates a high likelihood of amputation; ≤6 correlates with a salvageable limb.

Feature	Score
Skeletal soft tissue injury	
Low-energy injury	1
Medium-energy injury	2
High-energy injury	3
Very high-energy injury	4
Limb ischaemia	
Pulse reduced, but normal perfusion	1
Pulseless, reduced capillary refill	2
Cool, paralysed, insensate	3
Shock	
Systolic blood pressure >90mmHg	1
Transient hypotension	2
Persistent hypotension	3
Age	
<30 years	1
30-50 years	2
>50 years	3

An irreparable vascular injury as a result of trauma and an insensate foot due to tibial nerve injury are indications for amputation. The Mangled Extremity Severity Score (MESS) (Table 11.1) helps physicians to make an objective decision as to whether limb salvage is worthwhile.

A score of greater than 7 indicates a high likelihood of amputation. A score of 6 or less correlates with a salvageable limb. The decision to amputate or salvage is based on multiple factors, including the extent of the injury, the feasibility of reconstruction, the expected function after salvage, the cost and time involved in salvage and, importantly, the views of the patient.

Note

Johansen K, Daines M, Howey T, *et al.* Objective criteria accurately predict amputation following lower extremity trauma. *J Trauma* 1990; 30: 568-72. **A retrospective study of 25 patients and prospective application of the MESS in 26 patients. A score of more than 7 was 100% predictive of amputation.**

Burns are managed with immediate aggressive debridement and amputation as necessary. Frostbite is managed by rewarming and pain management in the initial stage. Amputation is delayed by 2-6 months until demarcation is clear.

Patient assessment

Locally, signs of impaired circulation are a weak or absent pulse, reduced skin temperature and reduced transcutaneous oxygen tension. The ankle-brachial index indicates the healing potential of lower limbs and an arteriogram will demonstrate the distal circulation.

A thorough evaluation of the general condition of the patient is carried out. Laboratory tests include a haematocrit, white cell count and serum albumin levels. The serum albumin level should be higher than 3.5g/dL and the total lymphocyte count higher than 1,500 cells/ml.

Glycaemic control is instituted and cardiac and renal functions are assessed. The nutritional condition of the patient should be assessed and deficiencies corrected as needed. Preoperative counselling and the use of support groups are helpful for early rehabilitation.

Surgical technique

The level of amputation is decided based on a balance between the preservation of useful limb and the removal of non-functional limb. A proximal level allows disease clearance, while a more distal level allows better function. Transtibial amputations allow better walking speed and greater energy efficiency than transfemoral amputations.

The optimum amputation level for the tibia is a minimum of 2.5cm for each foot of height of the patient. Commonly, it is 12.5-15cm below the medial joint line of the tibia. Amputations in the lower third of the leg have poor soft tissue cover and are avoided. Transfemoral amputations are planned in the middle third of the femur. A minimum of 15cm space should be allowed above the knee joint for fitting the prosthesis.

Transradial amputations are planned at the junction of the proximal two-thirds and distal third of the forearm. Transhumeral amputations are performed in the mid-third of the arm.

The skin flaps should be marked out, and the combined length of the flaps should be slightly more than the diameter of the planned stump. The base of the flaps should be level with the bone resection (Figure 11.1). The flaps should be full thickness. The scar should not adhere to the underlying bone.

In ischaemic limbs, the posterior flap in the leg is long and the anterior flap is kept short to maximise the blood supply to the suture line (Figure 11.2).

Neuromas can be reduced by avoiding injury to the nerves and dividing them with a sharp knife. The major vessels are ligated and haemostasis achieved. A suction drain is inserted and skin closure is achieved without tension.

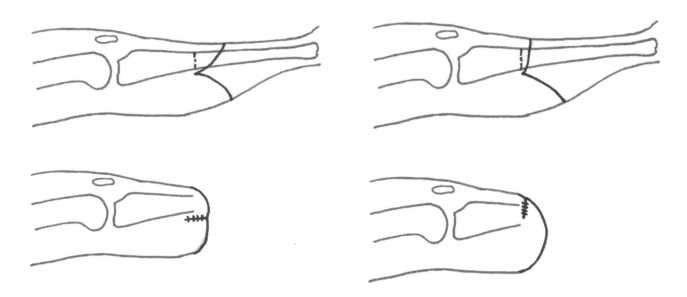

Figure 11.1. The base of the skin flaps are level with the bone resection and the lengths of the flaps should be sufficient to achieve closure.

Figure 11.2. Planning flaps in the ischaemic limb keeping a long posterior flap.

Postoperatively, compression dressings are provided and the avoidance of contractures is paramount through patient education and physiotherapy. Early prosthetic fitting is the goal, and a definitive cast for prosthesis can be provided once the stump is mature.

Complications

Early complications after amputation include haematoma, infection and necrosis of the skin margin. Infections are more common in those with diabetes and peripheral vascular disease.

Late complications are contractures, neuroma formation and phantom limb pain. Residual limb pain is often due to a poorly fitting cast and can be addressed by altering the cast to avoid pressure. Phantom sensation is very common and gradually resolves (known as 'telescoping'). Phantom pain is less common and is difficult to treat.

Children undergoing amputation may experience terminal bone overgrowth. This is due to appositional growth at the end of the bone. It is common in the humerus and the fibula and in severe cases may penetrate the skin, requiring excision.

Prosthetics

A prosthesis is a replacement of a body part. A limb prosthesis has the following components:

- Socket – the interface between the prosthesis and the stump.
- Suspension system – to hold the socket in place.
- Joint mechanism.
- Terminal device – for example, a foot or hand.

Chapter 12 Disorders in children

Legg-Calvé-Perthes disease

Legg-Calvé-Perthes (LCP) disease is idiopathic avascular necrosis (AVN) of the femoral head in childhood.

The condition was initially described by Professor Henning Waldenström in 1909, who thought the condition was a form of tuberculosis of the hip. Soon after, in 1910, Arthur Legg (from the USA), Jacques Calvé (France) and Georg Perthes (Germany) independently described the same disease, proposing that it was not tuberculosis.

Epidemiology

The annual prevalence is 5-10 per 100,000 children per year. There is a well-described regional variation in the UK: the prevalence is 5.5 per 100,000 in Wessex and 11.1 per 100,000 in Liverpool.

LCP disease is more common in the following:

- Temperate climates.
- White people, as opposed to black people.
- Passive smokers (odds ratio 5.3).
- Those with short stature.
- Those with delayed bone age.

Children aged 4-8 years are usually affected, but the age range can vary from 2 to 12 years. Boys are four to five times more commonly affected than girls.

The disease is bilateral in 10% of patients, although both sides usually do not present at the same time.

LCP disease is generally not related to irritable hip. Only 3% children with a single episode of irritable hip go on to develop LCP disease. Recurrent irritable hip may, however, constitute a risk factor, especially if associated with delayed bone age.

> **Note**
>
> Keenan WN, Clegg J. Perthes' disease after 'irritable hip': delayed bone age shows the hip is a 'marked man'. *J Pediatr Orthop* 1996; 16: 20-3. **This study looked at 13 children with recurrent irritable hip. Only those with more than 2 years delay in bone age were found to be in an early stage of Perthes disease.**

Aetiology

The underlying cause is ischaemia of variable duration. This is followed by a repair process that leads to femoral head deformity. Several causes of the initial ischaemia have been proposed:

In the thrombophilia theory, the ischaemia is believed to be the result of a coagulation disorder:

- Deficiency of protein C.
- Deficiency of protein S.
- Resistance to activated protein C.
- Increased activated partial thromboplastin time.

The vascular theory postulates that repeated occlusion of the lateral circumflex femoral artery leads to LCP disease. This may also explain the delayed bone age.

In the hormonal theory, it is thought that abnormal levels of insulin-like growth factor binding-protein 3 may be responsible for the disease.

> **Note**
>
> Hresko MT, McDougall PA, Gorlin JB, *et al.* Prospective reevaluation of the association between thrombotic diathesis and Legg-Perthes disease. *J Bone Joint Surg Am* 2002; 84-A: 1613-8. **This prospective study comprising consecutive patients found no relationship between thrombotic diathesis and Legg-Perthes disease.**

> **Note**
>
> Szepesi K, Pósán E, Hársfalvi J, *et al.* The most severe forms of Perthes disease associated with the homozygous factor V Leiden mutation. *J Bone Joint Surg Br* 2004; 86: 426-9. **This study found an association between homozygous factor V Leiden and the most severe form of LCP disease.**

Pathogenesis

The sequence of events is as follows:

- Initial stage – dense epiphysis, decalcified spots, flat uneven margins.
- Fragmentation – flat, divided, granular, dense epiphysis.
- Healing – homogenous, recalcification of epiphysis.
- Remodelling – normal growth and calcification resume in the deformed femoral head.
- Late disease – permanent residual features.

Pathology

Several pathologic changes occur:

- Inflamed synovium.
- Thickening of the articular cartilage on the medial side of the femoral head and acetabular floor.
- Distorted columns of growth-plate cartilage.
- Fragmented epiphysis.
- Metaphysis – sclerotic rimmed lesions of fibrocartilage.
- The growth plate ruptures into the adjacent tissue.
- Disruption of physis leads to a short neck and relative trochanteric overgrowth.

Natural history

After healing, the pain resolves. An elevated trochanter deformity leads to a limp. The leg-length shortening is usually less than 2cm. Most patients are symptomatic after the age of 40 years and 50% are expected to have significant arthritis by the age of 45 years.

Clinical features

- Pain in hip or knee.
- Limp – initially antalgic and later Trendelenburg due to trochanteric overgrowth and a flattened femoral head.
- On flexion, the hip goes into abduction and external rotation.
- The presence of adduction contracture is a sign of severe disease.

Differential diagnosis

If symptoms and signs are bilateral, consider hypothyroidism and spondyloepiphyseal or multiple epiphyseal dysplasia.

If the presentation is unilateral:

- Down's syndrome.
- Renal dysfunction.
- Infection – tuberculosis hip, subacute septic arthritis, osteomyelitis of the femoral neck.

- Blood disorders – sickle-cell disease, haemophilia, leukaemia.
- Eosinophilic granuloma.
- Gaucher's disease.
- Lymphoma.
- Steroid therapy, immunosuppressed patient.

Imaging

- Anteroposterior (AP) and frog-leg lateral – in abduction, flexion and external rotation of the hip. For follow-up, an AP view of the pelvis is adequate.
- AP of the wrist for bone age (optional).

- Ultrasound scan – persistent distension of the capsule for more than 6 weeks and thickened cartilage are suspicious features.
- Arthrography – to see the shape of the femoral head, containment.
- Pinhole collimated Tc-99m bone scan – to identify revascularisation.
- Magnetic resonance imaging (MRI).

Classification

Different classification systems have been proposed, of which the Catterall and Herring systems are commonly used (Table 12.1 and Figure 12.1).

Table 12.1. The Catterall and Herring classifications.

Catterall classification

I   Anterocentral:
- Visible in lateral view
- Only the anterior part of the femoral head is involved
- No collapse, loss of height, metaphyseal changes

II Centrosuperior:
- Collapse with dense sequestrum
- AP view – density between medial and lateral pillar
- Lateral view – V sign

III Centrosuperior lateral:
- Anteroposterior – head-within-head appearance on radiographs
- Broad femoral neck, metaphyseal changes

IV Whole femoral head:
- Epiphysis mushrooms anteriorly and posteriorly

Herring classification*

A   No density change or loss of height of lateral pillar
B   >50% height of lateral pillar maintained
C   <50% height of lateral pillar maintained

*   In the Herring system, the lateral pillar is defined as the lateral 15-30% of the femoral head in the anteroposterior view. The height of the lateral pillar serves as a guide to severity.

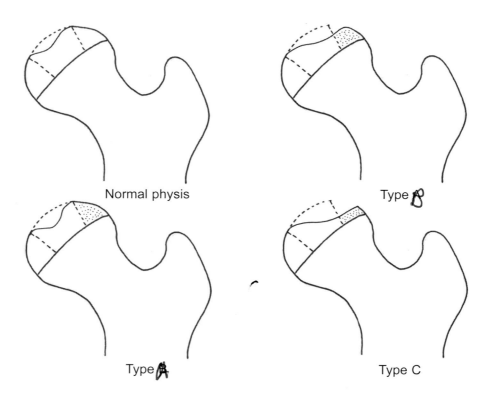

Normal physis

Type B

Type A

Type C

Figure 12.1. Herring classification for Legg-Calvé-Perthes disease.

Note

Herring JA, Kim HT, Browne R. Legg-Calvé-Perthes disease. Part I: Classification of radiographs with use of the modified lateral pillar and Stulberg classifications. *J Bone Joint Surg Am* 2004; 86-A: 2103-20. **The lateral pillar is demarcated from the femoral head by a radiolucent line of fragmentation and can be 5-30% of the head on the AP view. If there is no demarcation then the head is the lateral quarter.**

A borderline B/C group has also been defined for the Herring system:

- A very narrow lateral pillar (2-3mm) >50% height.

- A lateral pillar with very little ossification but >50% height.
- A lateral pillar exactly 50% height, depressed relative to the central pillar.

Another classification system has been proposed by Salter and Thompson, based on the crescent sign:

- Group A – less than 50% of the femoral head is involved (equivalent to Catterall groups I and II).
- Group B – more than 50% of the femoral head is involved (Catterall groups III and IV).

Stulberg has devised a classification to describe late changes in the hip joint. This system can also be used to predict arthritis (Table 12.2).

Note

Salter RB, Thompson GH. Legg-Calvé-Perthes disease. The prognostic significance of the subchondral fracture and a two-group classification of the femoral head involvement. *J Bone Joint Surg Am* 1984; 66: 479-89.

Note

Stulberg SD, Cooperman DR, Wallensten R. The natural history of Legg-Calvé-Perthes disease. *J Bone Joint Surg Am* 1981; 63: 1095-08.

Note

Herring JA, Kim HT, Browne R. Legg-Calvé-Perthes disease. Part I: Classification of radiographs with use of the modified lateral pillar and Stulberg classifications. *J Bone Joint Surg Am* 2004; 86-A: 2103-20. **Circle fit – 2mm. Less than 2mm on Mose sphericity. The widest diameter of the femoral head is drawn. The perpendicular to widest point is drawn and a circle drawn. The same diameter is used on the lateral view to examine sphericity.**

Mose proposed a sphericity measurement, whereby more than 2mm deviation from a perfect circle on the AP and lateral views is considered abnormal.

Prognostic factors

- Herring C – the strongest predictor of a poor outcome:
  - Herring A – almost all patients have a good result;
  - Herring B – two-thirds have a good result;

Table 12.2. The Stulberg classification of late changes in the hip joint and the predictability of arthritis.

Group	Description	Arthritis prediction
I	Normal articulation	Spherical head, congruous – no early arthritis
II	Spherical head but larger (coxa magna) or short neck (coxa brevis)	
III	Aspherical head – ovoid/mushroom shape + type II, not flattened	Aspherical head, congruous – moderate early arthritis
IV	Flat femoral head and abnormal neck and acetabulum	
V	Flat femoral head and normal neck and acetabulum, loss of congruence	Aspherical head, incongruous – severe early arthritis

- Herring B/C – a quarter have a good result;
- Herring C – one-eighth have a good result.
- Age of onset:
  - under 8 years – 8% have a poor result;
  - over 8 years – 26% have a poor result.
- Lateral extrusion over 20% of epiphysis indicates a poor prognosis.

Girls may have a poorer prognosis than boys, but this is not universally accepted.

Femoral head 'at-risk' signs

Clinical indicators of an at-risk femoral head include obesity, a decreasing range of movement and adduction contracture due to lateral subluxation of the head.

Radiological signs may also be seen (Figure 12.2):

- A lytic area in the lateral epiphysis and metaphysis (Gage sign) indicates hinged abduction.
- Calcification lateral to the epiphysis may be caused by ossification of the extruded head, which is mushroomed out.
- A diffuse metaphyseal reaction indicates non-ossified nests of cartilage.
- Lateral subluxation of the femoral head is caused by thick cartilage medially on the femoral head and acetabulum.
- A horizontal growth plate indicates the hip is lying in external rotation.

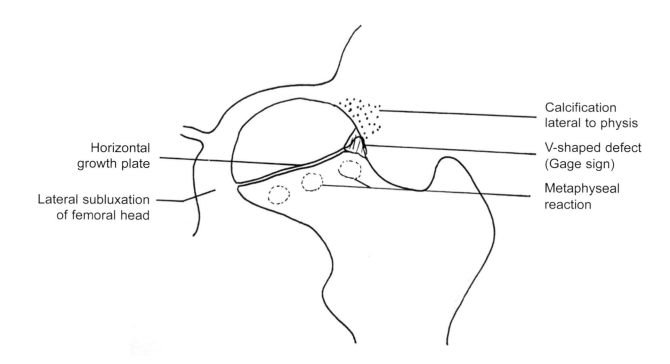

Horizontal growth plate

Lateral subluxation of femoral head

Calcification lateral to physis

V-shaped defect (Gage sign)

Metaphyseal reaction

Figure 12.2. Diagrammatic representation of radiologic femoral head 'at-risk' signs.

Management

Fifty to 60% of children have a good prognosis regardless of management. The rest will require hip replacement or hip salvage surgery when adults, usually in middle age.

The aim of management is to contain the femoral head.

Management of acute painful episodes is with short-term bed rest, traction, an abduction cast and anti-inflammatory medication (non-steroidal anti-inflammatory drugs, NSAIDs).

Bracing

Bracing (e.g., Atlanta Scottish rite brace) keeps the hip in over 30° abduction but allows flexion and extension. The brace should be worn at all times, with removal only for 1 hour for a bath and for a maximum of 3 hours for swimming in a day. An arthrogram is performed before bracing to check containment in abduction. The patient should be followed up with X-rays every 3-4 months. Bracing continues until the lateral column ossifies and sclerotic areas of epiphysis disappear.

Decreased hip movements indicate a worsening prognosis. The period in the brace varies from 3 months to 3 years. In modern practice, bracing is rarely advised.

> **Note**
>
> Herring JA, Kim HT, Browne R. Legg-Calvé-Perthes disease. Part II: Prospective multicenter study of the effect of treatment on outcome. *J Bone Joint Surg Am* 2004; 86-A: 2121-34. **Bracing was not effective in this study.**

Adductor tenotomy and Petrie cast

Adductor tenotomy addresses the tight adductors and improves abduction range. A Petrie cast keeps the knees flexed and the hips in internal rotation with a bar between the legs. Forty degree abduction is maintained at the hips. However, a cast is rarely used in modern practice.

Surgical containment

The recommendations for surgery are summarised in Table 12.3.

> **Note**
>
> Herring JA, Kim HT, Browne R. Legg-Calvé-Perthes disease. Part II: Prospective multicenter study of the effect of treatment on outcome. *J Bone Joint Surg Am* 2004; 86-A: 2121-34. **This prospective, multicentre study was started in 1984. A total of 438 patients, aged 6-12 years at disease onset, were enrolled. This amounted to 451 affected hips, and 345 hips were studied at maturity.**

Table 12.3. Recommendations for surgery based on the Herring classification.

Herring classification	Age <8 years	Age >8 years
A	No need for surgery	No need for surgery
B	No need for surgery	Surgery
B/C	No need for surgery	Surgery
C	Surgery has no effect	Surgery has no effect

Table 12.4. Comparison of femoral varus osteotomy and Salter's osteotomy.

Procedure	Indications	Notes
Femoral varus osteotomy	Age 8-10 years No leg-length discrepancy Uncovered femoral head on arthrogram Reduced angle of Wiberg	Causes additional shortening The varus remodels in 3 years The neck shaft angle should not be reduced below 115° A 20° abnormal angle is restored with growth
Salter's osteotomy	Age >6 years Full range of motion Round femoral head Reasonable congruence in abduction Subluxation in weight bearing >50% head involvement	No shortening Avoids varus

Redirectional procedures include femoral varus osteotomy and Salter's osteotomy (Table 12.4).

Note

Böhm P, Brzuske A. Salter innominate osteotomy for the treatment of developmental dysplasia of the hip in children: results of seventy-three consecutive osteotomies after twenty-six to thirty-five years of follow-up. *J Bone Joint Surg Am* 2002; 84-A: 178-86. In this study, the investigators performed Salter's osteotomy on 73 hips in patients with a mean age of 4 years at surgery and a 31-year follow-up; 21% had poor results.

Non-redirectional procedures include the shelf procedure and Chiari osteotomy. The latter is indicated in an enlarged incongruous epiphysis in an older patient.

Late sequelae

Hinge abduction is a late sequelae. It is managed with valgus osteotomy or cheilectomy:

- In valgus extension osteotomy, 20° valgus will relieve pain for a few years.
- An anterolateral approach is used in cheilectomy as the protuberance is usually anterolateral.

Note

Yoo WJ, Choi IH, Chung CY, *et al*. Valgus femoral osteotomy for hinge abduction in Perthes disease. Decision-making and outcomes. *J Bone Joint Surg Br* 2004; 86: 726-30. In this study of 21 hips, with a mean patient age of 9.7 years and a 7.1-year follow-up, the mean hip score improved from 66 to 92 following valgus femoral osteotomy.

Arthrodiastasis

Arthrodiastasis is a technique for distraction of the joint to maintain joint space. It should be conducted before epiphyseal collapse.

Note

Maxwell SL, Lappin KJ, Kealey WD, *et al*. Arthrodiastasis in Perthes disease. Preliminary results. *J Bone Joint Surg Br* 2004; 86: 244-50. This study recruited 15 children older than 7 years at symptom onset and compared them with historical controls. The children were classified as Herring group C and an at-risk femoral head was excluded. Orthofix was used for distraction and 20-70° flexion was allowed. The frame was left in place for 4 months and the children were followed up for 3 years. The authors concluded that distraction should be applied before epiphyseal collapse.

Developmental dysplasia of the hip

The term 'developmental dysplasia of the hip' (DDH) includes prenatal teratologic dislocation, postnatal instability and adolescent acetabular dysplasia.

Epidemiology

The male to female ratio of DDH is 7:1. The left side is more commonly affected than the right. Incidences are as follows:

- Positive Barlow or Ortolani test (see examination section, below) – one in 250 live births.
- Frank dislocation – one in 1,000 live births.
- Late dislocation, dysplasia – four in 1,000 live births.

Aetiology

The family history is positive in 34% of patients. Other factors associated with DDH are breech presentation, oligohydramnios, congenital dislocation of the knee, congenital torticollis and metatarsus adductus.

Pathology

- The femoral head and neck are anteverted and ossification of the femoral head is delayed.
- The acetabulum is flattened.
- The acetabular labrum is enlarged and may infold, preventing reduction of the femoral head.
- The ligamentum teres is lengthened, hypertrophic and redundant.
- The transverse acetabulum ligament blocks the lower portion of the acetabulum.
- The acetabulum fills with pulvinar, a fibrofatty tissue.
- The hamstring, glutei and psoas tendons are contracted. The psoas tendon causes an hourglass constriction in the joint capsule seen on arthrograms.

Natural history

Ninety percent of unstable hips stabilise within 2 months. If unreduced, the joint will develop osteoarthritic changes at ages 20-60 years.

Screening

An ultrasound examination at age 6 weeks or X-ray at age 4 months is performed for those at risk of DDH. This includes children with a family history, breech presentation, foot deformities or an abnormal hip examination.

The arguments against general screening are that it results in a higher treatment rate and has a negative cost-benefit analysis.

> **Note**
>
> Wirth T, Stratmann L, Hinrichs F. Evolution of late presenting developmental dysplasia of the hip and associated surgical procedures after 14 years of neonatal ultrasound screening. *J Bone Joint Surg Br* 2004; 86: 585-9. **General neonatal ultrasound screening was found to reduce surgical procedures and late presentations. The authors strongly recommended general screening. With selective screening, the splintage rate is 4-10 per 1,000 live births; with general screening, the rate is 49 per 1,000 live births.**

> **Note**
>
> Lewis K, Jones DA, Powell N. Ultrasound and neonatal hip screening: the five-year results of a prospective study in high-risk babies. *J Pediatr Orthop* 1999; 19: 760-2. **Selective ultrasound screening reduced late DDH cases from 2.2 to 0.34 per 1,000 live births. The authors recommended general screening.**

Clinical features

Examination focuses on the Barlow and Ortolani tests:

- Barlow – the examiner attempts to dislocate a reduced hip. The hip is flexed and adducted, and the thigh pushed axially in a proximal direction in an attempt to dislocate the hip. An unstable hip will be felt as a click as the femoral head slips out of the acetabulum.
- Ortolani – the examiner attempts to reduce a dislocated hip. The hip is flexed and adducted. The examiner's thumb is placed on the medial side of the thigh with the fingers around the greater trochanter. The hip is then abducted and an attempt made to gently reduce the hip. A clunk or sensation of reduction indicates a positive test.

Both of these tests are negative after 3 months because a dislocated hip (Ortolani-positive) cannot be reduced, and a hip that is reduced in a position of rest (Barlow-positive) tends to stabilise by 3 months.

These tests are 60% sensitive and 90% specific, so are poor screening tests.

Clinical features of DDH are as follows:

- Galeazzi sign – shortened femur.
- Asymmetry of the skin folds – a non-specific sign.
- Telescoping of the thigh.
- If the child is walking, clinical signs of DDH are excess lordosis, pelvic obliquity, Trendelenburg gait and hip flexion contracture.

A 'clicky hip' is not related to DDH. Rather, it has a soft tissue aetiology.

Note

Bond CD, Hennrikus WL, DellaMaggiore ED. Prospective evaluation of newborn soft-tissue hip 'clicks' with ultrasound. *J Pediatr Orthop* 1997; 17: 199-201. **This study looked at 50 infants over the age of 3 months with clicky hips. All had a stable hip on dynamic ultrasound examination.**

Imaging

X-ray

In a fixed irreducible hip dislocation, an X-ray of the pelvis in the AP view should be performed to assess the presence of teratologic dislocation.

Several parameters should be assessed on X-rays (Figure 12.3):

- Perkin's line – a vertical line at the superolateral margin of the acetabulum.
- Hilgenreiner's line – a horizontal line at the triradiate cartilage.

Based on these two lines, the femoral head should be in the inferomedial quadrant. The presence of the femoral head in the superolateral quadrant indicates hip dysplasia.

- Acetabular index – normally less than 30° at age 1 year.
- Shenton's line – a continuous curve from the inferior border of the femoral neck to the inferior border of the superior pubic ramus.
- Centre-edge angle – the angle should be more than 25° in children older than 8 years.

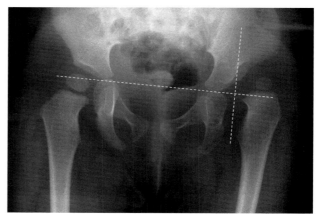

Figure 12.3. A radiograph showing developmental dysplasia of the left hip. The femoral physis is lateral to Perkin's line (vertical line through the superior margin of the acetabulum) and superior to Hilgenreiner's line (horizontal line through the triradiate cartilage). The acetabular index is high and the Shenton's line is discontinuous.

Ultrasound

Ultrasound is used to document and monitor reduction. It is useful before the age of 6-8 months because it can identify the non-osseous part of the femoral head, the acetabulum and soft tissue structures such as the labrum and capsule. It may, however, overdiagnose dysplasia.

In the static (Graf's) method, the hip is assessed in the coronal plane. A straight line of the ilium indicates the scan is through the centre of the acetabulum. The alpha angle is the angle between the outer cortex of the ilium and the bony acetabulum, and measures the depth of the acetabulum (Table 12.5 and Figure 12.4). It should be more than 60° in children older than 3 months.

The beta angle reflects the cartilaginous roof and the position of the femoral head.

In the dynamic (Harcke's) method, measurement is performed in the transverse plane and the joint is stressed while imaging.

Table 12.5. Grading based on the static (Graf's) method.

Type	Alpha angle	Description
I	>60°	Normal
II	43-59°	Normal if age <3 months Indicates delayed ossification if age >3 months
III	<43°	Dislocation
IV	<43°	Dislocated with the labrum interposed between the femoral head and acetabulum

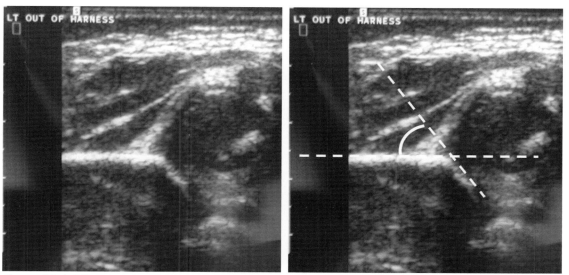

Figure 12.4. Ultrasound measurement of the alpha angle. The image on the left shows the view obtained when the lateral cortex of the ilium appears as a straight line. The angle measurement is shown in the image on the right.

Arthrography

Arthrography is the gold standard. The 'rose-thorn sign' indicates the labrum is not interposed between the femoral head and the acetabulum. The medial pooling should be less than 5mm and the image should demonstrate a deep concentric reduction.

Computed tomography scan

A computed tomography (CT) scan is useful to document a reduction in spica after open or closed reduction. A limited scan of the hip is sufficient to demonstrate reduction.

Magnetic resonance imaging

The role for MRI is uncertain at present.

Management

Closed reduction with a Pavlik harness

Closed reduction in a Pavlik harness is generally an option up to the age of 6 months, although it may be used satisfactorily up to 12 months. The harness works as a dynamic splint to maintain flexion and abduction. It can be used for a hip that is initially not reducible (negative Ortolani test), but this treatment must be abandoned if the hip does not reduce within 3 weeks.

Hip flexion is kept between 100° and 110°, and abduction between 50° and 70°. Excess abduction causes AVN, while excess flexion can damage the femoral nerve. Reduction is confirmed by ultrasound and the patient should be followed up again after 1 week to ensure the parents can manage the harness effectively. Follow-up is with ultrasound every 4-6 weeks. The harness is worn continuously until the hip is stable, and this is checked on ultrasound. Bracing is continued part time until acetabular remodelling is complete.

Bracing is effective in 90% of patients and the risk of AVN is less than 5% if bracing is started within 6 weeks of birth. The following factors are associated with a poor prognosis:

- Bracing started after age 7 weeks.
- A negative Ortolani test.
- Bilateral hip involvement.

Note

Nakamura J, Kamegaya M, Saisu T, et al. Treatment for developmental dysplasia of the hip using the Pavlik harness: long-term results. J Bone Joint Surg Br 2007; 89: 230-5. This study looked at 115 patients, with 130 complete dislocations of the hip, over 14 years of follow-up. A Pavlik harness was applied at age 1-12 months and the average duration was 6.1 months. Overall, 83% patients were treated with the harness alone and the rest required supplementary surgery. The outcome was satisfactory in 91.5% and AVN was seen in 12.3% of patients.

Closed reduction in traction

There is no evidence that traction is useful.

Closed reduction with hip arthrography

Closed reduction with hip arthrography is performed under general anaesthetic and image intensifier control. A medial approach is used. Using the medial groin crease as a landmark, the needle entry site is posterior to the adductor longus. A spinal 22G needle is aimed towards the ipsilateral shoulder or iliac spine, keeping the needle parallel to the table (horizontal). Once in the joint, 2-4ml of saline is injected. The saline should flow back. Needle placement is checked with an image intensifier, and then 1ml of iohexol 240mg/ml is injected.

The following are assessed on the arthrogram:

- The amount of medial pooling – should be less than 5mm.
- Deep concentric reduction indicates the hip is congruent.
- Rose-thorn sign – indicates the labrum has folded outwards and is associated with a good prognosis.
- The safe zone (of abduction) – percutaneous tenotomy of the adductor longus can be performed to increase the safe zone.

Obstruction to closed reduction can be caused by several characteristics:

- Hourglass contracture – due to the iliopsoas tendon.
- Constriction of the inferior capsule.
- Neolimbus – infolding and hypertrophy of the labrum.
- Thickened and superior migration of the transverse acetabular ligament.
- Elongation of the ligamentum teres.
- Proliferation of fibrofatty tissue (pulvinar).

Reduction is acceptable when the limbus is not interposed and there is less than 5mm contrast between the femoral head and the acetabulum.

A spica cast is applied in the human position: 90° flexion and 30-60° abduction. Congruence is checked with a CT scan. Spica is continued for 4 months, changed every 6 weeks and followed by night-time abduction bracing.

Note

Kiely N, Younis U, Day JB, Meadows TM. The Ferguson medial approach for open reduction of developmental dysplasia of the hip. A clinical and radiological review of 49 hips. *J Bone Joint Surg Br* 2004; 86: 430-3. **This study looked at 49 hips in patients aged 6-23 months, with a 4-year follow-up. Three redislocations occurred. AVN Kalamchi and MacEwen group I was seen in four hips, group II in two hips and group III in one hip.**

Open reduction

Open reduction is indicated where reduction is non-concentric.

Open reduction in the anterior approach can be performed at any age. It gives versatile, excellent exposure. Capsulorrhaphy and pelvic osteotomies can be performed through the same approach. A bikini incision is made from the middle of the iliac crest, centred on the anterior superior iliac spine. The interval between the sartorius and the tensor fascia lata is developed. The lateral femoral cutaneous nerve is protected and retracted medially.

The iliac apophysis is split. The sartorius is divided and retracted distally. The psoas tendon is recessed. Tenotomy of the rectus femoris is performed 1cm distal to the anterior inferior iliac spine and the muscle is retracted distally. A T-capsulotomy is performed excising the ligamentum teres. Multiple T-incisions are made in the hypertrophied labrum. Excision of the labrum may damage the lateral acetabular physis, resulting in dysplasia. The deep transverse acetabular ligament is divided and fat cleared from the acetabulum.

If the femoral head is stable, a double breast of the capsule is performed, suturing the lateral flap as far medially as possible. A postoperative CT scan will confirm reduction in spica.

The medial (Ludloff) approach is applicable for infants aged less than 1 year. If capital epiphysis is not seen on X-rays, a higher risk of AVN is present. There is no access to the labrum and capsulorrhaphy cannot be performed.

The anteromedial approach goes anterior to the adductor brevis, while the posteromedial approach is posterior to the adductor brevis.

The transverse incision is centred over the adductor longus. The adductor longus is divided. The plane of dissection is anterior to the adductor brevis, protecting the anterior division of the obturator nerve. The iliopsoas is divided, taking care to avoid damage to the medial circumflex femoral artery.

Femoral shortening

Femoral shortening is required in children older than 2 years. A lateral approach is used and the amount of overlap of the femur indicates the degree of resection. Excess anteversion and varus can be corrected and the osteotomy is fixed with a plate and screws.

In children older than 3 years, open reduction, femoral osteotomy and redirectional pelvic osteotomy can be performed simultaneously with good results. There is no increased risk of AVN.

Pelvic osteotomy

Pelvic osteotomies are considered in children older than 3 years. Acetabular remodelling is highest in those younger than 4 years, unpredictable between 4-8 years and non-existent in those older than 8 years. Maximal remodelling occurs within 1 year of hip reduction.

Pelvic osteotomy improves contact and reduces point loading. Osteotomies can be redirectional, reshaping or salvage.

Redirectional procedures involve complete cuts through the innominate bone and fixation:

- Salter osteotomy:
  - ideal for providing anterolateral coverage;
  - provides 20-25° lateral and 10-15° anterior coverage.
- Steel osteotomy:
  - used in older patients (age >8 years) with limited mobility of the pubic symphysis;
  - this is a triple osteotomy. Preoperatively, abduction, flexion and internal rotation of the hip should result in concentric reduction.
- Ganz periacetabular osteotomy:
  - this is an osteotomy of all three bones and vertical osteotomy of the posterior column;
  - the osteotomy is inherently stable as the posterior column is intact;
  - a periacetabular osteotomy is contraindicated if the triradiate cartilage is open;
  - technically, this is a demanding procedure.

Reshaping can be with the Pemberton or Dega procedures:

- Pemberton:
  - incomplete extracapsular cuts are made 1cm above the joint capsule;
  - this procedure can be performed in the age range of 2-10 years;
  - hinging of the periacetabular segment is at the triradiate cartilage;
  - this helps to decrease the volume of the acetabulum;
  - both the outer and inner table of the ilium are cut, beginning 5mm above the joint capsule.

- Dega:
  - cuts are through the outer table of the ilium only.

Salvage procedures:

- An extra-articular buttress of bone is fashioned over the subluxed femoral head. There is fibrocartilaginous metaplasia of the joint capsule. Examples of salvage procedures are the Chiari osteotomy and Staheli's shelf augmentation.
- Chiari osteotomy:
  - the ilium is divided inclined cephalad 20° through both outer and inner surfaces;
  - the osteotomy is between the joint capsule and the reflected head of the rectus;
  - the acetabulum is displaced medially.
- Staheli's shelf augmentation:
  - a corticocancellous bone shelf is made over the femoral head.

Note

Macnicol MF, Lo HK, Yong KF. Pelvic remodelling after the Chiari osteotomy. A long-term review. *J Bone Joint Surg Br* 2004; 86: 648-54. This study involved a long-term follow-up of 215 Chiari osteotomies at a mean of 18 years after surgery (range 5-30 years). Only 20% of procedures were converted to a total hip arthroplasty. The centre-edge angle improved from 2.5° to 41.8° postoperatively, and was maintained at 38.5° on follow-up. Remodelling did not reverse the medialisation produced by the osteotomy.

Complications

Failed reduction is generally due to inadequate capsular release or inadequate capsulorrhaphy, and a repeat open reduction. Poorer results and higher rates of AVN are seen with repeat attempts at reduction.

AVN can occur with any treatment method and the incidence is the same for open or closed treatment. It is caused by compression of the vascular supply due to excessive abduction or repeat surgery.

Radiological evidence of AVN:

- Failure of appearance of the ossific nucleus within 1 year.
- Increased radiographic density and fragmentation.
- Deformity of the femoral head and neck.
- Broadening of the femoral neck.

The changes may involve part or all of the femoral head. Kalamchi and MacEwen proposed a classification system for avascular changes:

- Group I – change affects the ossific nucleus.
- Group II – lateral physeal damage.
- Group III – central physeal damage.
- Group IV – total damage to the head and physis.

Note

Kalamchi A, MacEwen GD. Avascular necrosis following treatment of congenital dislocation of the hip. *J Bone Joint Surg Am* 1980; 62: 876-88. **Classification of avascular changes.**

Treatment options for AVN include proximal femoral varus osteotomy, trochanteric epiphysiodesis and distal transfer of the trochanter.

Clinical decision scenarios

Scenario 1

Newborn with hip positive for Ortolani test (hip is dislocated but reducible)
↓
Pavlik harness
↓
Re-examine at 2 weeks to ensure hip is reduced
↓
Discontinue brace when hip is stable

Scenario 2

Newborn with hip positive for Barlow test (hip is unstable)
↓
Review with ultrasound scan at 6 weeks
↓
Hip stable – no treatment
Hip unstable – Pavlik harness, as in Scenario 1

Scenario 3

3-month-old with a stable hip but reduced alpha angle on scan
↓
No treatment needed
X-ray at 6 months

Scenario 4

6-month-old with a dislocated hip
↓
Examination under anaesthesia, arthrogram ± adductor tenotomy
↓
Spica for 4 months
Change every 6-8 weeks

Scenario 5

6-month-old with a subluxed hip
↓
As for Scenario 4
Consider a Denis Browne splint

Scenario 6

6-month-old with dysplasia
↓
X-ray in 6 months
↓
Consider Salter's osteotomy at age 4 or 5 years

Scenario 7

1-year-old with a dislocated hip
↓
Examination under anaesthesia, arthrogram, adductor tenotomy/open reduction and spica

Scenario 8

2 years or older with a dislocated hip
↓
Examination under anaesthesia, arthrogram, adductor tenotomy/open reduction and spica
Femoral osteotomy

Scenario 9

8-year-old with a dislocated hip
↓
Examination under anaesthesia, arthrogram, adductor tenotomy, femoral osteotomy, Salter's osteotomy and spica for 2 months

Scenario 10

12-year-old with dysplasia
↓
Consider a periacetabular or
triple osteotomy or observe
If painful, perform an osteotomy
If painless, an operation is controversial

Slipped capital femoral epiphysis

Epidemiology

A slipped capital femoral epiphysis (SCFE) (or slipped upper femoral epiphysis) is more common in boys and Polynesian and Afro-Caribbean children. There is a link with obesity, and more than 60% of affected children are over the 90th percentile for weight. SCFE is also linked to short stature and delayed growth-plate closure.

Presentation is usually between the ages of 9 and 16 years.

Aetiology

The development of SCFE is multifactorial. Possible contributory factors include mechanical factors and hormonal influences.

Mechanical factors

- The orientation of the physis changes from horizontal to more oblique in early adolescence.
- Increased femoral retroversion causes more stress across the physis.
- Normal femoral anteversion is about 10°. In obese children, it has been reported to be as low as 0.4°.
- A deeper acetabulum may play a role. The centre-edge angle of Wiberg is 37° in children with SCFE compared with 33° in unaffected children.

Hormonal influences

Widening and closure of the physis is influenced by several hormones:

- Increased levels of growth hormone stimulate widening of the physis.
- Testosterone stimulates widening and then closure of the physis.
- Oestrogen stimulates closure of the physis.
- Thyroid hormone, vitamin D and calcium are also needed for closure.

In addition, there may be other hormonal causes of SCFE:

- General metabolic causes.
- Hypothyroidism.
- Hypogonadism.
- Renal osteodystrophy.
- Klinefelter syndrome.

Pathophysiology

- The slip occurs because of failure at the junction of the zone of hypertrophy and the zone of provisional calcification.
- A wide physis, deep acetabulum and increased retroversion increase stress across the physis.
- Interconnections of chondrocytes provide resistance to shear.
- Thinning of the perichondrial ring of la Croix is considered as a contributing factor to the occurrence of slip.

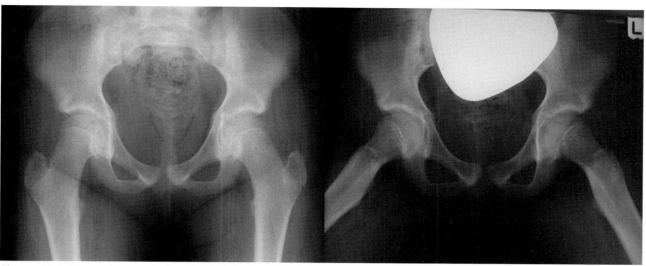

Figure 12.5. The anteroposterior view of the pelvis (left) does not show an obvious slip, while the frog-leg lateral view in the same patient (right) shows the mild slip.

Clinical features

Fifteen percent of patients have pain in the distal thigh and knee only, while 22% have bilateral slip. In bilateral slip, 60% of patients have a simultaneous slip, while the rest present on the other side in the following 18-24 months.

Eighty-five percent of slips are chronic, implying more than 3 weeks' duration. Chronic slip presents as an out-turning of the affected leg. Acute-on-chronic slip is diagnosed when there is a sudden change in pain with a chronic slip.

An unstable slip is present if the child is unable to bear weight. In a stable slip, the child can walk with or without crutches. There is a 50% risk of osteonecrosis in unstable SCFE, compared to 4% in stable SCFE.

'Preslip' is mild hip pain with no radiologic slip.

Examination will find the following:

- Pain on internal rotation.
- Increasing external rotation with flexion.
- Decreased hip flexion and internal rotation.

Imaging

In an early slip, widening of the physis on AP radiograph and periphyseal irregularity may be the only abnormalities (Figure 12.5).

Klein's line is drawn along the superior border of the femoral neck. In a normal hip, it should intersect with the lateral edge of the epiphysis. A line that passes lateral to the epiphysis (Trethowan's sign) indicates a slipped physis.

In later stages, new bone formation at the medial edge of the physis and rounding off of the exposed superior edge may be evident.

The accuracy of imaging for diagnosis is as follows:

- AP radiograph view – 66% sensitivity.
- AP radiograph and frog-leg lateral views – 80% sensitivity.
- Ultrasound scan – 95% sensitivity.
- MRI – the gold standard.

Grading of slip severity

The severity is graded shown in Table 12.6.

Two screws may be used for severe slip (Figure 12.6). This gives a 33% increase in shear resistance but a 10-fold increase in the complication rate.

Table 12.6. Grading of slipped capital femoral epiphysis.

Factor	Grade of slip	Description
Absolute displacement	-	Complete displacement of the physis
Percentage epiphyseal displacement	Mild	Displacement is less than a third of the neck width
	Moderate	Displacement is a third to a half of the neck width
	Severe	Displacement is more than half of the neck width
Slip angle on frog-leg lateral view	Mild	Slip angle <30°
	Moderate	Slip angle 30-50°
	Severe	Slip angle >50°

Management

The immediate management of mild and moderate SCFE is *in situ* pinning. A single cancellous screw is used to stabilise the slip and prevent progression (Figure 12.6). The location of the screw is marked preoperatively. The screw should be at least 5mm from subchondral bone. The anterolateral quadrant of the femoral head should be avoided as the artery of Brodetti may be damaged, causing AVN.

Transient pin penetration does not cause damage, but the screw should not penetrate into the hip joint. The screw position is checked thoroughly by rotating the image intensifier.

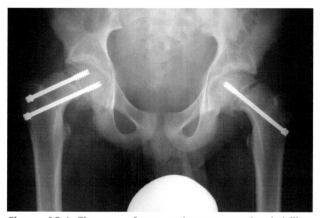

Figure 12.6. The use of one or two screws to stabilise a slipped epiphysis.

Note

Zionts LE, Simonian PT, Harvey JP Jr. Transient penetration of the hip joint during *in situ* cannulated-screw fixation of slipped capital femoral epiphysis. *J Bone Joint Surg Am* 1991; 73: 1054-60.

Screw removal is not routinely advised, although practices vary in different units.

The traditional view is that the slip should not be reduced prior to fixation. In severe slip, however, reduction may be attempted in specialist units. This aims to minimise the abnormal morphology of the femoral head and avoid problems due to impingement in adulthood.

Note

Peterson MD, Weiner DS, Green NE, Terry CL. Acute slipped capital femoral epiphysis: the value and safety of urgent manipulative reduction. *J Pediatr Orthop* 1997; 17: 648-54. **AVN was 7% with reductions performed within 24 hours of symptoms and 20% with reductions performed after 24 hours.**

Note

Carney BT, Birnbaum P, Minter C. Slip progression after *in situ* single screw fixation for stable slipped capital femoral epiphysis. *J Pediatr Orthop* 2003; 23: 584-9. **Slip progresses if fewer than five screw threads are in the epiphysis.**

Note

O'Brien ET, Fahey JJ. Remodeling of the femoral neck after *in situ* pinning for slipped capital femoral epiphysis. *J Bone Joint Surg Am* 1977; 59: 62-8. **This study reported on the remodelling potential of the proximal femur in SCFE. The proximal femur remodels and range of motion improves after pinning, but the hip develops arthritis earlier and arthroplasty is needed.**

Moderate and severe slips lead to degenerative disease. If the patient presents within 24 hours then gentle manipulation can be attempted. If not, skin traction is applied for 3 weeks and may reduce the slip to a mild slip, which allows pinning *in situ*. If a high-grade slip remains then osteotomy should be considered.

Note

Carney BT, Weinstein SL, Noble J. Long-term follow-up of slipped capital femoral epiphysis. *J Bone Joint Surg Am* 1991; 73: 667-74.

Note

Uglow MG, Clarke NM. The management of slipped capital femoral epiphysis. *J Bone Joint Surg Br* 2004; 86: 631-5.

Note

Guzzanti V, Falciglia F, Stanitski CL. Slipped capital femoral epiphysis in skeletally immature patients. *J Bone Joint Surg Br* 2004; 86: 731-6. **This study investigated the use of a modified screw with only three threads to maintain fixation without causing premature closure. Ten patients participated (age 10.6-12.6 years), with a 44-month follow-up. The smooth part of the screw was in the region of the physis. The threads were 9mm long and 6.4mm thick, and the screw head was left 2-3mm lateral to the femoral cortex. No difference was seen in epiphyseal closure between the involved and uninvolved sides, and there was continued growth and remodelling in all patients.**

Management of the contralateral hip

- If the hip is clinically and radiologically normal, simple observation is advised.
- If it is associated with renal osteodystrophy or endocrine abnormality, fixation is advised.
- If the hip is asymptomatic but there are changes on X-ray, fixation is advised.
- If symptomatic, fixation is advised.

Reconstructive osteotomies

In severe slips, the area of contact decreases and the chances of vascular injury increase with pinning. There may therefore be a role for subcapital osteotomy, which removes a wedge of bone just distal to the physeal plate. Subcapital cuneiform osteotomy has a 20-35% risk of AVN.

Note

Fish JB. Cuneiform osteotomy of the femoral neck in the treatment of slipped capital femoral epiphysis. *J Bone Joint Surg Am* 1984; 66: 1153-8. **Fish reported a 4.5% rate of AVN with cuneiform osteotomy.**

A base of neck osteotomy is best for moderate deformities. The degree of correction is limited, but the risk of AVN and chondrolysis is less than with subcapital cuneiform osteotomy.

An intertrochanteric (Southwick) osteotomy carries a 10% risk of AVN. The osteotomy can be fixed internally.

The Berne unit (see reference below) has described a capital reorientation procedure through a surgical dislocation approach for patients with moderate and severe slip.

Note

Ziebarth K, Zilkens C, Spencer S, *et al.* Capital realignment for moderate and severe SCFE using a modified Dunn procedure. *Clin Orthop Relat Res* 2009; 467: 704-16. **Forty patients underwent capital realignment and were followed for 1-3 years. No patient had osteonecrosis or chondrolysis. The slip angle was corrected to 4-8°. Articular cartilage damage, full-thickness loss and delamination were observed at the time of surgery.**

Long-term outcomes

Internal fixation helps alleviate the pain. The deformity of the proximal femur persists and results in an externally rotated leg. Patients with mild slips have good long-term results. The presence of an angular deformity at the neck leads to impingement and there is an increasing trend towards hip arthroscopy to alleviate this.

Note

Fraitzl CR, Käfer W, Nelitz M, Reichel H. Radiological evidence of femoroacetabular impingement in mild slipped capital femoral epiphysis: a mean follow-up of 14.4 years after pinning *in situ*. *J Bone Joint Surg Br* 2007; 89: 1592-6. **Mild slip was fixed *in situ* in 16 patients. All hips were abnormal radiologically. None of the hips had a normal head. The neck ratio and average alpha angle was 86° in the AP view and 55° in the lateral cross-table view.**

Complications

Chondrolysis is acute arthritis of unknown aetiology characterised by the rapid loss of articular cartilage. It can also occur after fracture, infection or inflammatory conditions, or after spica for SCFE or fracture. Patients present with hip pain and adduction contracture, and radiographs show reduced joint space and juxta-articular osteoporosis. Histologically, there is non-specific cartilage necrosis and joint synovitis. Management is with range of motion exercises and NSAIDs. Chondrolysis may improve over time but usually causes stiffness and pain. Half of all patients have a poor prognosis.

The risk of AVN is 50% in unstable SCFE and 3% in chronic SCFE. Incidental reduction of SCFE does not increase the risk. AVN presents with recurrence of hip pain several months after SCFE. The management plan relies on rest, NSAIDs and crutches. AVN may require an osteotomy or arthrodesis.

Pathologic fracture through the metalwork site is rarely seen.

Approximately 10% of patients develop osteoarthritis of the hip and a pistol-grip-shaped femoral head is found in 40% patients. Remodelling of up to 60° can occur in SCFE.

Congenital pseudarthrosis of the tibia

Epidemiology

The prevalence of congenital pseudarthrosis of the tibia is about one in 200,000 live births. Most cases (50-70%) are associated with neurofibromatosis type I, while 10% of patients with neurofibromatosis type I have pseudarthrosis of the tibia.

Clinical features

Pseudarthrosis of the tibia manifests as a short leg with an anterior bow in the distal third evident at birth. Rarely, it is bilateral. Café-au-lait spots or neurofibromas may be present. The foot is in a calcaneus position.

Differential diagnosis

- Fibrous dysplasia.
- Osteogenesis imperfecta.
- Rickets.
- Campomelic dysplasia.

Classification

Boyd's classification is used (Figure 12.7).

Management

Prior to fracture
- Ankle-foot orthosis.
- Onlay graft. Realignment osteotomy should not be performed due to an extremely high risk of non-union.

Post-fracture
- Resection, bone grafting and Williams intramedullary telescoping nail has 90% success. A rod can be inserted retrograde through the foot if the distal fragment is small.
- Free fibular grafting using contralateral normal fibula. There is a risk of refracture.
- Ring fixators (Ilizarov or Taylor spatial frame) can achieve union in up to 80% of patients. They correct angulation and restore length. A risk of refracture remains.
- Below-knee amputation can be considered for failed reconstructions.

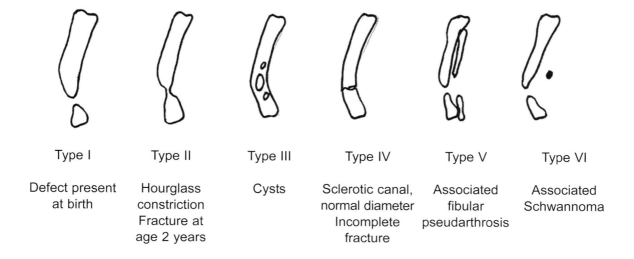

Type I	Type II	Type III	Type IV	Type V	Type VI
Defect present at birth	Hourglass constriction Fracture at age 2 years	Cysts	Sclerotic canal, normal diameter Incomplete fracture	Associated fibular pseudarthrosis	Associated Schwannoma

Figure 12.7. Boyd's classification of congenital pseudarthrosis of the tibia.

Bone grafting and plating has almost a 100% failure rate.

Note

Boero S, Catagni M, Donzelli O, *et al*. Congenital pseudarthrosis of the tibia associated with neurofibromatosis-1: treatment with Ilizarov device. *J Pediatr Orthop* 1997; 17: 675-84. **In 21 patients treated with an Ilizarov external fixator, 66% had good results at 2 years or more after the treatment. The prognosis was better for children aged 5 years or older.**

Congenital posteromedial bow of the tibia

Congenital posteromedial bow is a benign condition compared to anterolateral bowing of the tibia.

Aetiology

It is thought to be a 'uterine packing disorder' caused by the position of the foetus in the uterus.

Clinical features

- The foot is in a calcaneovalgus position.
- There is excessive dorsiflexion.
- The posteromedial bow is at the junction of the middle and distal one-third of the tibia.
- The condition is almost always unilateral.

Differential diagnosis

- Calcaneovalgus foot – this has no tibial bow and resolves spontaneously.
- Fibular hemimelia – this has a valgus limb but less ankle dorsiflexion. There may be hypoplasia of the lateral rays of the foot.

- Distal motor paresis (L5 myelomeningocele) – a dorsiflexed foot, but the tibia is straight.
- Congenital vertical talus – deformity at the midfoot.

Imaging

The bones have a normal appearance with no sclerosis of the canal. There may be some cortical thickening on the concave cortex.

Management

The natural course is spontaneous correction before the age of 2 years in 50% of patients. If correction does not occur by the age of 4 years then it is unlikely to correct spontaneously thereafter. Patients may have limb shortening of up to 4cm at skeletal maturity.

Patients without spontaneous correction should be followed up and undergo epiphysiodesis for limb-length discrepancy. Limb lengthening should be performed with deformity correction.

Blount's disease

Blount's disease is characterised by reduced growth at the medial and posterior aspects of the proximal tibial physis resulting in abrupt angulation of the medial proximal tibial metaphysis.

It is associated with obesity, female sex and Afro-Caribbean ethnicity. The family history is positive in up to 40% patients. Histologically, there is disordered endochondral ossification.

Clinical features

- Internal tibial torsion.
- Shortening of the tibia.
- Progressive varus deformity of the knee.
- Pronation of the feet.

In normal physiological development, the knees have varus alignment at birth and become neutral at age 18 months. A physiological valgus develops at 30-36 months. Varus that persists at the age of 24 months indicates a genu varum deformity.

The varus angulation in Blount's disease is sharp and there may be a thrust while walking. This thrust is absent in physiological bowing.

Differential diagnosis

- Physiologic bowing – bowing occurs both in the femur and tibia.
- Rickets.
- Osteomyelitis.
- Trauma.
- Ollier's disease.
- Focal fibrocartilaginous dysplasia – shows indentation on the medial side of the tibia at the junction of the metaphysis and diaphysis. It improves spontaneously.

Imaging

Imaging is of the lower limb with the hip and ankle on the same plate (long-leg view). The radiographic features are as follows:

- Beaking of the medial wall with a straight lateral cortex.
- Drennan's angle is between a line joining the metaphyseal beaks and the long axis of the tibia. It represents the metaphyseal-diaphyseal angle, and an angle of more than 16° is diagnostic for Blount's. Six-monthly monitoring is advised with an angle of 11-16°.
- The upper tibial epiphysis slopes medially, while the physeal plate is narrow medially and wide laterally.

Classification

Three types are recognised:

- Infantile, age under 3 years.

- Juvenile, ages 3-8 years.
- Adolescent, age over 8 years.

The infantile form has a similar appearance to physiologic bowing. However, in physiologic bowing the varus occurs equally in the distal femur and proximal tibia.

Infantile Blount's disease is bilateral in 60% of patients and will sometimes resolve spontaneously. The adolescent type is usually unilateral and may be associated with femoral varus.

Langenskiöld proposed six radiological types. Type 6 has a bony bar and a vertical tibial physis.

> **Note**
>
> Langenskiöld A. Tibia vara. A critical review. *Clin Orthop Relat Res* 1989; (246): 195-207.

Management

Bracing is effective for infantile disease in Langenskiöld stages I-II. It is advised if the metaphyseal-diaphyseal angle (Drennan's angle) is more than 16°. Bracing is also advised if Drennan's angle is more than 11° in the presence of female sex, obesity, progression or laxity. The brace is a knee-ankle foot orthosis worn during weight bearing. The efficacy of bracing is 65-90%.

> **Note**
>
> Richards BS, Katz DE, Sims JB. Effectiveness of brace treatment in early infantile Blount's disease. *J Pediatr Orthop* 1998; 18: 374-80. **Bracing was effective in 65% of 37 stage II limbs.**

Tibial osteotomy is indicated for progressive deformity. An oblique or dome osteotomy can be performed. Overcorrection is performed to 5-10° of valgus. Osteotomy should be performed before the age of 4 years; there is a high risk of recurrence after this point.

Note

Chotigavanichaya C, Salinas G, Green T, *et al*. Recurrence of varus deformity after proximal tibial osteotomy in Blount disease: long-term follow-up. *J Pediatr Orthop* 2002; 22: 638-41. **Children younger than 4 years had a lower recurrence of varus after corrective osteotomy.**

For stage IV disease or higher, an MRI scan is performed to view the medial bar. If the bar is present, it should be excised or an epiphysiodesis performed on the lateral side to avoid recurrent deformity. The effectiveness of epiphysiodesis is questionable and this should be used only for mild deformities.

An external fixator and hemicallotasis is useful for those with moderate to severe deformity.

Lateral hemiepiphysiodesis can be performed in adolescents, if sufficient growth remains. The growth of the medial side is unpredictable.

The use of external fixation (e.g., an Ilizarov ring fixator or Taylor spatial frame) allows correction of the deformity without compromising bone length.

Internal torsion of the tibia or femur

Torsional deformities of the lower limb are generally due to uterine moulding and resolve with time.

After formation of limb buds, the upper limb undergoes external rotation and the lower limb undergoes internal rotation in utero at 8 weeks. Abnormal rotation in this phase causes torsional abnormalities.

Internal torsion results in in-toeing. With the child standing erect with the patella facing forward, the feet will turn inward. The reverse is seen with external tibial torsion.

Clinical features

The following features should be assessed:

- Hip rotation in a prone position. Internal rotation of more than 70° indicates medial femoral torsion.
- Foot progression angle. This is the angle between the long axis of the foot and the line of walking. Internal torsion of the femur or tibia will lead to internal rotation of the foot.
- Thigh-foot angle. This is the angle between the axis of the foot and the longitudinal axis of the thigh. It is best assessed in the prone position with the knee bent to 90°. The foot points medially in newborns and gradually achieves a 10° lateral thigh-foot angle. The thigh-foot angle indicates tibial torsion and deviations from the norm are a measure of the severity of deformity.

In persistent femoral anteversion, the patella points inwards when the child is standing with the feet parallel to each other. There is increased internal rotation of the hip with a consequent reduction in external rotation. Secondary tibial torsion may be present in these children.

The Ryder test measures the rotational angle (anteversion) of the femur. In the prone position with the knee flexed, the leg is rotated until the greater trochanter is felt prominently. The angle between the leg and the horizontal plane indicates the angle of femoral anteversion.

Imaging

CT scans provide the most accurate measurement of rotational alignment.

Management

The femoral deformity corrects with age. Derotation femoral osteotomy is indicated for deformities that persist after the age of 10 years. The osteotomy can be performed at the subtrochanteric, diaphyseal or supracondylar level. An excessive (>35°) external rotation deformity of the tibia will be accentuated while correcting internal rotation of the femur, and this should be taken into consideration.

Tibial torsion also tends to resolve with age. Supramalleolar osteotomy is required in patients with a medial thigh-foot angle of more than 10° or a lateral thigh-foot angle of more than 35°.

Fibular hemimelia

Fibular hemimelia is longitudinal deficiency of the fibula. It can be partial or complete.

Associated conditions

- Proximal femoral focal deficiency.
- Absence of cruciate ligaments.
- Equinovarus foot.
- Ball-and-socket ankle.
- Tarsal coalition.
- Absence of lateral rays of the foot.

Imaging

Standard radiographs are diagnostic.

Management

Management is based on correcting the deformity and equalising the leg-length discrepancy. Prosthetics allow optimum mobility.

Genu varum and valgum

Genu varum and valgum are physiologic change in knee alignment. Angular deformities at the knee are common in children.

The alignment of the knee is varus at birth and becomes neutral by the age of 18 months. There is an increase in valgus up to the age of 3 years, after which the alignment returns to physiologic valgus (Figure 12.8). This pattern of development was first proposed by Salenius and Vankka.

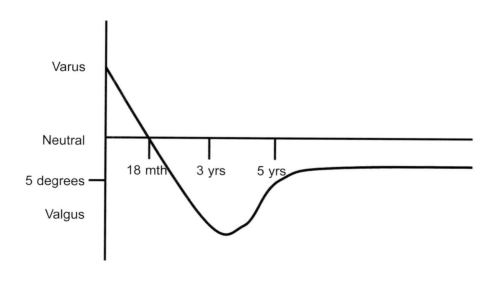

Figure 12.8. Changes in knee alignment with age.

Note

Salenius P, Vankka E. The development of the tibiofemoral angle in children. *J Bone Joint Surg Am* 1975; 57: 259-61.

The causes of genu varum and valgum are shown in Table 12.7.

Congenital knee dislocation

Congenital dislocation of the knee can be an isolated entity or associated with breech presentation, Larsen syndrome, arthrogryposis, myelodysplasia, clubfoot or congenital hip dislocation.

Patients have fibrosis of the quadriceps and anterior subluxation of the tibia. The suprapatellar

Table 12.7. Causes of genu varum and valgum.	
Genu varum	**Genu valgum**
Physiologic	Primary genu valgum
Asymmetric growth:	Trauma
• Tibia vara – Blount's disease	
• Partial physeal arrest due to trauma, infection or tumour	Tumour
	Infection
Metabolic:	
• Renal disease	Metabolic:
• Rickets	• Renal osteodystrophy
Bone dysplasia:	Developmental:
• Achondroplasia	• Dysplasia
• Multiple epiphyseal dysplasia	• Absent fibula
• Enchondromatosis	• Contracture of the iliotibial band
Osteopenia:	
• Juvenile rheumatoid arthritis	
• Osteogenesis imperfecta	

Management of genu valgum is based on the age of the child and degree of deformity. Mild deformity can simply be monitored periodically, while a deformity of more than 12-15° indicates surgical correction (proximal tibial osteotomy, distal femoral osteotomy or lateral epiphysiodesis). Most patients do not require surgery.

pouch is absent and the patella is underdeveloped. The cruciate ligaments may be absent. The knee is hyperextended and flexion of the knee is restricted.

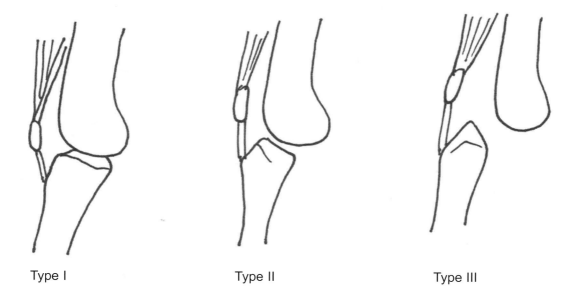

Type I   Type II   Type III

Figure 12.9. Types of congenital dislocation of the knee.

Congenital knee dislocation can present with varying severity. Three types are described (Figure 12.9):

- Type I – a hyperextended knee.
- Type II – anterior subluxation of the tibia.
- Type III – anterior dislocation of the tibia.

Type I resolves spontaneously, but type II requires serial casting. A Pavlik harness is quite helpful once adequate knee flexion is achieved to maintain and improve flexion. Type III carries the worst prognosis and quadricepsplasty and open reduction are needed to realign the knee. This should be performed before the age of 6 months. Isolated knee dislocation carries a better prognosis.

Congenital patellar dislocation

Congenital patellar dislocation is anterolateral displacement of the extensor mechanism. The patella is fixed to the lateral aspect of the distal femur with contracture of the iliotibial band and the lateral capsule. The vastus medialis is atrophic and the trochlea is shallow. An external rotation and valgus deformity of the tibia may be evident.

Congenital patellar dislocation is not reducible and requires surgical correction before the age of 1 year. The lateral structures are released and the medial structures are reefed. Associated syndromes are myelodysplasia and arthrogryposis.

Bipartite patella

Bipartite patella is usually an incidental finding. It is more common in boys.

Saupe's classification is used (Figure 12.10):

- Type I – the fragment is located at the inferior pole.
- Type II – the fragment is at the lateral patellar margin.
- Type III (most common) – the fragment is at the superolateral margin.

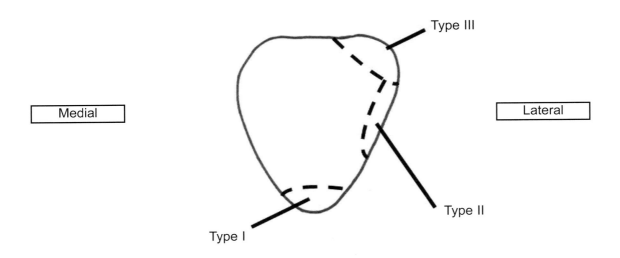

Figure 12.10. Types of bipartite patella.

Symptoms may arise from repetitive overuse or trauma. The differential diagnosis includes acute fractures. Sinding-Larsen disease may mimic inferior pole bipartite patellae.

Thrombocytopenia with absent radius (TAR) syndrome

Thrombocytopenia and absent radii are the features of this syndrome. Knee abnormalities are in the form of meniscal hypoplasia, instability and ball-and-socket medial tibiofemoral articulation.

Nail patella syndrome

Nail patella syndrome comprises nail dysplasia, patellar absence or hypoplasia, radial head instability and iliac horns. It is often associated with nephritic syndrome.

Larsen syndrome

Patients with Larsen syndrome have bilateral congenital knee dislocation along with hip dislocation, clubfoot, cervical kyphosis and laryngeal flaccidity. Deformities usually require operative correction.

Osgood-Schlatter disease

Osgood-Schlatter disease is the result of submaximal repeated avulsion fractures of the patellar tendon from the tibial tubercle. The resulting inflammation causes pain, swelling and local tenderness. It is more common in boys and is bilateral in a quarter of patients.

Patients experience intermittent pain related to activity and the tibial tubercle is enlarged in size and tender. Ossification within the tendon may be seen on radiographs, but more than half of patients have normal radiographs. Fragmentation of the ossicle may be a normal variant and is not diagnostic of Osgood-Schlatter disease.

Management is symptomatic. The symptoms resolve with bone maturity and surgery is rarely needed. If required, surgical intervention aims to enucleate the ossicle and debulk the tubercle. However, this should not be performed before skeletal maturity.

Sinding-Larsen-Johansson disease

Sinding-Larsen-Johansson disease is similar to Osgood-Schlatter disease and affects the inferior pole of the patella. Radiographs may show ossification in the patellar tendon and the condition should be differentiated from bipartite patella. Management is symptomatic.

Baker's cyst

Baker's cyst develops in the popliteal fossa, commonly between the semi-membranosus and the gastrocnemius muscles. It is painless but is noticed because of the visible swelling. The cyst is transilluminant. Aspiration can be diagnostic but is not therapeutic. Most cysts resolve spontaneously and excision is not indicated. There is a high recurrence rate following excision.

Congenital radial head dislocation

Congenital dislocation is characterised by a dysplastic trochlea and lack of concavity in the proximal articular surface of the radial head. Function is generally good and relocation is not indicated. Development of arthritis of the humeroulnar joint is a possibility.

Metatarsus adductus

In metatarsus adductus, the forefoot is adducted and the lateral border of the foot is convex. The heel is unaffected, which differentiates this condition from clubfoot. A few children (1-5%) have associated DDH. Metatarsus adductus can also present as a residual deformity following the correction of clubfoot. Metatarsus adductus can be of varying severity:

- In the mild form (85% of cases), the forefoot is passively abducted beyond the midline of the foot.
- In the moderate type, the forefoot is abducted up to the midline but not beyond.
- In the severe type, no abduction is possible.

Differential diagnosis

A skew foot is associated with lateral translation of the midfoot and hindfoot valgus in addition to forefoot adduction. It is difficult to correct by casting and surgery is more difficult.

Management

If the deformity is passively correctable then passive stretching exercises are advised. Serial manipulation and casting are conducted in patients with rigid deformity. Treatment should preferably start before the age of 2 years.

Kite has proposed three criteria for determining the adequacy of correction:

- The convexity of the lateral border of the foot is corrected.
- Prominence at the base of the fifth metatarsal is corrected.
- The active abduction is as strong as the active adduction.

In the older child (age >4 years), multiple tarsometatarsal osteotomies and medial release of the abductor hallucis and medial capsule are an option. Metatarsal osteotomy is associated with a risk of damage to the physis of the first metatarsal. Dome-shaped osteotomies are performed after the age of 4 years.

A closing-wedge osteotomy of the cuboid and opening wedge of the first cuneiform, as described by McHale and Lenhart, gives good results.

> **Note**
>
> McHale KA, Lenhart MK. Treatment of residual clubfoot deformity – the 'bean-shaped' foot – by opening wedge medial cuneiform osteotomy and closing wedge cuboid osteotomy. Clinical review and cadaver correlations. *J Pediatr Orthop* 1991; 11: 374-81.

Clubfoot

Clubfoot is congenital malalignment of the talocalcaneal-navicular and calcaneocuboid axis of the foot. It is associated with calf atrophy.

Aetiology

Genetics
There is significant evidence for a role of genetics in the aetiology of clubfoot:

- A second child has a one in 30 chance of having clubfoot if the first child is affected.
- A second child has a one in four chance of having clubfoot if the first child and a parent are affected.
- A monozygotic twin has a one in three chance of having clubfoot if the other twin is affected.
- A dizygotic twin has a 3% chance of having clubfoot if the other twin is affected.
- Males are 2.5 times more likely to be affected.
- An affected female child increases the risk for both male and female subsequent children.
- Patients have a family history in 25% of cases.
- The incidence of clubfoot is 0.39% in those of Chinese descent, 1.2% in whites and 6.8% in those of Polynesian descent.

Histologic
Possible underlying factors are as follows:

- An increase in the type I to type II muscle fibre ratio (possible primary nerve abnormality).
- A germplasm defect of bone.
- Increased collagen synthesis.
- Deformity of the talus.
- Reduced cell number and cytoplasm in the posterior tibial tendon sheath (regional growth disturbance).

Vascular
There may be hypoplasia of the anterior tibial artery.

Anomalous muscles
An anomalous flexor muscle in the calf, possibly an accessory soleus muscle, has been proposed as a cause.

Intrauterine factors
- Intrauterine pressure is not considered to be an aetiologic factor.
- Arrested foetal development has been proposed, but there is little evidence for this.
- Amniocentesis and fluid leakage can cause clubfoot.
- Intrauterine retroviral infection may be a cause.

Pathoanatomy

The underlying abnormality is a deformed talus with the anterior part flexed and medially deviated. The navicular often articulates with the medial malleolus. Posteromedial structures are shortened. The talus forces the calcaneus into plantar flexion. The calcaneus rotates into varus and the cuboid and navicular move medially.

Examination

Examination reveals the following:

- A short, wide foot.
- A plantar crease at the midfoot and a crease at the posterior aspect of the ankle.
- A small and drawn-up calcaneus and empty heel pad.
- An adducted and supinated midfoot and forefoot.
- A dorsolaterally palpable talar head.
- An atrophied calf.

Assessment of equinus is performed in flexion and extension, while assessment of varus is performed at the subtalar joint. The lateral border of the foot is measured and compared with the medial border.

Prenatal diagnosis

The false positive rate on ultrasound is 40%.

Differential diagnosis

Postural clubfoot due to intrauterine malposition must be differentiated from congenital clubfoot. Postural clubfoot is a benign, self-correcting condition.

Associated conditions

- Proximal femoral focal deficiency.
- Arthrogryposis.
- Amniotic-band syndrome.
- Myelodysplasia.
- Diastrophic dwarfism.
- Pierre Robin syndrome.
- Larsen syndrome.
- Möbius syndrome.
- Freeman-Sheldon syndrome.

Imaging

Radiographs are obtained in the position of best correction and weight bearing or simulated weight bearing. The beam is focused on the hindfoot.

AP radiograph
- AP talocalcaneal angle – less than 20° in clubfoot.

- Talar-first metatarsal angle – normally 30° valgus, but varus in clubfoot.
- Medial displacement of the cuboid ossific nucleus on the calcaneus is seen.

Lateral radiograph
Performed in maximum dorsiflexion but with no pronation. The plate is placed laterally.

- Lateral talocalcaneal angle – less than 25° in clubfoot.
- Plantar flexion of the forefoot on the hindfoot indicates clubfoot.
- A tibia-calcaneal angle of more than 90° indicates equinus contracture.

Classification

There is poor interobserver reliability among the different scoring systems. The Dimeglio classification (Table 12.8) has an interobserver k of 0.83.

Table 12.8. The Dimeglio 20-point scale for the classification of clubfoot.

Feature	Points
Equinus	4 points
Heel varus	4 points
Internal torsion	4 points
Adduction	4 points
Posterior crease	1 point
Medial crease	1 point
Cavus	1 point
Poor muscle condition	1 point

Grade	
I (score 1-5)	Mild or postural, not requiring surgery
II (score 5-10)	Considerable reducibility
III (score 10-15)	Resistant but partially reducible
IV (score 15-20)	Teratologic

Management

Non-operative management of clubfoot, if successful, leads to a more supple foot. Historically, plaster-cast treatment was proposed by Guerin in 1836, while Kite emphasised the importance of gentle manipulation in 1932. More recently, the widespread use of the Ponseti method has dramatically reduced the rate of operative interventions for clubfoot deformity.

In the Ponseti method, the talonavicular joint is reduced by placing the thumb in the sinus tarsi over the head of the talus and pushing the navicular onto the talus with the index finger of the same hand. Lateral pulling of the forefoot corrects adduction. The foot is externally rotated and an above-knee cast applied. Serial casting produces stress relaxation and helps elongation by viscoelasticity.

Equinus is corrected after forefoot adduction and varus, otherwise a rocker-bottom foot will result. Percutaneous tendo-Achilles lengthening is often needed to correct equinus.

Ponseti reported good or excellent results at 30 years in 89% of cases. Seventy percent of children had Achilles tenotomies and the duration of cast treatment was 2-4 months, with weekly cast changes. A Denis Browne splint is applied until the child is walking and night splintage continues until the age of 2-4 years. Recurrence is increased with non-compliance with foot orthosis.

Note

Herzenberg JE, Radler C, Bor N. Ponseti versus traditional methods of casting for idiopathic clubfoot. *J Pediatr Orthop* 2002; 22: 517-21. **Posteromedial soft tissue release was required in 3% of patients following treatment with the Ponseti method versus 94% of patients without serial casts. Tendo-Achilles lengthening was required in 91% of Ponseti patients.**

Note

Dobbs MB, Rudzki JR, Purcell DB, *et al.* Factors predictive of outcome after use of the Ponseti method for the treatment of idiopathic clubfeet. *J Bone Joint Surg Am* 2004; 86-A: 22-7. **The cases of 51 patients with 86 idiopathic clubfeet were examined retrospectively. Recurrence was related to parent compliance and education level. The severity of the deformity and age at treatment initiation were not related to recurrence.**

Other non-operative measures

Historical measures included daily manipulation by a physiotherapist and taping for 30 minutes for 8 months, as proposed by Bansahel. Dimeglio recommended daily manipulation and continuous passive motion for 8 hours a day and then splintage in the remaining time.

The French method involved a regimen of stretching exercises. Delgado used the French technique along with botulinum toxin-A injection into the gastrocnemius soleus and tibialis posterior muscles. These methods are rarely used in modern practice.

Operative management

The extent of surgery depends on the residual deformity.

Timing
Early surgery at the age of 4-6 months is associated with greater remodelling potential. However, surgery at the age of 9-12 months age is easier and the anatomy is more obvious. In addition, walking helps with spontaneous correction. Simons suggested the foot should be 8cm long at the time of surgery, which makes it easier to identify the anatomy.

Note

Simons GW. The diagnosis and treatment of deformity combinations in clubfeet. *Clin Orthop Relat Res* 1980; 150: 229-44.

Incisions

Various incisions have been described:

- Hockey Stick posteromedial incision (Turco) – this crosses the medial skin crease. It may be difficult to reach the lateral structures (calcaneofibular ligament and plantar fascia).
- Cincinnati – a circumferential posterior incision. Exposure of the Achilles tendon is difficult and there may be problems with skin closure but not wound healing. The eventual scar is good, even if the skin edges are not approximated primarily.
- Carroll – a two-incision technique: one posterior and one medial.

Medial release

The abductor hallucis is released from the calcaneus and reflected distally. Attachment of the abductor hallucis to the sustentaculum tali is also released. The motor branch from the medial plantar nerve can be cut. The laciniate ligament is divided, exposing the medial plantar neurovascular bundle. The lateral plantar bundle is identified. Neurovascular structures are protected by a Penrose drain. The origin of the plantar fascia and short toe flexors is divided.

The flexor hallucis longus (FHL) and flexor digitorum longus (FDL) are identified from the ankle joint to the master knot of Henry. The retinaculum under which the FHL passes under the sustentaculum tali is divided. The peroneus longus is protected as it passes around the lateral border of the foot at the level of the calcaneocuboid joint.

The calcaneocuboid joint is released plantarly and medially. The spring ligament is divided, helping to identify the medial portion of the talonavicular joint. The talocalcaneal capsule is released.

The deep deltoid ligament is not divided and damage to the sustentaculum tali is avoided.

Z-plasty of the tibialis posterior is performed above the ankle joint. Slips of the tibialis posterior extending to the cuneiforms and metatarsals are divided, if needed.

The talonavicular joint capsule is completely divided dorsally, plantarly and medially.

Posterior release

Z-plasty of the Achilles tendon is performed, dividing the medial part distally. The sural nerve is protected. The talocalcaneal joint is released posteriorly and laterally. The calcaneofibular ligament is divided to allow the calcaneus to rotate back. The cuboid is reduced onto the calcaneus and stabilised with a pin.

Assessment

If the toe cannot be brought back to the neutral position, the FHL and FDL can be lengthened.

The foot should be plantigrade and the thigh foot axis should be deviated 20° externally.

Closure

The skin can be closed and the foot kept in equinus for 1-3 weeks to relieve tension on the closure. The cast is then changed to neutral. Alternatively, a gap of up to 2-3cm may be left between the skin margins. This still leads to good healing and minimal scarring. A bivalved above-knee cast is applied.

Postoperative management

Pain relief is with caudal block or an epidural. A wound check and change of cast is performed after 1 week. The cast is changed after 4-6 weeks, and then pins are removed.

Recurrence

Recurrence (commonly forefoot adduction and supination) occurs in 25% of patients.

Residual forefoot adduction

Forefoot adduction is the most common residual deformity. It is caused by failure to release the calcaneocuboid joint.

Age less than 2 years

Repeat soft tissue release can be performed.

Age 2-4 years

Calcaneocuboid joint cartilage is excised and the joint fused along with medial release. Enucleation of the cuboid is an option.

Age older than 4 years

- The distal part of the calcaneus is excised and the calcaneocuboid joint fused.
- Evans (1961) – calcaneocuboid wedge resection. This may overcorrect and lead to decreased growth of the lateral border of the foot.
- Fowler (1959) – open-wedge osteotomy of the medial cuneiform, plantar release and transfer of the tibialis posterior to the dorsum of the first metatarsal for children aged over 8 years.
- McHale and Lenhart (1991) – open-wedge osteotomy of the medial cuneiform and closing-wedge osteotomy of the cuboid ('flip-flop' procedure).
- Metatarsal osteotomies – when the deformity is distal to the navicular.
- Lateral transfer of the tibialis anterior to the third cuneiform or split transfer to the fourth metatarsal.

Residual cavus

Release of the plantar fascia from the calcaneus can be performed to correct varus. In children aged over 6 years, options include Japas midfoot osteotomy or Jahss osteotomy at the level of the tarsometatarsal joint.

Heel varus

In children aged over 4 years, a Dwyer lateral closing-wedge osteotomy can be performed.

Heel valgus

In those aged 4-10 years, an extra-articular Grice procedure is recommended.

Salvage procedures

In patients aged over 10 years, triple arthrodesis helps to correct the foot deformity. Distraction histogenesis using Ilizarov principles or the Taylor spatial frame can be performed.

Transfer of the tibialis anterior is an option for supple recurrent clubfoot. Prerequisites for this procedure are as follows:

- Age over 6 years.
- Passively correctable deformity.
- Weak peroneals on electromyography.
- No active abduction or eversion.

Supramalleolar osteotomy or talocalcaneal osteotomy can be performed for residual toe-in.

Dorsal bunions result from plantar contracture of the first metatarsophalangeal joint and dorsiflexion contracture of the tarsometatarsal joint. The underlying cause is a strong FHL and tibialis anterior and weak peronei and Achilles. Treatment is with the reverse Jones procedure – transfer of the FHL to the head of the first metatarsal.

An overcorrected foot can result from the release of deep deltoid or interosseous subtalar ligaments. Management is as follows:

- Over 4 years, correctable – ankle-foot orthosis.
- Over 4 years, rigid – soft tissue release.
- Over 10 years – triple arthrodesis.

Tarsal coalition

Tarsal coalition results from congenital failure of differentiation and segmentation of the primitive mesenchyme. It is the most common cause of a rigid flat foot.

Epidemiology

Tarsal coalition is inherited as an autosomal dominant condition with almost full penetrance. It affects 1% of the population.

It may be associated with fibular hemimelia, Apert syndrome or Nievergelt-Pearlman syndrome.

Talocalcaneal and calcaneonavicular coalition are the most common types, comprising 90% of all coalitions. The condition is bilateral in 50-80% of patients.

Pathology

Initially there is fibrous coalition, transforming to synchondrosis or synostosis. This leads to progressive valgus of the hindfoot and flattening of the medial arch. About 25% of feet with coalition are symptomatic.

Calcaneonavicular coalitions become symptomatic by 8-12 years and talocalcaneal coalition presents around 12-16 years. The onset of symptoms coincides with metaplasia from cartilage to bone.

Clinical features

Pain may be aggravated by activity and relieved by rest. Pain may be due to ligament sprain, muscle spasm, subtalar joint irritation or impingement in the sinus tarsi.

Examination

Talocalcaneal coalition is associated with a flat foot and lack of subtalar motion. In calcaneonavicular coalition, the flat foot is less rigid. There is adaptive shortening of the peroneal tendons due to hindfoot valgus, but actual spasm of the muscle is debatable.

Due to rigidity, the arch does not appear on toe-standing or toe-raising tests.

Imaging

AP, lateral, oblique and axial views are obtained on X-ray:

- 'C sign' describes the continuous curve formed by the talar dome and the inferior border of the sustentaculum tali on a lateral heel radiograph in talocalcaneal coalition.
- The 'anteater nose sign' describes an elongated process of the anterior calcaneus. It indicates calcaneonavicular coalition.
- Dorsal beaking of the talar head represents a traction spur due to the pull of the dorsal talonavicular ligament.
- A broad and round lateral process of the talus and narrow posterior talocalcaneal facet may be seen in talocalcaneal coalition.

On a CT scan, coronal slices demonstrate the coalition. MRI can help detect fibrous coalitions.

Management

Asymptomatic coalitions require no treatment.

Non-operative measures include activity modification, NSAIDs and shoe inserts. A walking below-knee cast for 4-6 weeks can be worn if the pain does not settle.

The aim of surgery is pain relief. For calcaneonavicular coalition, surgery involves resection of coalition and interposing the extensor digitorum brevis in the defect. In talocalcaneal coalition, resection can be performed if less than half the width of the subtalar joint is involved and there are no degenerative changes in the adjoining joints. Arthroscopic resection has been described. Triple arthrodesis is effective for persistent pain or arthritis.

In patients with severe pain, minimal arthritis and a severe valgus deformity, Evans calcaneal lengthening osteotomy or medial closing-wedge osteotomy of the posterior part of the calcaneus can be considered.

Cavus foot

Several anatomical abnormalities are associated with a cavus foot:

- Plantarflexion of the first metatarsal.
- Pronation of the forefoot.
- Contracture of the plantar fascia.

- Plantarflexion of the talonavicular or naviculocuneiform joint.
- Hindfoot varus.
- Calcaneus deformity.

Causes

- Charcot-Marie-Tooth disease.
- Dejerine-Sottas disease.
- Refsum disease.
- Spina bifida.
- Tethered cord.
- Polio.

Symptoms

The main symptoms are pain and difficulty with wearing shoes due to the altered shape of the foot.

Examination

- Arch in standing and walking.
- Colman block test.
- Range of motion of ankle and subtalar joint.
- Hindfoot varus.
- Clawing of toes.

Indications for surgery are pain and difficulty with wearing shoes.

Management

Non-operative management includes shoe modifications, moulded orthoses and stretching exercises.

Surgical options include the following:

- Plantar fascia release.
- Tibialis posterior transfer to the dorsum of the foot.
- Dorsal closing-wedge osteotomies of all metatarsals.
- Tarsometatarsal wedge osteotomies.
- Triple arthrodesis.

Accessory navicular

An accessory navicular can present as a small ossicle in the tendon of the tibialis posterior, or as a prolongation of the medial end of the navicular with a thin zone of fibrocartilage interposed between the two.

These are usually asymptomatic and the findings are incidental. A Tc-99m bone scan will show increased uptake in symptomatic patients and an MRI can demonstrate an accessory navicular before it ossifies and becomes visible on plain radiographs.

Management is largely symptomatic and most patients are symptom-free on skeletal maturity. Excision of the ossicle and repair of the tibialis posterior tendon to the navicular is performed for those with persistent pain.

Congenital vertical talus

Congenital vertical talus is a congenital dislocation of the talonavicular joint whereby the talus is plantarflexed and the navicular articulates with the dorsum of the talus. Clinically, it gives the appearance of a flat, valgus foot, which is known as a 'rocker-bottom foot'.

Congenital vertical talus can present as an isolated entity. It can also be associated with arthrogryposis multiplex congenita, neurologic anomalies such as myelomeningocele, tethered cord and sacral agenesis, Larsen syndrome, nail patella syndrome, neurofibromatosis and chromosomal anomalies.

Clinical features

- The talonavicular joint is not reducible by manipulation.
- The hindfoot is in equinus with contracture of the Achilles tendon.
- The midfoot is in valgus with contracture of the peroneal tendons.
- The forefoot is dorsiflexed with contracture of the extensor tendons.
- The talar head is palpable on the sole of the foot.

Differential diagnosis

- Oblique talus – the talonavicular joint is reducible on plantar flexion.
- Flexible flat foot – the arch of the foot is reduced but deformity is correctible.
- Rigid flat foot.
- Peroneal spastic flat foot.

Imaging

A lateral radiograph of the foot in dorsiflexion and plantarflexion is obtained. This demonstrates the dislocated talonavicular joint, fixed hindfoot equinus and lack of correctability on plantarflexion. The AP view shows an increased talocalcaneal angle.

Management

The initial management is aimed at stretching the contracted tissues with serial casts, which will aid open reduction. Surgery is needed to lengthen the contracted tendons and reduce the talonavicular joint.

Untreated dislocation in the older child requires talectomy or fusion.

Sever's disease

Sever's disease is inflammation of the calcaneal apophysis. It affects skeletally immature children and causes tenderness around the calcaneal tuberosity.

Differential diagnosis includes Achilles tendonitis, plantar fasciitis, stress fracture, tarsal tunnel syndrome, cysts and tumours. Radiographs are helpful to rule out other causes of pain. Sclerosis of the apophysis is not consistently related to symptoms.

Acute symptoms are managed by rest or a short period in a cast. Once symptoms settle, Achilles tendon stretching exercises are commenced.

Polydactyly

Polydactyly is usually an isolated, autosomal dominant condition, but may occur as part of genetic abnormality syndromes. It is occasionally associated with syndactyly. The accessory digit can be preaxial or postaxial. Management involves excision of the accessory digit.

Macrodactyly

Macrodactyly is hypertrophy of one or more toes. It may be associated with neurofibromatosis or haemangiomatosis. Management aims to achieve cosmetic correction and enable shoe fitting.

Treatment options include soft tissue debulking with osteotomy or epiphysiodesis, or ray amputation.

Curly toes

'Curly toe' describes a flexion deformity of the metatarsophalangeal and interphalangeal joints of the small toes due to contracture of the FHL muscle. The affected toe is deviated under the adjoining medial toe. It commonly involves the third toe.

Most of these resolve and do not interfere with walking. Percutaneous tenotomy of the FHL corrects the deformity.

Torticollis

Congenital muscular torticollis or 'wry neck' is associated with unilateral shortening of the sternomastoid due to fibrosis.

Trauma to the sternomastoid at the time of birth leads to fibrosis and contracture. Other possible aetiologies are vascular injury, infection or intrauterine positioning. A nodule or muscle enlargement may be palpable. The mass is palpable within 2 weeks of birth and can disappear by the age of 1 year. Persistent thickening predisposes to congenital muscular torticollis.

The condition may be associated with metatarsus adductus, clubfoot and dysplastic hips.

Treatment in infancy is with passive stretching. Deformities persisting beyond the age of 1 year are managed by release of the sternomastoid muscle. In mild deformities, a unipolar release (distal only) is sufficient. More severe deformities require bipolar (proximal and distal) release. Endoscopic release has also been described.

Rigid torticollis results from atlanto-occipital injuries or congenital disorders.

Klippel-Feil syndrome

Klippel-Feil syndrome is characterised by a triad of fusion of two or more cervical vertebrae, short neck and low hair line. Restricted cervical movement is evident on examination.

Associated findings include facial asymmetry, torticollis, Sprengel's shoulder and neck webbing. Neurologic compromise may be present.

Radiographs and MRI scans aid the diagnosis. Non-operative management is with avoidance of contact sports and analgesia as required. Decompression or fusion is performed for neurologic compromise or cervical instability.

Sprengel's shoulder

Sprengel's shoulder is an abnormal superior position of the scapula, which is hypoplastic and misshapen. It is associated with Klippel-Feil syndrome, cervical ribs, scoliosis and diastematomyelia.

The omovertebral bone is a quadrangular accessory bone extending from the superior angle of the scapula to the cervical vertebrae. It is present in about one-third of patients and must be excised at the time of correction.

In mild disease, the limitation is minimal. In severe disease, however, there is a cosmetic as well as functional disability.

Management is based on release of the vertebral scapular muscles, excision of the supraspinous part of the scapula, moving the scapula down and repairing the inferior muscles to retain the scapula in the corrected position. This was first described by Green. Associated scarring of the soft tissues may compromise the results of surgery.

The Woodward procedure involves the transfer of the trapezius inferiorly on the spinous process.

The operation to correct the deformity should be performed around the age of 3 years. Injury to the brachial plexus is a risk in older children.

Congenital pseudarthrosis of the clavicle

Congenital pseudarthrosis of the clavicle is present at birth and affects the middle third of the clavicle. Failure of the two ossification centres to fuse may be related to pressure from the underlying subclavian artery.

Functional limitation, pain and cosmetic deformity indicate operative intervention, which is internal fixation by plate and bone grafting. The operation is performed between the ages of 3 and 5 years and the plate can be removed after 1-2 years. The potential for healing is better than for pseudarthrosis of the tibia.

Congenital dislocation of the radial head

Congenital dislocation of the radial head is suspected when there is no associated ulna injury. The radial head lacks the proximal concavity and appears misshapen. The radial shaft is longer.

Attempts at reduction are futile because there is an insufficient soft tissue envelop to retain the head in place and the bony anatomy is abnormal. Excision of the head is an option to relieve pain, once skeletal growth is complete.

Congenital pseudarthrosis of the radius and ulna

Congenital pseudarthrosis of forearm bones is extremely rare. It may be related to neurofibromatosis. The radial non-union is in the distal third and is managed by dual-onlay bone grafting or a free vascularised fibular transfer. Pseudarthrosis of the ulna is more resistant to treatment. Options include bone grafting with internal fixation, creation of a one-bone forearm, a free vascularised fibula graft or the use of ring fixators and bone transport.

Congenital radioulnar synostosis

Synostosis of the radius and ulna usually affects the proximal third of the diaphysis. Wilkie has described two types:

- In type I, the fusion is extensive and the medullary canals of the radius and ulna are connected.
- In type II, the fusion is limited and the proximal end of the radius is dislocated.

Resection of the fusion to restore pronation and supination is not successful. Operative intervention is indicated to correct the hyperpronation deformity if it is greater than 90°.

Madelung deformity

Madelung deformity results from premature fusion of the ulnar half of the distal radial growth plate. The deformity can be congenital or the result of trauma. Congenital deformities present in the early teenage years with pain and cosmetic impairment. Ulnar deviation of the wrist is seen.

Radiologically, there is widening of the radioulnar distance, the ulna is long compared with the radius and the distal radial epiphysis appears triangular.

Treatment is by shortening the ulna and performing a dorsolateral closing-wedge osteotomy of the radius.

Osteogenesis imperfecta

Epidemiology

Osteogenesis imperfecta affects one in 25,000 people.

Pathogenesis

A mutation in the *COL1A1* gene on chromosome 17 or in the *COL1A2* gene on chromosome 7 leads to osteogenesis imperfecta. These genes code for pro-alpha chains, which form type I procollagen. The mutations are generally point mutations resulting in the substitution by glycine, which compromises the stability of the helix.

Patients with type I disease have an 80% quantitative reduction in collagen due to presence of a null allele. This is the mildest form of the disease. Patients with type II, III and IV disease have abnormal collagen.

Clinical features

- Multiple fractures.
- Osteopenia.
- Skeletal deformities.
- Blue sclera.
- Dentinogenesis imperfecta.
- Joint laxity.
- Middle-ear deafness.
- Microcephaly, triangular facies.
- Short stature.
- Chest-wall deformities, kyphoscoliosis.
- Spinal curves of greater than 60° may result in a forced vital capacity below 50%, which can lead to respiratory compromise.
- Post-traumatic intracranial bleeding is common.

Antenatal diagnosis

Osteogenesis imperfecta types II and III can be diagnosed by the age of 16-20 weeks. Types I and IV cannot be diagnosed in the antenatal period. Chorionic villus sampling is useful if there is a positive family history.

Classification

Osteogenesis imperfecta is classified according to Sillence (Table 12.9).

Note

Sillence D. Osteogenesis imperfecta: an expanding panorama of variants. *Clin Orthop Relat Res* 1981; (159): 11-25.

Telescoping rods have been designed to allow lengthening with bone growth and may increase the time span between repeat surgeries. However, some studies have reported a higher complication rate with these rods.

Spinal deformity causes respiratory compromise. The presence of six biconcave vertebrae predicts the development of severe scoliosis. Fusion is considered for curves of more than 50°.

Basilar invagination is the cause of death in patients with types III and IV osteogenesis imperfecta. Symptoms are headache, cranial nerve dysfunction, hyperreflexia, ataxia and nystagmus. Occipitocervical fusion may not be able to halt progression and a long-term Minerva brace may be needed.

Medical treatment is with bisphosphonates, which may help to reduce bone fragility.

Table 12.9. Sillence classification of osteogenesis imperfecta.

Type	Inheritance	Colour of sclera	Features
I	AD	Blue	Type IA – normal teeth Type IB – dentinogenesis imperfecta Type IC – a severe form of IA
II	AD	Blue	Lethal *in utero* or perinatal, beaded ribs
III	AR	White	Multiple fractures at birth, dentinogenesis imperfecta
IV	AD	White	Type IVA – normal teeth Type IVB – dentinogenesis imperfecta

AD = autosomal dominant; AR = autosomal recessive

Management

The aim of management is to maximise function and prevent fractures. Acute fractures are usually managed non-surgically. Surgery, if required, is with an intramedullary nail and realignment osteotomy.

Gene therapy and bone marrow transplantation are not yet in clinical use.

Note

Saldanha KA, Saleh M, Bell MJ, Fernandes JA. Limb lengthening and correction of deformity in the lower limbs of children with osteogenesis imperfecta. *J Bone Joint Surg Br* 2004; 86: 259-65. **This study compared distraction histogenesis with monolateral and Ilizarov frames in osteogenesis imperfecta. Six children were included, with a mean age of 14.3 years. The average lengthening achieved was 6.26cm. Fixators were well tolerated and regenerate bone formed normally.**

Leg-length discrepancy

Causes

Congenital
- Femur:
  - proximal femoral focal deficiency;
  - congenital short femur;
  - hypoplastic femur.
- Leg:
  - fibular hypoplasia;
  - tibial hypoplasia.
- General:
  - hemihypertrophy, hemiatrophy;
  - Klippel-Trénaunay-Weber syndrome;
  - Proteus syndrome;
  - neurofibromatosis.
- Bone diseases:
  - diaphyseal aclasis;
  - dysplasia;
  - enchondromatosis;
  - congenital coxa vara;
  - chondrodysplasia punctata.

Acquired
- Inflammatory:
  - juvenile rheumatoid arthritis;
  - haemophilia.
- Infection:
  - physeal arrest;
  - meningococcal septicaemia.

- Trauma:
  - physeal injury;
  - compensatory overgrowth of diaphyseal fractures;
  - radiation;
  - burns.
- Neurologic:
  - cerebral palsy;
  - congenital hemiplegia;
  - polio.

Assessment

Standing
- Look for scoliosis, pelvic obliquity and contracture of the hip and knee joints. Flexion contractures of the hip and knee can cause apparent leg-length inequality.
- Look for hairy patches, vascular markings, muscle wasting and neurofibromas.
- Stand the patient on premeasured blocks and reassess for scoliosis or pelvic obliquity.
- Symmetry of lateral flexion.
- Assess the patient's gait.

Sitting
Scoliosis that corrects in the sitting position indicates a functional cause.

Supine
In Galeazzi's test, the patient places the heels together with the knees flexed. This test can be used with shortening in either the thigh or leg.

Measurement of true leg lengths is performed with the pelvis square (a line joining the anterior superior iliac spine is perpendicular to the trunk) and both legs in an identical position. Measurement is performed from the anterior superior iliac spine to the medial malleolus. The true length indicates the actual difference in leg length. Segmental leg lengths should be measured to compare the lengths of the supratrochanteric region (the anterior superior iliac spine to the tip of the greater trochanter), femur (the tip of the greater trochanter to the lateral joint line) and tibia (the medial joint line to the tip of the medial malleolus).

Apparent leg length is measured with the patient asked to lie straight with the legs parallel to each other. Measurement is performed from a fixed point in the midline (umbilicus). On comparing this with the true length, pelvic tilt and flexion contractures of the hip and knee may be assessed.

Movements of the hip and knee joints should be assessed.

In patients with hemihypertrophy, screening with abdominal ultrasound and alpha-fetoprotein is performed till the age of 6 years to screen for Wilms' tumour.

The block method is the most accurate clinical test and also takes into account the foot height. The pelvis is made level by placing blocks of appropriate height under the short leg.

Imaging

- A scanogram shows the entire extremity on a single film. An X-ray tube moves linearly to show all of the bone structure.
- An orthoroentgenogram is a multiple-exposure radiograph. It shows an AP view of the hips, knees and ankle.
- A CT scanogram is the most accurate imaging modality to assess leg-length differences.

Prediction of leg-length discrepancy

The Menelaus 'rule of thumb' is applicable in girls and boys older than 8 and 10 years, respectively. The rule states that the distal femoral physis grows at the rate of 10mm/year and contributes 70% of femoral growth. The proximal tibial physis grows at the rate of 6mm/year and contributes 60% of tibial growth. The total adult height is twice the height at the age of 2 years. Skeletal growth ceases at 14 years in girls and 16 years in boys.

In the Menelaus 'rule of thumb', the current discrepancy is measured and the time remaining for growth (girls: 14 years minus current age; boys: 16 years minus current age) is calculated:

Total discrepancy at maturity =
[current discrepancy + (years remaining x discrepancy per year)]

Green Anderson growth-remaining charts can also be used to predict leg-length discrepancy, as can the Moseley straight-line graph. The latter method relies on at least three measurements over 4-month intervals. It is useful in predicting the effect of epiphysiodesis.

The Greulich and Pyle atlas for bone age was compiled in the 1940s and is still occasionally used for determining bone age.

> **Note**
>
> Moseley CF. A straight-line graph for leg-length discrepancies. *J Bone Joint Surg Am* 1977; 59: 174-9.

Management

- Discrepancy of 0-2cm – generally no treatment is needed. A shoe lift is adequate, if the patient is symptomatic (limp).
- Discrepancy of 2-5cm – epiphysiodesis, physeal bar resection, distraction lengthening or acute shortening.
- Discrepancy of 5-18cm – distraction lengthening.
- Discrepancy of more than 18cm – multiple distraction lengthening, contralateral epiphysiodesis or amputation.

The current discrepancy and the final expected discrepancy should be predicted accurately. The procedure should not result in different knee heights. Weight bearing is allowed as tolerated postoperatively. Surgery can be performed as an open or closed procedure.

Epiphysiodesis
Contraindications to epiphysiodesis include inadequate growth remaining and short stature (a relative contraindication).

Acute shortening of the femur

This is performed as the child nears skeletal maturity so that the correction is not lost. The correction achieved is 2-5cm. Problems include oedema, muscle weakness, compartment syndrome and neurovascular compromise.

Shortening can be conducted as an open procedure (subtrochanteric osteotomy) or by closed intramedullary nailing. In the latter, a segment of the femur is divided into halves and separated, and the remaining proximal and distal fragment is fixed by the nail after acute docking. An intramedullary saw is used to divide the femur.

Lengthening

Lengthening is indicated in patients with shortening of more than 5cm or shortening of less than 5cm with severe deformity.

Tissue distraction techniques are used. The correction is 1mm per day, achieved in three or four turns of the distraction screw. Monolateral or ring fixators can be used. Monolateral frames are easier to apply, have fewer pin sites, are less bulky and cause less muscle transfixion. Ilizarov and other circular frames are more versatile and can correct severe deformities, but are bulky.

Physeal bar resection

Physeal bar resection is indicated if the child has significant growth remaining. CT and MRI help to define the bar. Resection is advisable only for bars involving less than 50% of the physis. Peripheral bars can be resected but the recurrence rate is higher than with central bars. Central bars are resected through a metaphyseal window and fat is interposed. The physis may not achieve normal growth and osteotomy may be needed.

Amputation or rotationplasty

Amputation or rotationplasty may be performed for Aitken C or D proximal femoral focal deficiency (see below).

Lengthening for short stature
Indications:

- Achondroplasia.
- Hypochondroplasia.
- Familial short stature.

Arthritic/unstable joints (e.g., diastrophic dysplasia, pseudoachondroplasia, epiphyseal dysplasias) are a contraindication.

Bilateral tibial lengthening is performed to increase height.

Proximal femoral focal deficiency

Proximal femoral focal deficiency is malformation of the proximal femur.

Classification

The Aitken classification is used (Figure 12.11). Proximal femoral focal deficiency may be associated with fibular hemimelia, absent lateral rays of the foot and tarsal coalition.

Management

In patients with type A and B, varus corrective osteotomy will help restore alignment. The gross shortening of the extremity due to loss of growth at the proximal end of the femur can be compensated for with knee fusion and a prosthetic limb. Rotationplasty is an option.

Types C and D respond poorly to surgery; a prosthesis is a viable option.

The limping child

The assessment of a limping child can be divided based on age group.

Age 1-3 years with a painful limp

Causes include the following:

- Septic arthritis.
- Transient synovitis.
- Discitis.
- Fracture.
- Inflammatory disorders.
- Neoplasm.

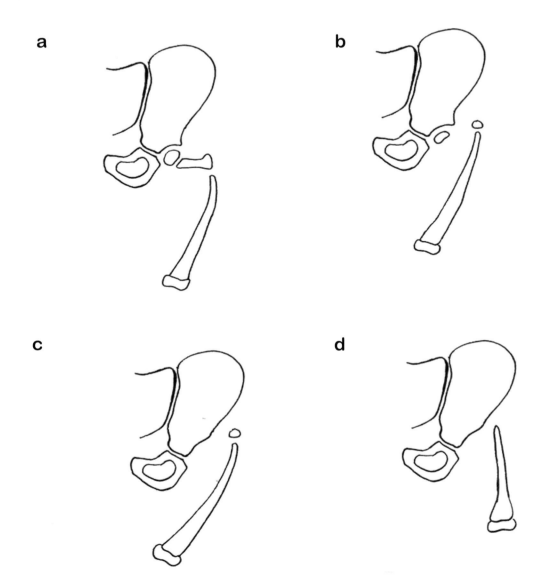

Figure 12.11. Diagrammatic representation of the Aitken classification. (a) Type A: gap at the proximal half of the femur, which ossifies by skeletal maturity. **(b)** Type B: as for Type A, with a hypoplastic femoral head and shallow acetabulum. **(c)** Type C: an absent femoral head and proximally migrated femoral shaft remnant. **(d)** Type D: complete absence of the femoral head and acetabulum.

Children with septic arthritis present with fever, local swelling, tenderness, reduced range of motion and an increased erythrocyte sedimentation rate (ESR) and C-reactive protein (CRP) level. An ultrasound scan shows effusion and X-rays may show increased joint space. A bone scan shows increased local uptake and an MRI will demonstrate bone marrow changes. Aspiration is diagnostic, and over 80,000 white blood cells/mm^3 and more than 75% polymorphs indicate infection. Culture of aspirate helps to identify the causative organism, which is usually *Staphylococcus* and rarely *Streptococcus*.

Transient synovitis is more common in children older than 3 years and presents with pain, a limp and reduced range of motion. Fever is not a feature and ESR and CRP levels are near normal. Aspirate has 5000-15,000 white blood cells/mm^3 with less than 25% polymorphs. Transient synovitis generally resolves spontaneously over 7-10 days.

Discitis can present between the ages of 6 months and 4 years. The child will have pain on bending forwards. ESR and CRP levels are raised and a bone scan will be positive after 1 week. X-rays are positive after 2-6 weeks. The usual causative organism is *Staphylococcus aureus*.

Fractures of the tibia, fibula, calcaneum or metatarsals can present with a painful limp.

Juvenile arthritis can present at 2 years of age with swelling, raised local temperature and multiple joint involvement. The most common joints involved are the knee, ankle and subtalar joint.

Acute leukaemias may present with a limp. The usual age group is 2-6 years. Clinical features are local pain, raised temperature and enlarged lymph nodes, liver and spleen. Myeloblasts are seen in blood film. X-rays may show metaphyseal bands.

Age 1-3 years with a painless limp

- Developmental dysplasia of the hip causes a painless limp with increased lumbar lordosis, shortening and a positive Galeazzi sign. X-rays are diagnostic.
- Congenital coxa vara presents with poor abduction and a painless limp. X-rays are diagnostic.
- Cerebral palsy is sometimes noticed when a child starts walking. The tone is increased and hyperreflexia is seen. The limp is accentuated when the child runs. There may be a history of problems at the time of birth.
- Muscular dystrophy.

Age 4-10 years

Causes include the following:

- Transient synovitis.
- LCP disease.
- Discoid lateral meniscus.
- Limb-length discrepancy.

Age 11-15 years

The causes are related to the hip (SCFE, dysplasia of the hip, idiopathic chondrolysis), knee (overuse syndromes such as Osgood-Schlatter disease or jumper's knee, or osteochondritis dissecans) or foot (tarsal coalition).

Cerebral palsy

Cerebral palsy describes a group of permanent disorders of the development of movement and posture causing activity limitation(s) that are attributed to non-progressive disturbances that occurred in the developing foetal or infant brain.

> **Note**
>
> Rosenbaum P, Paneth N, Leviton A, *et al*. A report: the definition and classification of cerebral palsy April 2006. *Dev Med Child Neurol Suppl* 2007; 109: 8-14.

Although the neurological insult is non-progressive, the increasing functional demands of the growing child may make the neurological manifestations of the condition appear to progress.

Incidence

Cerebral palsy has an incidence of 1-7 per 1,000 live births. This incidence has not changed in the last 10 years. Improvements in neonatal care have resulted in the increased survivorship of preterm infants, with associated long-term sequelae.

Aetiology

A large number of causes have been identified, although no risk factors can be identified in 30% of patients. The causes can be grouped as follows:

- Prenatal – congenital malformation, intrauterine infection (cytomegalovirus, toxoplasmosis).
- Perinatal – birth trauma/asphyxia, kernicterus.
- Postnatal – infection, non-accidental injury, cerebral haemorrhage.

Neuropathology

Children with cerebral palsy exhibit upper motor neuron signs. The management of the child should address both the negative and positive features of the condition.

> **Note**
>
> Kerr Graham H, Selber P. Musculoskeletal aspects of cerebral palsy. *J Bone Joint Surg Br* 2003; 85: 157-66. **A description of the constellation of positive and negative features that interact to produce the musculoskeletal manifestations of cerebral palsy.**

Cerebral palsy results in several problems for the child:

- Muscle weakness.
- Spasticity.
- Muscle contractures.
- Lengthened muscles.
- Bony deformities – torsional problems, subluxation and dislocations.
- Premature degenerative changes.

Spasticity is a velocity-dependent increase in tone that is caused by the loss of central inhibitory control on anterior horn cells within the spinal cord.

Neurological classification

Spastic

Spastic cerebral palsy is the most common type, accounting for 80% of all cases. Thirty percent of patients with other forms of cerebral palsy will have a spasticity element to their condition. Children have a generalised increased tone as a result of damage to the pyramidal system, corticospinal tract or motor cortex.

Spastic cerebral palsy is further classified by the distribution of body involvement:

- Monoplegia – paralysis of a single limb, usually an arm. This is the mildest form of cerebral palsy and can affect just one muscle group or muscle. Children generally have a good prognosis.
- Diplegia – paralysis of the lower extremities with little or no upper-body spasticity. This is the most common of the spastic forms. Children are usually fully ambulatory, but may require assistive devices and have a scissor-type gait. Flexion contractures of the knees and hips to varying degrees are common. Hip dislocations and strabismus (three-quarters of those with spastic diplegia) can also be present. The children are usually of normal intelligence.
- Hemiplegia – one side of the body is affected. Children with spastic hemiplegia are typically ambulatory, although there may be dynamic equinus on the affected side.
- Quadriplegic/whole-body involvement – all four limbs are affected equally. Children with spastic quadriplegia are the least likely to be able to walk, if they are ambulatory. Often their muscles are too tight and children require a large energy expenditure to ambulate.

Ataxia

Ataxic-type symptoms are attributed to cerebellar damage. Ataxic cerebral palsy accounts for 10% of cases. Fine motor skills and balance are affected, especially while walking. Children may also be hypotonic, but hip dysplasia is rare.

Athetoid/dyskinetic

Athetosis or dyskinesia accounts for 10-20% of cerebral palsy cases and is notably difficult to treat. The damage occurs to the extrapyramidal motor system and basal ganglia. In the past kernicterus was a cause of athetoid cerebral palsy, with untreated high bilirubin levels in the blood of newborn infants resulting in damage to the basal ganglia.

Patients have abnormal movement. Children have trouble holding themselves in an upright, steady position for sitting or walking, and often show involuntary movements. Because of the mixed tone and trouble maintaining a steady position, they may not be able to hold objects (e.g., a toothbrush or pencil).

Hypotonia

Children appear limp and have generally poor mobility.

Mixed

Some children exhibit a mixed pattern of neurological compromise. The individual functional deficits will determine management.

Gross Motor Function Classification System

The Gross Motor Function Classification System for cerebral palsy is a useful system for describing the usual functional levels of an affected child. It gives generalised descriptions of five functional levels:

- Level I – walks without limitations.
- Level II – walks with limitations.
- Level III – walks using a hand-held mobility device (e.g., walker, crutches, cane).
- Level IV – self-mobility with limitations; may use powered mobility.
- Level V – transported in a manual wheelchair.

Each of these levels further contains a separate description for the age groups: less than 2 years, 2-4 years, 4-6 years, 6-12 years and 12-18 years.

Note

Palisano R, Rosenbaum P, Walter S, *et al.* Development and reliability of a system to classify gross motor function in children with cerebral palsy. *Dev Med Child Neurol* 1997; 39: 214-23.

Specific gait abnormalities in cerebral palsy

Several specific gait abnormalities are commonly seen in children with cerebral palsy:

- Toe walking – commonly seen in hemiplegic cerebral palsy as a consequence of dynamic equinus and spasticity in the gastrosoleus complex.
- Crouch gait – increased knee flexion in stance due to hamstring spasticity.
- Scissoring gait – caused by adductor spasticity.
- Jump gait – involves a decrease in flexion at the hip and knee from initial contact to late stance, with equinus in late stance, giving the appearance that the child is jumping up and down.
- Stiff knee gait – decreased knee flexion during swing associated with rectus femoris tightness.
- Foot drop – excessive equinus in swing caused by weakness of the tibialis anterior or gastrosoleus contracture.

Examination

General inspection

A general inspection will contribute a major part of the complete assessment. The examination should be tailored to the age and functional abilities of the child. Consider the following points:

- Is the child ambulant or chair-bound?
- Does the child use any walking aids?
- Is the child able to communicate either verbally or using aids?
- Does the child have good head control?

- Does the child make any involuntary movements?
- Is the child positioned adequately in his/her chair?
- Does the child use any splints, orthotics, special footwear or Lycra suits?

Gait

Watch the child walk and attempt to follow a straight line. Does the child have a recognisable gait pattern? If the child can run, do the upper limbs elevate? If so, this is a characteristic of diplegic cerebral palsy.

Spine

Assess for a scoliosis. If present, determine if it is postural (due to leg-length discrepancy). Consider whether the curve can be corrected by holding in a brace or seating modification.

Upper limbs

Check the general tone and passive movements of the joints. Are deformities fixed or correctable?

Lower limbs

Again, check the general tone and passive movements of the joints. Is the hip painful or in abduction? Measure any leg-length discrepancy. Conduct a Thomas test for hip flexion contracture, a Gage or Staheli's test for the rotational profile and Ely's test for a tight rectus femoris. Assess hamstring tightness and the popliteal angle.

Foot and ankle

The Silfverskiöld test differentiates an isolated gastrocnemius from a gastrosoleus contracture when there is increased dorsiflexion of the foot between an extended and flexed knee.

Management principles

Each management regimen should be individualised to the child, including his/her functional requirements and neurological deficits. A multidisciplinary approach is necessary to rationalise the number of hospital attendances.

- Define the long-term management objectives.
- Identify the patient's problems, both immediate and future.
- Analyse the potential effects of growth.
- Consider all management alternatives, including non-treatment.
- Treat the whole child, not just the motor skeletal parts.

Management of spasticity

Management aims to limit the joint contractures associated with chronic spasticity. Control of generalised spasticity is non-surgical, with popular agents including baclofen and diazepam. These can be administered orally, although there is a role for intrathecal baclofen in children with severe generalised spasticity. Botulinum toxin-A (BTX-A) and phenol are indicated for the control of localised spasticity in muscle groups.

BTX is a potent neurotoxin produced from the bacterium *Clostridium botulinum*. It is commercially available as two preparations: Dysport and Botox. The mechanism of action is binding of the neurotoxin to the cholinergic nerve endings, inhibiting the release of presynaptic vesicles containing acetylcholine. Its effects are dose-dependent and last for approximately 3 months, due to the growth of new nerve terminals. The beneficial effects of BTX-A for both upper and lower limb spasticity are well established within the literature.

> **Note**
>
> Hoare BJ, Wallen MA, Imms C, *et al.* Botulinum toxin A as an adjunct to treatment in the management of the upper limb in children with spastic cerebral palsy (UPDATE). *Cochrane Database Syst Rev* 2010; 1: CD003469. **This Cochrane review found high-level evidence supporting the use of BTX-A as an adjunct to managing the upper limb in children with spastic cerebral palsy. The review recommended that BTX-A should be accompanied by occupational therapy.**

Surgical treatment with selective dorsal rhizotomy aims to reduce spasticity by interrupting the stretch reflex. Sectioning the dorsal rootlets between L1 and S1 reduces the stimulatory input from muscle spindles, helping to balance muscle tone.

Management of orthopaedic problems

Spine
Posterior and/or anterior spinal fusion is performed for severe rigid deformities.

Shoulder
Adduction and internal rotation is caused by subscapularis and pectoralis major transfer. This is addressed by muscle lengthening or release and humeral derotation osteotomy.

Elbow
Flexion contracture is caused by contracture of the biceps, brachialis and brachioradialis. It is treated by serial casting, BTX-A injections or surgical release.

Pronation of the forearm is caused by contracture of the pronator teres and quadratus. These can be released surgically.

Wrist
Wrist flexion contracture is caused by a tight flexor carpi ulnaris or radialis, which can be released. In severe flexor spasticity, the flexor carpi ulnaris can be transferred to the extensor compartment (Green's transfer). Wrist fusion is an option.

Hand
Adductor pollicis contracture causes thumb-in-palm. Contractures can be released and unstable joints stabilised. For finger clawing, the flexor carpi ulnaris or radialis can be transferred to the extensor compartment. Spasticity of the finger flexors can be corrected by fractional lengthening of flexor digitorum superficialis and profundus in the forearm. Proximal row carpectomy is an option.

Swan-neck deformities can be managed by splinting or surgical correction.

Hip
Hip dislocation occurs in 1% of patients with spastic hemiplegia, 5% of those with spastic diplegia and 35-55% of those with quadriplegia. Contributory factors include muscular imbalance, acetabular dysplasia, pelvic obliquity, excess femoral anteversion, coxa valga and the absence of weight bearing. Problems are a continuum for the hip at-risk, progressing through to subluxation and dislocation. Reimer's migration index is a useful guide to the progression of the uncovered hip (Figure 12.12). A progression of more than 15% in 30 months predicts dislocation in 50% of hips.

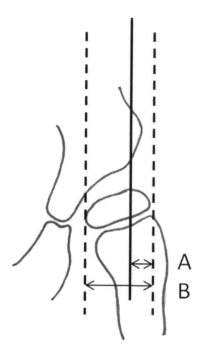

Figure 12.12. The Reimer's migration index. A vertical line is drawn from the superolateral margin of the acetabular roof (Perkin's line). The index is the ratio of the femoral head lateral to Perkin's line (A) and the total width of the femoral head (B).

Indications for surgical treatment include pain, perineal hygiene-associated scoliosis, difficulty sitting and to enable transfers. The principles of surgery include soft tissue release or lengthening in combination with a proximal femoral varus osteotomy and/or a pelvic osteotomy to redirect or augment the posterior-superior deficiency of the acetabulum. Other options involve excision or arthrodesis of the proximal femur.

Flexion contractures of the hip are managed by release of the psoas. In-toeing is the result of increased femoral anteversion and this can be addressed by derotation femoral osteotomy. Adduction contractures cause scissoring, and can be managed by BTX-A injection or release.

Hip subluxations are managed by a femoral varus derotation osteotomy with or without a pelvic osteotomy. Hip dislocations can be managed similarly. In severe cases, hip arthrodesis or replacement using constrained implants is considered. Proximal femoral resection helps in achieving abduction in wheelchair-bound patients with chronic hip dislocation.

Knee

Flexion contractures of the knee are managed by release of the posterior capsule and hamstrings or distal femoral extension osteotomy.

Ankle

Equinus at the ankle results from an overactive gastrosoleus and weak tibialis anterior. This is managed by BTX-X injections or lengthening of the Achilles tendon. Spastic tibialis anterior is managed by transfer of the muscle or SPLATT (split anterior tibial tendon transfer).

Foot

A planovalgus foot is managed by calcaneal osteotomy or subtalar fusion. An overactive adductor hallucis can lead to hallux valgus, which can be managed with soft tissue release or osteotomy.

Chapter 13 Trauma

Scapular fracture

General

Classification

Four types of scapular fractures are described in the anatomic classification (Table 13.1).

Management

Most scapular fractures are managed with a sling and early mobilisation. Surgery is indicated for glenoid rim fractures and coracoid fractures with acromioclavicular (AC) separation (see below).

Glenoid fracture

Classification

The classification of glenoid fractures was proposed by Ideberg:

- Type I – fracture of the rim.

Table 13.1. Types of scapular fractures.

Type	Subtype	Description
I	IA	Fracture of the acromion
	IB	Fracture of the spine of the scapula
	IC	Fracture of the coracoid process
II	IIA	Fracture of the neck of the scapula, lateral to the base of the acromion
	IIB	Fracture of the neck extending to the base of the acromion or the spine of the scapula
	IIC	Transverse fracture of the neck of the scapula
III	-	Intra-articular glenoid fracture
IV	-	Fracture of the body of the scapula

- Type II – transverse or oblique fracture of part of the glenoid.
- Type III – fracture involving the base of the spine and coracoid, with the inferior half of the glenoid remaining attached to the body of the scapula.
- Type IV – fracture across the glenoid and body exiting from the medial border.
- Type V – combined type II and IV injuries.

Note

Ideberg R, Grevsten S, Larsson S. Epidemiology of scapular fractures. Incidence and classification of 338 fractures. *Acta Orthop Scand* 1995; 66: 395-7.

Management

Operative stabilisation is generally required to achieve shoulder stability for glenoid rim fractures. An anterior deltopectoral or posterior Judet approach is used. Results are generally good.

Surgery is considered for glenoid neck fractures if the angulation is more than 40° or displacement is more than 1cm.

Note

Goss TP. Fractures of the glenoid neck. *J Shoulder Elbow Surg* 1994; 3: 42-52. **This study reported that type I fractures (90% of glenoid neck injuries) are not significantly displaced and can be managed non-operatively. Type II injuries have more than 1cm displacement or over 40° angulation and should be reduced and fixed.**

Coracoid fracture

Classification
- Type I – fracture of the tip.
- Type II – fracture between the coracoacromial and coracoclavicular ligaments.

- Type III – fracture of the base of the coracoid.

Management
Most coracoid injuries can be managed non-operatively. Type I injuries in high-demand individuals or athletes can be considered for operative stabilisation.

Floating shoulder

A floating shoulder is a combination of clavicle fracture or grade III or more AC joint injury along with fracture of the neck of the scapula.

The results in the literature appear to be similar whether management is with non-operative methods, open reduction and internal fixation (ORIF) of both bones or ORIF of the clavicle only.

Most of the reported studies have been small. In general, significant displacement at any site should prompt consideration of ORIF.

Note

Owens BD, Goss TP. The floating shoulder. *J Bone Joint Surg Br* 2006; 88: 1419-24. **The authors recommended considering fixation of the clavicle, scapula or both if there is significant displacement.**

Acromioclavicular joint dislocation

Classification
Three types were first described by Tossy, Mead and Sigmond. This was later expanded to six types by Rockwood:

- Type I – sprain, but intact AC ligaments.
- Type II – rupture of the AC ligaments, sprain of the coracoclavicular ligaments.
- Type III – disruption of the AC and coracoclavicular ligaments.
- Type IV – posterosuperior button-holing of the clavicle through the trapezius.
- Type V – tear of the deltoid and trapezius, marked superior dislocation.

- Type VI – the clavicle is trapped under the coracoid process.
- Type VII – total clavicular dislocation with disrupted AC and sternoclavicular joints.

Nguyen V, Williams G, Rockwood C. Radiography of acromioclavicular dislocation and associated injuries. *Crit Rev Diagn Imaging* 1991; 32: 191-228.

Pathology

A superior shoulder suspensory complex has been described by Goss. This comprises the superior part of the glenoid, the coracoid process, coracoclavicular ligament, distal end of the clavicle, AC joint and acromion process. Disruption of one part of this ring is often associated with injury to another part – the so-called 'double disruptions'. Injuries to one component of the complex usually respond well to non-operative management, but double disruptions require operative stabilisation.

Goss TP. Double disruptions of the superior shoulder suspensory complex. *J Orthop Trauma* 1993; 7: 99-106.

Diagnosis

The clinical diagnosis is based on local swelling and tenderness. The distal end of the clavicle is prominent in types III and IV. The clavicle feels mobile (piano-key sign).

In the scarf test, adduction of the arm across the chest reproduces the pain. Pain localised to the AC joint on O'Brien's test (see Chapter 16 – shoulder examination) is also specific for injuries to the joint.

Radiographs are normal in types I and II.

Management

- Types I and II – non-surgical management is adequate, with a sling for 1 week for comfort.
- Type III – the management of type III is debatable. Most patients respond well to non-operative management.
- Types IV, V and VI – surgical treatment is generally recommended.

Phillips AM, Smart C, Groom AF. Acromioclavicular dislocation. Conservative or surgical therapy. *Clin Orthop Relat Res* 1998; 353: 10-7. **This meta-analysis found no difference in the results of surgical and non-surgical management.**

Spencer EE Jr. Treatment of grade III acromioclavicular joint injuries. A systematic review. *Clin Orthop Relat Res* 2007; 455: 38-44. **This review found that operative management was not better than non-operative management. In addition, operative management was associated with a higher complication rate, longer recovery and delayed return to work and sport.**

Fixation methods include screws, cerclage wire or sutures (e.g., Tightrope). Other options include reconstruction of the coracoclavicular ligament and transfer of the tip of the coracoid to the clavicle to function as a dynamic transfer. Excision of the lateral end of the clavicle is a further option.

Weaver and Dunn described the classic procedure of transfer of the coracoacromial ligament, whereby the ligament is detached from the acromion and transferred to the lateral end of the clavicle. This is combined with excision of the lateral 5-10mm of the clavicle. Various modifications have been described since.

Note

Weaver JK, Dunn HK. Management of acromioclavicular injuries, especially complete acromioclavicular separation. *J Bone Joint Surg Am* 1972; 54: 1187-94. **Description of transfer of the coracoacromial ligament.**

Clavicle fracture

Clavicle fractures are one of the most common bone injuries. Middle-third fractures account for most clavicular fractures (85%), with the remaining fractures involving the medial third (5%) and the lateral third (10%) (Allman's classification).

Note

Allman FL Jr. Fractures and ligamentous injuries of the clavicle and its articulation. *J Bone Joint Surg Am* 1967; 49: 774-84.

Non-operative management is generally adequate and, despite healing in an overlapped position, functional results are acceptable. More recently, there has been an increasing trend towards fixation of fractures displaced 100% and shortening over 2cm in active, high-demand individuals. Displaced multifragmentary fractures of the mid-portion of the clavicle carry a 10-15% risk of non-union.

Indications for open reduction and internal stabilisation are as follows:

- Neurovascular injury.
- Open fractures.
- A widely displaced fracture in a high-demand patient.
- Non-union.
- Fracture of the distal third with injury to the coracoclavicular ligament.
- Soft tissue interposition.
- A floating shoulder (fracture of the clavicle and the surgical neck of the scapula).

Note

Robinson CM, Court-Brown CM, McQueen MM, Wakefield AE. Estimating the risk of nonunion following nonoperative treatment of a clavicular fracture. *J Bone Joint Surg Am* 2004; 86: 1359-65. **A total of 581 middle-third clavicle fractures were treated non-operatively. Lack of cortical apposition and comminution correlated with a higher risk of non-union.**

Note

Robinson CM. Fractures of the clavicle in the adult. Epidemiology and classification. *J Bone Joint Surg Br* 1998; 80: 476-84.

Options for internal fixation include the following:

- Smooth Steinmann pin bent at 90° under the skin to prevent migration.
- Two threaded Kirschner (K) wires.
- A Rockwood threaded pin.
- A reconstruction plate or contoured locking clavicular plates.

Reconstruction plates have a high risk of breakage. Contoured locking clavicular plates provide the most secure fixation.

The surgical approach can be through two different incisions:

- Along the subcuticular border of the clavicle gives easy access.
- Alternatively, a vertical incision centred over the fracture site can be used to avoid injury to the supraclavicular cutaneous nerves.

Note

Hill JM, McGuire MH, Crosby LA. Closed treatment of displaced middle-third fractures of the clavicle gives poor results. *J Bone Joint Surg Br* 1997; 79: 537-8. A total of 52 completely displaced fractures of the middle third in adults were studied. Fifteen percent resulted in non-union and the results were unsatisfactory in 31%. An initial shortening of more than 2cm was associated with a higher risk of non-union and a final shortening of more than 2cm was associated with a higher incidence of poor function.

Distal third (lateral third) fracture of the clavicle

Classification

The Neer and Rockwood classification is used:

- Type I – fracture lateral to an intact coracoclavicular ligament.
- Type II – fracture medial to the coracoclavicular ligament.
- Type III – an intra-articular AC joint fracture.

Note

Neer CS, 2nd. Fractures of the distal third of the clavicle. *Clin Orthop Relat Res* 1968; 58: 43-50.

Management

Types I and III are treated non-operatively.

Type II injuries have marked deformity and displacement, and up to a 30% non-union rate. Surgery is often needed. Non-absorbable sutures or slings, such as a tightrope passed though the medial fragment and the coracoid, can be used to stabilise the fragment.

A hook plate has been used for these injuries, but is associated with a high rate of impingement due to presence of metalwork in the subacromial space. Plate removal is required to resolve these symptoms.

Sternoclavicular joint dislocation

Dislocation can be anterior or posterior.

Anterior dislocation

Anterior dislocation is evident clinically from a history of trauma and prominence of the medial end of the clavicle. Serendipity views are the preferred radiographs. Computed tomography (CT) scanning is the best imaging modality for diagnosis. Closed reduction is possible and functional limitation is minimal if the joint is irreducible or unstable.

Posterior dislocations

Posterior dislocations risk causing pressure on the mediastinal structures. Manipulation under anaesthetic and reduction by holding the fragment with a sharp towel clip or bone-holding forceps is needed. If unstable, soft tissue reconstruction can be planned. The reconstruction involves using a tendon graft from the semitendinosus or palmaris longus passed through the medial end of the clavicle and manubrium.

Alternatively, the medial 1-2cm of the clavicle can be excised and the remaining part stabilised to the first rib. The results of excision without soft tissue stabilisation are unsatisfactory.

Dislocation of the glenohumeral joint

Dislocation of the glenohumeral joint is a common injury. The underlying mechanism is an abduction and external rotation force that dislocates the humeral head anterior to the glenoid. The vast majority are anterior dislocation. Posterior dislocations are rare and are sometimes missed on radiographs. From a mechanistic point of view more than 95% of these dislocations are classed as 'traumatic', but a minority can occur without significant trauma and demonstrate glenohumeral laxity.

Almost 90% of patients with anterior dislocation have a Bankart's lesion. The inferior glenohumeral ligament is avulsed, usually from the glenoid. Occasionally the ligament may be detached from the humeral attachment. This is known as HAGL (humeral avulsion of the glenohumeral ligament). Other associated injuries include rotator cuff tears and SLAP (superior labral anterior and posterior) lesions.

Clinical features

Patients with dislocation present with pain around the shoulder and a restricted range of motion. In anterior dislocation, the deltoid contour is lost due to the absence of the humeral head lateral to the glenoid. The acromion appears prominent and the anterior axillary fold is lower on the affected side.

Axillary nerve neurapraxia occurs in up to one-third of patients. Circulation in the arm should be checked.

Imaging

Plain radiographs are performed to assess for associated injuries: fracture of the neck of the humerus, greater tuberosity or glenoid rim. Fractures of the greater tuberosity are found in up to 30% of anterior dislocations. Glenoid rim fractures are found in up to 5% of anteroinferior shoulder dislocations.

The West Point axillary view is assessed for fractures of the glenoid rim. The Stryker notch view will show Hill-Sachs lesions (posterolateral humeral head defects).

Management

Isolated dislocations of the humeral head are reduced by closed means under sedation and analgesia. The techniques described for reduction are as follows:

- Hippocratic method – the foot is placed against the proximal end of the humerus and longitudinal traction is applied to the upper extremity.
- Kocher's manoeuvre – comprises traction and external rotation of the arm, followed by

adduction and internal rotation. Although highly successful, this technique is associated with neurovascular complications and humeral head fractures, and is currently not favoured.

- Stimson method – the patient is prone and a 10lb (4.5kg) weight is suspended from the arm. This effects a reduction in a few minutes.
- Rockwood's method – the patient is supine with a sheet placed around the chest to apply countertraction. The arm is carefully pulled in the direction of the deformity and gentle rotational movements help disengage the humeral head.

Once reduction is achieved, radiographs will confirm the congruence as well as any fractures of the proximal humerus.

The arm is immobilised in adduction and internal rotation in a broad arm sling (e.g., Polysling). The duration of immobilisation after reduction, or the presence of a Hill-Sachs lesion, is not related to the risk of recurrence. A sling is advised for comfort and pendulum exercises are started early to minimise stiffness.

Note

Hovelius L, Augustini BG, Fredin H, et al. Primary anterior dislocation of the shoulder in young patients. A ten-year prospective study. J Bone Joint Surg Am 1996; 78: 1677-84. This 10-year prospective study from Sweden looked at 245 patients aged 12-40 years. In 52% there was no further dislocation. With two recurrences within 1 year, 25% of patients were stable in the long term. A quarter of all patients needed stabilisation. The initial management had no effect on recurrence.

Bracing in external rotation (the gunslinger position) was proposed to reduce the risk of recurrence, but further studies have shown that this is no more effective than using the traditional sling in internal rotation.

Note

Itoi E, Hatakeyama Y, Kido T, *et al.* A new method of immobilization after traumatic anterior dislocation of the shoulder: a preliminary study. *J Shoulder Elbow Surg* 2003; 12: 413-5. **This study proposed bracing in external rotation.**

Note

Finestone A, Milgrom C, Radeva-Petrova DR, *et al.* Bracing in external rotation for traumatic anterior dislocation of the shoulder. *J Bone Joint Surg Br* 2009; 91: 918-21. **This was a prospective randomised study in 51 patients. No advantage to bracing in external rotation was found.**

The risk of recurrence following traumatic anterior dislocation is high in young people.

Note

te Slaa RL, Wijffels MP, Brand R, Marti RK. The prognosis following acute primary glenohumeral dislocation. *J Bone Joint Surg Br* 2004; 86: 58-64. **In this study of 105 patients with 4-year follow-up, the overall recurrence was 26%. The recurrence rate was 64% in those aged less than 20 years compared with 6% in those aged more than 40 years.**

Posterior dislocation

Posterior dislocations represent approximately 2% of all shoulder dislocations. These dislocations are often missed at the initial evaluation, leading to permanent disability. Posterior dislocations occur as a result of adduction and axial loading of the shoulder. Violent muscle contraction during seizures and electrocutions are associated with posterior dislocations.

Closed reduction is successful under suitable anaesthesia. The arm is immobilised in external rotation and extension. Open reduction is usually performed through an anterior approach. If the impression fracture (reverse Hill-Sachs) is more than 20% of the humeral head, either subscapularis tendon or the lesser tuberosity is transferred into the defect.

Fracture of the proximal humerus

Four parts of the proximal humerus fracture were first described by Codman and later included in the classification by Neer:

- Humeral head – covered by the articular cartilage and hence has a poor blood supply.
- Lesser tuberosity – with attachment of the subscapularis.
- Greater tuberosity – with attachment of the remaining three rotator cuff muscles.
- Humeral shaft – separated from the proximal humerus by fracture of the surgical neck.

Note

Neer CS, 2nd. Displaced proximal humeral fractures. Part I. Classification and evaluation. By Charles S. Neer, I, 1970. *Clin Orthop Relat Res* 1987; 223: 3-10.

The main blood supply of the humeral head is derived from the anterior circumflex humeral artery, a branch of the third part of the axillary artery. The arcuate artery arises from the anterior circumflex and enters the head from the metaphysis. The posterior circumflex artery provides a small contribution and is in itself unable to maintain vascularity. Fracture of the lesser tuberosity implies a significant risk of loss of blood supply to the humeral head.

Classification

- Avulsion fracture of the tuberosities.
- Impaction fracture.

- Articular surface impression fracture.
- Displaced fractures or fracture dislocations.

The Neer classification for displaced fractures is based on displacement of segments instead of actual fracture lines (see above). A segment is considered displaced if it is more than 45° or more than 1cm translated. This classification has poor interobserver reliability.

> **Note**
>
> Edelson G, Kelly I, Vigder F, Reis ND. A three-dimensional classification for fractures of the proximal humerus. *J Bone Joint Surg Br* 2004; 86: 413-25. **The authors proposed a CT-based three-dimensional classification. The types are two-part, three-part, shield fracture, isolated greater tuberosity fracture and fracture dislocation.**

Fragment stability is an important consideration. A compression fracture will heal faster than a shear fracture.

Management

Impacted/undisplaced fractures

These fractures can be managed in a sling for 2 weeks, with mobilisation starting within 14 days – initially with pendulum exercises followed by active range of motion exercises.

Impacted fractures with unacceptable displacement in active patients require operative correction and stabilisation.

Displaced two-part fractures

Impacted, stable fractures of the surgical neck in elderly patients can be managed in a sling.

Displaced shear fractures in young patients are best managed with internal fixation.

For operative treatment, the choices are reduction and stabilisation with a proximal humeral locking plate, intramedullary nail or percutaneous pins. The locking plate provides rigid fixation and is stable enough to allow early mobilisation, with consequent early rehabilitation.

Greater tuberosity fractures should be reduced and fixed if displaced more than 5mm. A tension-band wire or heavy suture or screw fixation can be used to achieve stability. The displaced fracture may block abduction or external rotation, and hence operative stabilisation is indicated. These fractures are sometimes associated with anterior dislocation.

Lesser tuberosity fractures may be associated with posterior dislocation of the humeral head. Displaced fractures require rotator cuff repair and stabilisation.

Anatomical neck fractures in young patients are managed with fixation with screws. Fixation will not prevent avascular necrosis (AVN), but the head may revascularise before collapse if the fracture heals. In elderly low-demand patients, hemiarthroplasty is the treatment of choice.

Displaced three-part fractures

Fixation of surgical neck fractures and stabilisation of the greater tuberosity is performed with a locking proximal humeral plate. The deltopectoral approach is commonly used. A delay before surgery makes reduction and fixation difficult. Almost one in four patients develops AVN. This is frequently asymptomatic as it involves only a part of the head.

Displaced four-part fractures

In valgus impacted fractures, minimal lateral displacement of the humeral head is associated with intact medial epiphyseal arteries and a viable head. The tuberosities maintain some blood supply to the humeral head. If the head is not mechanically blocking abduction, these patients can be managed non-operatively.

The results of early arthroplasty are better than the results of arthroplasty after failed internal fixation. Neer reported 100% poor results with fixation and recommended hemiarthroplasty for all patients.

> **Note**
>
> Neer CS, 2nd. Four-segment classification of proximal humeral fractures: purpose and reliable use. *J Shoulder Elbow Surg* 2002; 11: 389-400.

Hemiarthroplasty for three- and four-part fractures

> **Note**
>
> Kralinger F, Schwaiger R, Wambacher M, *et al*. Outcome after primary hemiarthroplasty for fracture of the head of humerus. A retrospective multicentre study of 167 patients. *J Bone Joint Surg Br* 2004; 86: 217-9. **Hemiarthroplasty was performed for three- and four-part fractures. Following the procedure, 41.9% of patients were unable to flex beyond 90°. Healing of the tuberosity was found to influence the Constant score. Older patients were at higher risk for non-union of the tuberosity.**

> **Note**
>
> Antuña SA, Sperling JW, Cofield RH. Shoulder hemiarthroplasty for acute fractures of the proximal humerus: a minimum five-year follow-up. *J Shoulder Elbow Surg* 2008; 17: 202-9. **A total of 57 patients (44 women), with an average age of 66 years (range 23-89 years) were followed up for a minimum of 5 years and a mean of 10.3 years. The mean elevation was 100° at final follow-up. On follow-up, 16% had moderate or severe pain and two patients required implant removal. Overall, the pain relief was satisfactory but shoulder function was less predictable.**

> **Note**
>
> Bosch U, Skutek M, Fremerey RW, Tscherne H. Outcome after primary and secondary hemiarthroplasty in elderly patients with fractures of the proximal humerus. *J Shoulder Elbow Surg* 1998; 7: 479-84. **Thirty-nine patients were followed up for a mean of 42 months. Early hemiarthroplasty patients did better than those who underwent delayed operations.**

Fixation of three- and four-part proximal humerus fractures

> **Note**
>
> Solberg BD, Moon CN, Franco DP, Paiement GD. Surgical treatment of three and four-part proximal humerus fractures. *J Bone Joint Surg Am* 2009; 91: 1689-97. **This study looked at 122 patients, all aged more than 55 years. Thirty-eight patients had a locking plate and 48 had hemiarthroplasty. There was a minimum 2-year follow-up. Those with locked plates had a better outcome than those with hemiarthroplasty, but a higher complication rate. Initial varus angulation of the head correlated with poor outcome with a locked plate, while those with a valgus impacted pattern did better with fixation.**

> **Note**
>
> Moonot P, Ashwood N, Hamlet M. Early results for treatment of three- and four-part fractures of the proximal humerus using the PHILOS plating system. *J Bone Joint Surg Br* 2007; 89: 1206-9. **Thirty-two patients were followed up for a mean of 11 months. There was one non-union and one screw breakage.**

Note

Südkamp N, Bayer J, Hepp P, *et al*. Open reduction and internal fixation of proximal humeral fractures with use of the locking proximal humerus plate. Results of a prospective, multicenter, observational study. *J Bone Joint Surg Am* 2009; 91: 1320-8. **From 187 patients 34% experienced a complication, of which 40% were related to incorrect surgical technique. The reoperation rate was 19% within 1 year.**

Fracture dislocation

Closed or open reduction of the humeral head may be used. ORIF is indicated in three-part fracture dislocations. In four-part dislocations, an effort should be made to preserve the humeral head in young patients. In older patients, hemiarthroplasty may be the best option.

Articular surface impression defects are generally associated with dislocations of the glenohumeral joint with the glenoid making the impression on the head. Treatment options are as follows:

- For anterior defects – transfer of the subscapularis with or without the lesser tuberosity into the defect.
- For posterior defects – proximal humeral retroversion osteotomy.
- For large defects (>40%) – prosthetic replacement or autografting.

With humeral head splitting fractures, there is a high risk of AVN in fragments. Prosthetic replacement is often needed.

Surgical approach

The deltopectoral approach provides extensile exposure. The deltoid can be reflected from the clavicle as an osteoperiosteal flap. This can be combined with an acromion osteotomy for further exposure of the proximal fragments. The acromion osteotomy is fixed back with screws.

For limited access, a deltoid splitting approach is an option.

Humeral shaft fracture

Humeral shaft fractures are commonly low-energy injuries. In one study (see below), the incidence was 14.5 per 100,000 per year and increased with age. Humeral shaft fractures account for 3% of all fractures.

Note

Ekholm R, Adami J, Tidermark J, *et al*. Fractures of the shaft of humerus. An epidemiological study of 401 fractures. *J Bone Joint Surg Br* 2006; 88: 1469-73. **Radial nerve palsy was seen in 8% of 401 fractures. Two percent of fractures were open and 8% were pathological.**

Management

Most humeral shaft fractures are managed non-operatively. Bracing achieves healing in more than 90% of cases and can be preceded by a period of 1-2 weeks in a cast splint. However, it often takes up to 12 weeks of immobilisation to achieve solid bony union. It can also be difficult to control fracture alignment in some patients. The current trend is towards an aggressive approach with a low threshold for internal fixation, particularly in young, active patients.

Note

Klennerman L. Fractures of the shaft of the humerus. *J Bone Joint Surg Br* 1966; 48: 105-11. **Twenty-degree anterior angulation, 30° varus angulation and up to 3cm of shortening is well tolerated with little functional deficit.**

The indications for surgery are as follows:

- Open fractures.
- Vascular injury.
- Pathologic fractures.
- Polytrauma.
- Segmental fractures.
- Irreducible fracture or unacceptable alignment with non-operative management (includes long spiral fractures, which often have soft tissue interposition).
- Spiral fracture of the distal third (Holstein Lewis) with radial nerve palsy.
- Floating elbow.
- Patient unable to tolerate or adhere to non-operative management.
- Associated chest-wall trauma or bilateral fractures.
- Radial nerve palsy developing secondary to manipulation of the fracture.

The posterior approach allows exposure of 15cm of the humerus above the lateral epicondyle (20cm above the medial epicondyle) before the radial nerve is encountered. The recommended approach is to identify the nerve between the long and lateral head of the triceps (approximately 9cm from the tip of the acromion) and trace its course.

There are several indications for exploring the radial nerve:

- Open fractures.
- Nerve palsy occurring after closed reduction.
- Holstein and Lewis fracture – closed spiral fracture at the distal third of the humerus where the radial nerve is at high risk of being trapped between the two fragments. If nerve palsy develops after closed reduction, exploration and internal fixation is indicated.

> **Note**
>
> Ekholm R, Ponzer S, Törnkvist H, *et al.* The Holstein-Lewis humeral shaft fracture: aspects of radial nerve injury, primary treatment, and outcome. *J Orthop Trauma* 2008; 22: 693-7. **This retrospective multicentre study looked at 27 patients with a Holstein-Lewis fracture. The risk of radial nerve injury was 22% compared with 8% for humeral fractures in general. Seven patients were managed operatively. Six patients had radial nerve injury (two managed non-operatively and four operatively). There was no relationship between radial nerve recovery and operative management.**

In other situations, it may be advisable to wait for up to 3 months and observe the recovery of nerve function. In most instances the nerve will recover. If there is no recovery then nerve conduction studies are undertaken, followed by nerve repair/graft or tendon transfer.

Fixation options

Plating

Locking plates or dynamic compression plates are used. Fixation extending to eight cortices on either side of the fracture is desirable. A 96% union rate with 2% incidence of radial nerve palsy has been reported. A broad plate with staggered holes is preferable to avoid the possibility of fissuring (longitudinal splitting) of the shaft.

In the upper two-thirds, plates are applied on the anterior or anterolateral surface to avoid injury to the radial nerve. The humeral shaft is exposed after splitting the brachialis, which carries a dual nerve supply. In the distal third, plates are easier to apply on the flat posterior surface.

The relationship of the radial nerve and plate should be recorded in the notes.

Note

McCormack RG, Brien D, Buckley RE, *et al.* Fixation of fractures of the shaft of the humerus by dynamic compression plate or intramedullary nail. A prospective, randomised trial. *J Bone Joint Surg Br* 2000; 82: 336-9. **This study randomised 44 patients with a 6-month follow-up. Six patients with fixation by an intramedullary nail experienced shoulder impingement, seven needed secondary surgery and 13 had a complication. Only three patients with a plate experienced a complication.**

Intramedullary nail

In antegrade humeral nailing, the rotator cuff should be repaired at the entry site and the proximal end of the nail should be under the surface of the bone. The intramedullary canal ends 2-3cm above the olecranon fossa. The nail should be statically locked. Distal locking carries a risk of injury to the nerves around the elbow, but improves stability.

In retrograde nailing, the entry point is located posteriorly, 2.5cm above the olecranon fossa. A triceps splitting approach is used. There is a risk of iatrogenic fracture and myositis ossificans in the triceps, leading to elbow stiffness.

Nailing is preferable for segmental fractures and pathologic fractures.

Note

Crates J, Whittle AP. Antegrade interlocking nailing of acute humeral shaft fractures. *Clin Orthop Relat Res* 1998; 350: 40-50. **From 73 acute fractures, the authors recorded non-union in 6%, transient radial nerve palsies in 3% and infection in 2%. Ninety percent of patients regained normal shoulder function and 96% regained normal elbow function.**

External fixation

Uniplanar lateral fixators are generally used. The radial nerve is at risk of injury during pin insertion. The main indication is temporary stabilisation in polytrauma victims and patients with open fractures.

Periprosthetic humeral fracture

Periprosthetic humeral fractures involve fracture of the humerus in the presence of a shoulder or elbow replacement prosthesis.

In well-fixed components, the aim is to achieve healing of the fracture with fixation rather than revision of the humeral stem. A shaft fracture can be stabilised with a compression plate supplemented with cable, strut graft or bone grafting. Revision of the prosthesis is considered if the components are loose.

Removal of plates from the humerus runs the risk of radial nerve injury. Adequate healing of the fracture should be confirmed before plate removal. Patients should abstain from heavy lifting for 6-8 weeks following plate removal to reduce the risk of fracture through the screw holes.

Fracture of the distal humerus

Anatomy of the distal humerus

The distal humeral articular surface comprises the trochlea and the capitellum. The articular surface is angled anteriorly in the sagittal plane by 30° in relation to the shaft. Additionally, the articular surface is tilted laterally (valgus) in the coronal plane, giving the carrying angle of the elbow. The normal angle is 10-15° in males and 12-16° in females.

Types

Supracondylar fracture in adults

These can be managed non-operatively with a hanging cast. Alternatively, ORIF can be used with crossed compression screws in the medial and lateral pillars. Contoured plates can be applied for comminuted fractures.

Transcondylar fractures

The fracture line in transcondylar fractures is intra-articular and runs across the condyles. These are unstable injuries and the callus itself may restrict motion. Percutaneous cannulated screws can enable early motion and restoration of function.

Intercondylar fractures

A commonly used classification has been given by Riseborough and Radin:

- Type I – an undisplaced fracture between the trochlea and capitellum.
- Type II – a displaced fracture, but no rotation of fragments.
- Type III – rotation of fragments.
- Type IV – a comminuted fracture.

Note

Riseborough EJ, Radin EL. Intercondylar T fractures of the humerus in the adult. A comparison of operative and non-operative treatment in twenty-nine cases. J Bone Joint Surg Am 1969; 51: 130-41.

The AO group has proposed a classification for distal humeral fractures:

- Type A – extra-articular fracture:
  - 1 – apophyseal avulsion;
  - 2 – metaphyseal simple;
  - 3 – metaphyseal multifragmentary.
- Type B – partial articular fracture:
  - 1 – sagittal lateral condyle;
  - 2 – sagittal medial condyle;
  - 3 – frontal.
- Type C – complete articular fracture:
  - 1 – articular simple, metaphyseal simple;
  - 2 – articular simple, metaphyseal multi-fragmentary;
  - 3 – articular multifragmentary.

Planning should be conducted preoperatively on radiographs. CT scans are also useful in planning. Intraoperative traction radiographs can be helpful in defining various fragments.

Fracture of the medial or lateral humeral condyle in adults

Displaced fractures are fixed by medial or lateral incision. These are intra-articular injuries and require stable anatomic fixation and early mobilisation.

Fracture of the lateral epicondyle

These are generally associated with elbow dislocations. The fragment usually reduces once the elbow is reduced. If satisfactory alignment is achieved, the injury can be managed non-operatively. If rotated, internal fixation is advisable.

Fracture of the medial epicondyle

This is rare in adults and is usually the result of a direct injury or an avulsion fracture. Small, undisplaced fractures do not need surgery.

Indications for surgery include a fragment displaced into the elbow joint and displaced fractures in high-demand patients. Fixation is achieved with a screw and the ulnar nerve should be protected from damage.

Management

The choice of treatment depends on the patient's age, functional demand, degree of osteoporosis, type of fracture, degree of displacement, extent of joint involvement and the presence of compression fractures of joint surfaces.

Undisplaced fractures can be managed non-operatively. An initial cast is followed by gradual mobilisation.

Displaced fractures require ORIF. Total elbow arthroplasty is an option in comminuted fractures in elderly patients.

Surgery is preferably performed within 48 hours. An open fracture, associated vascular injury and other associated injuries are indications for emergent surgery. Open fractures should be debrided and internally fixed to reduce the risk of sepsis. In the presence of gross contamination and delayed presentation, spanning fixators can be used for temporary stabilisation.

As a treatment, traction imposes a long period in hospital, results in stiffness and does not restore anatomical alignment. Intra-articular fractures of the distal humerus are treated with anatomic reduction, rigid internal fixation and early active mobilisation. The elbow joint does not tolerate long periods of immobilisation and residual stiffness often results.

Surgical approach

The incision is posterior in the midline of the arm and ends distal to the olecranon, curving medially around the point of the elbow. Curving the incision medially is cosmetically more acceptable and gives easy access to the ulnar nerve. The ulnar nerve should always be isolated and protected. Most fractures with intra-articular displacement or comminution are best visualised with a transolecranon approach.

Campbell's posterior approach involves elevation of a distally based U-flap of the triceps aponeurosis to expose the distal humerus. The ulnar nerve should be identified and protected.

In olecranon osteotomy, extra-articular osteotomy provides only restricted exposure.

Intra-articular olecranon osteotomy can be transverse or chevron. The transverse osteotomy does not provide rotational stability. A chevron pattern with the apex pointing distally is the preferred option.

Osteotomy is performed 2cm from the tip of the olecranon. A drill hole and tap should be made prior to osteotomy to help with fixation after fixing the humeral fracture. Using an oscillating saw through three-quarters of the olecranon and fracturing the remaining with an osteotome helps to prevent iatrogenic injury to the articular surface. The osteotomy can be fixed securely with a combination of an intramedullary, partially threaded cancellous screw and a tension-band wire. Olecranon osteotomy is relatively contraindicated if a total elbow replacement is possible.

Note

Jacobson SR, Glisson RR, Urbaniak JR. Comparison of distal humerus fixation: a biomechanical study. *J South Orthop Assoc* 1997; 6: 241-9. **In this study, a medial reconstruction plate with posterolateral dynamic compression plate provided maximum stiffness.**

Principles of surgery

Careful preoperative planning is essential to decide the fixation method and approach. The patient should be in a lateral position to give access to the posterior aspect of the arm and elbow. The draping should allow free movement of the extremity. Reconstruction of the articular fragments is performed first, and then the articular block is fixed to the diaphysis. Provisional stabilisation can be gained by K-wires or the guide wire of a cannulated screw system. Soft tissue attachments of the fragments should be preserved.

The metalwork is placed on the medial and lateral columns and should not encroach on the olecranon fossa, coronoid fossa or radial fossa. Two plates, 90° to each other, should be used for maximum mechanical stability. One plate is applied to the medial border and the other posterolaterally. In the lateral view, the longitudinal axis of the lateral condyle is angled 60° anterior to the axis of the shaft and this relationship should be restored on fixation.

Postoperatively, supervised active motion can be started after 48-72 hours if stable fixation has been achieved. Immobilisation for 3 weeks in a cast leads to stiffness.

Complications

- Infection.
- Non-union.
- Malunion.
- Heterotopic ossification.
- Nerve injury.
- Failure of fixation.

Doornberg JN, van Duijn PJ, Linzel D, et al. Surgical treatment of intra-articular fractures of the distal part of the humerus. Functional outcome after twelve to thirty years. J Bone Joint Surg Am 2007; 89: 1524-32. **This study conducted a long-term follow-up of 30 patients with an AO type C fracture. The average flexion arc was 106° and the average pronation-supination arc was 165° at final follow-up. Overall, 26 patients had a good or excellent result, and the rest had a fair or poor result.**

ORIF is not contraindicated in elderly patients. Total elbow arthroplasty is an option for comminuted fractures. Where internal fixation may be unsatisfactory due to osteoporotic bones, constrained elbow replacement (Coonrad-Morrey) should be considered.

Cobb TK, Morrey BF. Total elbow arthroplasty as primary treatment for distal humerus fractures in elderly patients. J Bone Joint Surg Am 1997; 79: 826-32. **In this study of 20 patients with an average age of 72 years, 15 had excellent results and five had good results at 3 years.**

Capitellum fracture

The mechanism of a capitellum fracture is a shearing injury, because the centre of the capitellum is 12-15mm anterior to the humeral shaft axis.

Classification

- Type I – complete fracture (Hahn-Steinthal fracture), large fragment of bone and cartilage.
- Type II – superficial fracture of the subchondral bone and articular cartilage (Kocher-Lorenz fracture).
- Type III – comminuted fracture.
- Type IV – coronal shear of the capitellum and part of the trochlear ridge (described by Mckee et al). Coronal shear fracture of the capitellum is indicated by a double-arc sign on lateral X-ray.

More complex articular fractures involving the lateral condyle and extending to the trochlea have been described by Ring.

McKee MD, Jupiter JB, Bamberger HB. Coronal shear fractures of the distal end of the humerus. J Bone Joint Surg Am 1996; 78: 49-54.

Ring D, Jupiter JB, Gulotta L. Articular fractures of the distal part of the humerus. J Bone Joint Surg Am 2003; 85-A: 232-8.

Management

The anterior aspect of the capitellum articulates with the radial head in the flexed elbow. The posterior surface of the capitellum is non-articular. The osteochondral fragment often displaces superiorly into the radial fossa of the distal humerus.

Type I fractures are managed with closed reduction or ORIF. A lateral approach is taken between the anconeus and the extensor carpi ulnaris. Fixation is performed with Herbert screws or a posteroanterior lag screw. The screw is countersunk.

Type II and III fractures are managed with early excision. Small fragments are difficult to fix due to high shear forces and excision may provide the best chance for minimising disability.

Type IV fractures and other complex fractures with trochlear extension are best treated with internal fixation. These injuries can be clearly defined with preoperative CT scans. Most type IV fractures can be stabilised through a lateral approach, but some with medial extension warrant a posterior approach and lateral columnar plate fixation.

Complications

Complications include AVN, non-union, malunion and elbow stiffness.

Elbow dislocations

Anatomy

The elbow centre of rotation is 12-15mm anterior to the humeral shaft axis. The articular surface on the radial head covers an arc of 240°. There is a bare area on the lateral side of the radial head of 110°, which is a safe area for fixation devices. The proximal ulna forms an arc of 60-80°, which articulates with the radius.

Elbow dislocation can be posterior, anterior, medial, lateral or divergent, based on the position of the forearm in relation to the distal humerus. Combinations are possible and common. In divergent dislocation there is disruption of the radioulnar joint with separation of the radius and ulna.

Clinical assessment

The direction of dislocation is assessed. Posterior or posterolateral dislocations are most common.

Injury to the median, ulnar or anterior interosseous nerve is evaluated. Most nerve injuries are neurapraxia due to stretch and resolve spontaneously.

Injury to brachial artery is also assessed. Intimal damage is due to stretching. This may cause acute vascular occlusion or delayed occlusion as a result of thrombosis. A vein graft is required if vascular insufficiency is not restored after reduction.

Management

Simple elbow dislocations without associated fractures are managed with prompt relocation and early active mobilisation. Close follow-up with X-rays is required to detect dislocation recurrence.

Open reduction is required if closed reduction is unsuccessful. A posterior approach gives access to both medial and lateral structures. The lateral approach may be useful if the dislocation is associated with a radial head fracture and ligament injury.

The elbow is immobilised for 7-10 days before active motion is started. Further immobilisation is unlikely to improve stability, but may result in stiffness.

Fracture dislocations are screened for instability under anaesthesia. If unstable at or beyond 30° of extension, fixation of coronoid and radial head fractures and lateral ligament complex reconstruction may be required.

> **Note**
>
> Maripuri SN, Debnath UK, Rao P, Mohanty K. Simple elbow dislocation among adults: a comparative study of two different methods of treatment. *Injury* 2007; 38: 1254-8.

> **Note**
>
> Harrington IJ, Sekyi-Otu A, Barrington TW, *et al*. The functional outcome with metallic radial head implants in the treatment of unstable elbow fractures: a long-term review. *J Trauma* 2001; 50: 46-52. **From 20 patients with a 12.1-year follow-up, excellent results were reported in 12 patients, good results in four, fair results in two and poor results in two.**

Indications for nerve exploration

Exploration is considered if there is no recovery from nerve injury 3 months after dislocation. The onset of nerve palsy signs after reduction is a further indication for exploration.

Complications

- Stiffness, commonly with loss of 5-10° of terminal extension.
- Post-traumatic arthritis – in elbow fracture dislocations.
- Heterotopic ossification – this can cause significant stiffness. It may appear radiologically within 4 weeks. It is related to soft tissue damage and possibly passive elbow mobilisation. Preventative measures include local radiation therapy, which is often impractical considering the presence of a fracture or surgical incision. Indomethacin can be given orally.

- Ectopic calcification in the collateral ligaments and capsule is common and does not require treatment.

Terrible triad

The 'terrible triad' describes dislocation of the elbow, coronoid fracture and radial head fracture. The lateral ulnar collateral ligament is often torn in this pattern. This may lead to recurrent posterior subluxation or dislocation with a poor outcome. Most series report uniformly poor results in patients with the terrible triad. Radial head excision in this situation is contraindicated as it often leads to redislocation and instability. A consistent treatment algorithm consisting of fixation of coronoid or anterior capsular avulsion, radial head fixation or replacement and repair of lateral ligament repair, carried out in a sequential manner (Figure 13.1), has been shown to improve outcomes.

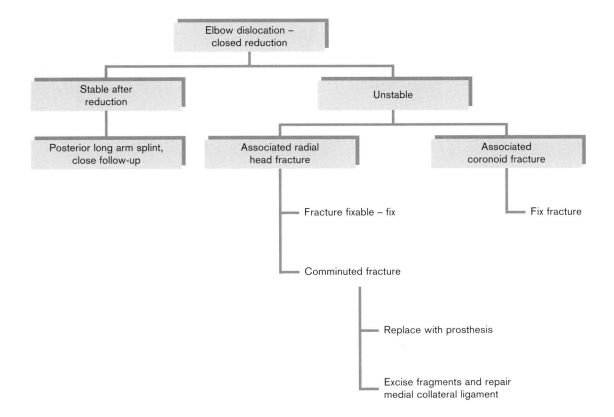

Figure 13.1. An algorithm for the management of fracture dislocations of the elbow.

Note

Pugh DM, Wild LM, Schemitsch EH, *et al*. Standard surgical protocol to treat elbow dislocations with radial head and coronoid fractures. *J Bone Joint Surg Am* 2004; 86-A: 1122-30. **In 36 patients with the terrible triad, the radial head was fixed or replaced, the coronoid was fixed and capsular injury repaired. At a mean of 34 months postoperatively, the mean flexion extension arc was 112° and forearm rotation was 136°.**

A hinged elbow external fixator can be applied to provide stability while the soft tissues heal. The hinge allows flexion and extension and the axis of the hinge is aligned with the axis of rotation of the elbow joint.

Recurrent elbow dislocation

Injury to the lateral collateral ligament leads to chronic posterolateral instability of the elbow. Clinically this causes pain, swelling, instability and clicking. A pivot shift test of the elbow is positive. Management is based on reconstructing the ligament using tendon grafts.

Coronoid fracture

Classification

Classification is from Regan and Morrey:

- Type I – avulsion of the tip of the coronoid.
- Type II – fracture of less than 50% of the coronoid.
- Type III – fracture of more than 50% of the coronoid.

Note

Regan W, Morrey B. Fractures of the coronoid process of the ulna. *J Bone Joint Surg Am* 1989; 71: 1348-54.

A compression fracture of the anteromedial facet of the coronoid has also been described. The mechanism is mainly varus force with concomitant injury to the lateral collateral ligament. These fractures are fixed with an anteromedial buttress plate along with lateral ligament repair to protect against posteromedial rotatory instability of the elbow.

Management

Types I and II are managed with closed treatment with early mobilisation. If the injury is associated with elbow dislocation, the brachialis is reattached with non-absorbable sutures passed through drill holes in the proximal ulna.

Type III fracture is managed with reduction and fixation with early mobilisation. These fractures are often associated with elbow dislocations. An interfragmentary screw is used to fix the fracture.

Olecranon fracture

Mechanism of injury

The usual mechanism is a fall on the point of the elbow or a fall on an outstretched hand with the elbow in flexion.

Classification

The classification of olecranon fractures is shown in Table 13.2.

Management

The aim of management is to restore the articular surface, preserve the extensor mechanism and maintain elbow stability.

Type I fractures (Colton classification) are managed with splinting with the elbow flexed to 90°. The position of the patient is either supine with the arm in a trough across the chest or prone.

Table 13.2. Classification of olecranon fracture.

Type		Description
Anatomical classification		
I		Fractures involving the proximal one-third of the articular surface of the olecranon notch
II		Fractures involving the middle one-third of the articular surface of the olecranon notch
	IIA	No comminution
	IIB	Articular comminution or depressed fracture
III		Fractures involving the distal one-third of the articular surface of the olecranon notch
Colton classification		
I		Undisplaced: <2mm displacement with an intact extensor mechanism
II		Displaced
	IIA	Avulsion fractures
	IIB	Oblique and transverse
	IIC	Comminuted
	IID	Fracture dislocations

Type II fractures (Colton classification) are managed with tension-band wiring with two knots. If associated with a coronoid fracture, open reduction and stabilisation by plating helps to fix the coronoid fracture as well as the olecranon.

Olecranon fractures associated with radial head fractures indicate ligament injury. The radial head fracture should be reduced and fixed or the radial head replaced to restore stability.

Tension-band wiring with a figure-of-eight loop is the most common method of fixation. The superficial surface of the olecranon is the tension surface and placing the figure of eight on this surface provides compression across the fracture site as the elbow flexes. The figure of eight is supplemented with an intramedullary screw or K-wires. Two 1.6mm wires are passed into the canal and not through the anterior cortex of the ulna. The K-wires resist rotational and angular forces across the fracture site.

Active range of motion exercises can be started after 7 days and splinting is discontinued within the following 2 weeks.

Plating of the olecranon is preferred for comminuted fractures, particularly of the compression side and fractures extending beyond the trochlear notch; 3.5mm reconstruction plates are suitable for this. Precontoured, low-profile locking plates are available, and provide comprehensive fixation options.

Plates are commonly applied to the posterior surface, which can be prominent and palpable under the skin. Plates on the medial or lateral surface are biomechanically less strong, but absolve the problem of prominent hardware.

Radial fracture

Radial head fracture

Fractures of the radial head are a common injury and about 10% of elbow dislocations are associated with radial head fracture. The radial head resists valgus stress.

Thirty percent of radial head fractures are associated with coronoid fractures, medial collateral injury or ulnar nerve neurapraxia. A medial collateral ligament injury with a radial head fracture results in an unstable elbow.

The mechanism of injury is a fall on the hand with a pronated forearm.

Classification
Classification is by Mason:

- Type I – segmental undisplaced fracture of the radial head.
- Type II – segmental radial head displaced fracture.
- Type III – comminuted radial head.
- Type IV – radial head fracture associated with elbow dislocation (added by Broberg and Morrey).

Note

Mason ML. Some observations on fractures of the head of the radius with a review of one hundred cases. *Br J Surg* 1954; 42: 123-32.

Note

Broberg MA, Morrey BF. Results of treatment of fracture dislocations of the elbow. *Clin Orthop* 1987; 216: 109-19.

Management
Management is based on the classification:

- Type I – non-operative with early active motion. One-third of patients experience restriction of full extension. The risk of non-union is 5%. Non-union is managed with excision of the fragment.
- Type II – if the radial head is displaced less than 2mm and the patient has normal pronation and supination, then non-operative management is preferred. If there is a block to motion or displacement is more than 2mm, internal fixation with screws and plate is performed. The block to motion can be assessed after infiltration of local anaesthetic in the elbow.
- Type III – if there is no forearm pain (indicates absence of significant interosseous membrane injury), the coronoid is intact and the elbow is stable in valgus strain in 30° flexion, the radial head should be excised. If not, replacement of the radial head is considered to provide stability.
- Type IV – restore stability by repairing ligaments and replacing the radial head.

Indications for surgery
- Loose intra-articular fragments.
- Associated olecranon fracture or medial collateral ligament injury.
- Block to motion from a displaced fragment.
- Axially unstable radius because of injury to the interosseous membrane or the distal radioulnar joint.

The radial head has a bare area of approximately 110° opposite to the articulation with the sigmoid notch. This is a non-articular part of the radial head and is suitable for the placement of fixation metalwork.

In radial head fractures with associated medial collateral ligament injury, the radial head should be preserved if possible by internal fixation. If the fracture is not fixable, a radial head replacement is the option. Late excision is acceptable, but early excision (within 3 weeks) will impair the healing of the medial ligament.

Radial head excision is performed through a posterolateral approach between the anconeus and extensor carpi ulnaris. The annular ligament is removed and all fragments are excised. The radial neck is divided just proximal to the radial tuberosity. Motion is started at 1 week and the sling is discarded at 3 weeks.

Early motion reduces pericapsular scarring and increases range of motion. Excision of the radial head may lead to proximal migration of the ulna and posterolateral instability of the elbow.

Radial head replacement
The radial head can be replaced with silicone or metal implants. Silicone implants have a high incidence of synovitis, while metal implants provide more stability. Lateral epicondyle osteotomy may be needed to insert the implant.

> **Note**
>
> Frank SG, Grewal R, Johnson J, *et al.* Determination of correct implant size in radial head arthroplasty to avoid overlengthening. *J Bone Joint Surg Am* 2009; 91: 1738-46. **The authors determined that incongruity of the lateral ulnohumeral joint is a reliable indicator of over-lengthening of the radius.**

> **Note**
>
> Ikeda M, Sugiyama K, Kang C, *et al.* Comminuted fractures of the radial head. Comparison of resection and internal fixation. *J Bone Joint Surg Am* 2005; 87: 76-84. **This study found no difference in range of motion between fixation and excision groups. The fixation group had significantly higher strength and functional scores.**

> **Note**
>
> Ring D, Quintero J, Jupiter JB. Open reduction and internal fixation of fractures of the radial head. *J Bone Joint Surg Am* 2002; 84-A: 1811-5. **In this study, fixation in comminuted radial head fractures with more than three fragments yielded unsatisfactory results.**

Radial neck fracture

Classification
Classification is similar to that of radial head fractures:

- Type I – undisplaced radial head.
- Type II – displaced radial head with one large fragment.
- Type III – comminuted radial head.

Management
Management options are internal fixation by T-plate, interfragmentary screws and excision of the radial head.

Essex-Lopresti fracture dislocation

Essex-Lopresti fracture dislocation is fracture of the radial head or neck with disruption of the distal radioulnar joint.

The mechanism of injury is a fall on an outstretched hand. The distal radioulnar joint is disrupted, along with tearing of the interosseous membrane and fracture of the radial head or neck. The membrane normally stabilises the radius and prevents its proximal migration. If the radial head is excised in this injury, the radius will migrate proximally due to an incompetent interosseous membrane. This will lead to radiocapitellar impingement at the elbow and ulnar carpal impingement at the wrist.

The diagnosis is indicated by radial head fracture along with pain along the forearm and at the distal radioulnar joint.

Management
Radial head excision is contraindicated in Essex-Lopresti fracture dislocation.

If the radial head is fixable, internal fixation is performed along with stabilisation of the distal radioulnar joint with a K-wire across the distal radius and ulna. The K-wire is removed after 6 weeks.

In comminuted fractures, the radial head is replaced and the distal joint stabilised with a K-wire.

Fracture of the radius and ulna

Monteggia lesions

Mechanism of injury
Hyperpronation-hyperextension injury.

Classification
Classification was proposed by Bado:

- Type I – anterior dislocation of the radial head with an anterior angulated fracture of the ulna.
- Type II – posterior dislocation of the radial head with a posterior angulated fracture of the ulna.
- Type III – lateral dislocation of the radial head with fracture of the proximal ulna.

- Type IV – anterior dislocation of the radial head with a proximal third fracture of the radius and ulna.

Radiographs
Clinicians should have a high index of suspicion for radial head dislocation in proximal ulna fractures. If the radial head is not dislocated, it must line up with the capitellum in all views of the elbow.

Management
An algorithm for the management of Monteggia lesions is shown in Figure 13.2.

Reconstruction of the annular ligament can be performed using a strip from the forearm fascia or

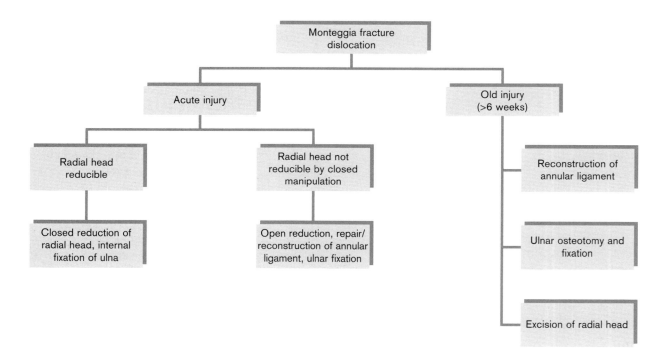

Figure 13.2. Treatment algorithm for Monteggia fracture dislocation.

triceps aponeurosis. This is used to make a loop around the radial head

If the ulnar fracture is associated with a fracture of the radial head, the radial head should either be fixed or replaced with a radial head prosthesis to restore stability at the time of ulnar fixation.

Pronation and supination exercises can be started under supervision at 4 weeks. Close follow-up with radiographs is advisable to ensure the radial head does not sublux or dislocate postoperatively.

Galeazzi lesion

A Galeazzi lesion is a fracture anywhere in the radial shaft, with or without fracture of the ulna with distal radial joint injury.

X-ray shows the following:

- Signs of distal radioulnar joint injury.
- Ulnar styloid fracture.
- Widening of joint space on the anteroposterior (AP) view.
- Dislocation of the radius on the lateral view.
- Radial shortening of more than 5mm.

Management
Management is ORIF by a dynamic compression plate. The distal radioulnar joint reduces when the radial fracture is reduced. If the joint is unstable, it can be stabilised with a K-wire.

Fracture of the radius and ulna midshaft

Angulation of more than 10° in either bone restricts forearm function. Internal fixation is indicated with angulation of more 10° or displacement of more than 50% at the fracture site.

Management
In adults, this injury is best managed with anatomic reduction, rigid internal fixation and early mobilisation. Fixation may be achieved with intramedullary rods or dynamic compression plates.

Closed treatment is indicated with undisplaced fractures and with less than 10° angulation in an isolated distal ulna fracture. External fixation is an alternative to internal fixation in severe soft tissue injury.

Complications with intramedullary implants include poor rotational control, loss of radial bow, shortening and non-union.

Plate fixation achieves union in 96-98% of cases. The radial bow should be restored. Fixation is recommended in six cortices in each fragment. Plate fixation allows early mobilisation and no postoperative cast is required.

The dorsal approach (Thompson) carries a risk of injury to the posterior interosseous nerve. Henry's approach carries a risk of damage to the superficial branch of the radial nerve.

Complications
Complications include malunion, synostosis and stress fracture. Osteotomies performed within 12 months regain better rotation.

Cross-union between the radius and ulna occurs in up to 5% of patients. Factors which predispose to the increased incidence of synostosis are delayed ORIF, severely comminuted fractures and placement of a bone graft near the interosseous membrane.

The Vince and Miller classification is used, which is based on the site of synostosis:

- Type I – distal intra-articular part of the radius and ulna.
- Type II – non-articular distal and middle third of the radius and ulna.
- Type III – proximal third of the radius and ulna.

Resection and interposition of a silicone sheet or fat is successful in 50% of cases. This should be performed 1-3 years after injury. The worst prognosis is in type I and the best in type II.

A stress fracture can occur at the end of the plate, which is the junction of bone supported by the plate with the unsupported bone. Plate removal can be performed after 2 years but is not routinely advised. Indications for plate removal include irritation from a subcutaneous location of the plate. In addition, plate removal may be advised in athletes participating in contact sports. Following plate removal, the forearm should be protected in a splint for 6-8 weeks.

Fracture of the distal radius

Epidemiology

The incidence of this injury is 1 in 500 persons per year. It follows a bimodal distribution – one peak in the second decade of life and a second in the seventh decade.

Anatomy

The normal ulnar inclination of the distal radial articular surface is 23° in the AP view. The normal volar inclination of the distal radial articular surface (lunate fossa) is 11° in the lateral view.

Radial length is measured as the distance between a line drawn through the tip of the radial styloid perpendicular to the long axis of the radius and another line drawn through the distal articular surface of the ulna. Typically this distance is 12mm. The distal radial articular surface is generally 1mm distal to the distal ulnar articular surface.

Classification

AO:

- A – extra-articular.
- B – partial articular.
- C – complete articular.

Other classification systems have been proposed by Frykman and Malone.

The universal classification is simple and descriptive and is commonly used:

- Type I – undisplaced extra-articular.
- Type II – displaced extra-articular.

- Type III – undisplaced intra-articular.
- Type IV – displaced intra-articular.

Types II and IV are further divided into reducible and stable, reducible and unstable, irreducible, and complex.

Evaluation

The posteroanterior view, lateral view and oblique radiographs are used to assess the lunate fossa, scaphoid fossa and sigmoid notch.

CT scans can be used to see the joint surface step or metaphyseal comminution. Magnetic resonance imaging (MRI) will demonstrate the soft tissue injuries.

Radial shortening (3-6mm) may lead to a poor clinical result with symptoms of ulnar-sided pain, decreased forearm rotation, diminished grip and ulnar carpal impaction.

Dorsal tilt leads to increased load transmission through the ulna. This can cause dorsal intercalated segment instability and extrinsic midcarpal instability.

Loss of ulnar inclination leads to increased load transmission onto the lunate fossa.

An intra-articular step greater than the thickness of the articular cartilage leads to poor remodelling and increased contact stresses. The intra-articular step-off should be less than 2mm.

> **Note**
>
> Barton T, Chambers C, Bannister G. A comparison between subjective outcome score and moderate radial shortening following a fractured distal radius in patients of mean age 69 years. *J Hand Surg Eur Vol* 2007; 32: 165-9. In this study, 60 patients were managed with K-wiring. Shortening of 8mm did not correlate with poor outcome. The Frykman classification correlated with outcome.

Note

Knirk JL, Jupiter JB. Intraarticular fractures of the distal end of radius in young adults. *J Bone Joint Surg Am* 1986; 68: 647-59. **This retrospective study showed a higher incidence of wrist arthritis in patients where accurate reduction was not achieved. The authors reported a total of 43 fractures with 6.7-year follow-up.**

Management

The aim of management is to restore the alignment of the distal radial articular surface and congruence of the radiocarpal and distal radioulnar joints.

Management is summarised in Table 13.3.

For fractures that cannot be reduced closed, open reduction, internal fixation and bone grafting are performed.

Cast

There is no demonstrable advantage of a long-arm cast over a short-arm cast. Furthermore, there is no benefit in remanipulation in patients older than 60 years.

The predictors of instability are as follows:

- Initial displacement.
- Age.
- Dorsal comminution.
- Intra-articular fractures.

Manipulation and K-wire stabilisation

Wiring is acceptable for stable fractures without significant comminution. A cross K-wire technique has been described, in which one 1.6mm K-wire is

Table 13.3. Summary of management options for fracture of the distal radius, based on the universal classification.

Type	Management
I	Cast
II	Manipulation under local/regional anaesthetic and cast
	If unstable, K-wires can be used
	If an irreducible or complex fracture, use ORIF and a dorsal or volar plate
III	Cast
	If there is displacement on follow-up, use K-wires to stabilise
IV	Reducible, stable: K-wire, interfragmentary screws, plates or external fixator
	Reducible, unstable: if >2mm step or >5mm shortening, use a K-wire, bone graft or external fixator with a limited open approach
	Use a maximum of 1mm distraction of the radiocarpal joint to prevent overdistraction
	Use an external fixator for 6 weeks

inserted through the radial styloid and another from the dorsal metaphysis, or through the dorsal fracture site. Wires are removed 5-6 weeks after injury.

A limited open reduction to reduce the dorsal fragment is a useful adjunct to percutaneous pinning. The fragment is reduced under image-intensifier control by levering and a 1.6mm K-wire is passed adjacent to the subchondral bone to support the fragment.

Metaphyseal bone defects may be managed with bone grafting: autograft, allograft or bone substitutes.

> **Note**
>
> Kapandji A. Intrafocal pinning of fractures of the distal end of radius; 10 years later. *Ann Chir Main* 1987; 6: 57-63. **Kapandji suggested using three separate pins to lever the fragment and then driving the pins through the volar cortex to allow early motion. This is known as intrafocal pinning, where the K-wires act as a buttress.**

External fixation
Reduction is by ligamentotaxis.

Limited open exposure is performed to place the pins, avoiding injury to the cutaneous branches of the radial nerve. Drilling is performed before pin insertion. Two pins are placed in the radius and two in the dorsoradial aspect of the index finger metacarpal. The radiocarpal joint should not be more than 1mm wider than the midcarpal joint. This is an indicator of overdistraction and may lead to stiffness. Ligamentotaxis does not reduce dorsal fragments, as volar ligaments tighten first. For these, limited open reduction can be used. The fixator can be retained for 6-8 weeks. The benefit of early dynamisation is debatable.

In a non-bridging external fixator, the distal pins are placed into the distal fragment instead of the metacarpal. This is very effective for extra-articular fractures and fractures with simple intra-articular

extension. Comminution and osteopenia may compromise fixation in the distal fragment.

> **Note**
>
> Hayes AJ, Duffy PJ, McQueen MM. Bridging and nonbridging external fixation in the treatment of unstable fractures of the distal radius. A retrospective study of 588 patients. *Acta Orthop* 2008; 79: 540-7. **A non-bridging external fixator is preferable, if it is possible to insert pins in the distal fragment.**

Dynamic mobile fixators have been proposed. These allow movement at the wrist while maintaining tension across the fracture site, but their benefit is debatable.

Open reduction and internal fixation
Open reduction and plate osteosynthesis are indicated for intra-articular shearing-type injuries. These include volar and dorsal Barton injuries.

Complications

Potential complications include a stiff wrist, pin-site infection, extensor pollicis longus tendon rupture, median nerve compression, stiffness, post-traumatic arthritis, neuropathy, complex regional pain syndrome, malunion and non-union.

Prophylactic release of the carpal tunnel is not required.

> **Note**
>
> Odumala O, Ayekoloye C, Packer G. Prophylactic carpal tunnel decompression during buttress plating of the distal radius - is it justified? *Injury* 2001; 32: 577-9. **This study reported no benefit of prophylactic carpal tunnel decompression at the time of plating of the distal radius.**

Note

Ng CY, McQueen MM. What are the radiological predictors of functional outcome following fractures of the distal radius? *J Bone Joint Surg Br* 2011; 93: 145-50. **Predictors of good outcome are less than 2mm of step or gap in the articular surface, less than 2mm of shortening and restoration of normal carpal alignment.**

Dorsal plates on the distal radius (also known at Pi plates because of their shape) have been used for comminuted fractures of the distal radius that require either a dorsal approach or a combined volar and dorsal approach. Concerns have been raised about the high complication rate with these plates. Potential complications include tendon adherence, wrist stiffness, tendon irritation and rupture.

Note

Grewal R, Perey B, Wilmink M, Stothers K. A randomized prospective study on the treatment of intra-articular distal radius fractures: open reduction and internal fixation with dorsal plating versus mini open reduction, percutaneous fixation, and external fixation. *J Hand Surg Am* 2005; 30: 764-72. **This study compared dorsal plates with percutaneous fixation and external fixation in patients with AO type C intra-articular fractures. Plate fixation resulted in higher levels of pain and reduced grip strength.**

Volar Barton fracture

Volar Barton fracture is a marginal fracture of the anterior margin of the distal radial articular surface with dislocation of the carpus. It is best managed with ORIF with a volar buttress plate.

Ulnar styloid fracture

Ulnar styloid fractures are commonly associated with distal radius fractures. In most cases, the ulnar styloid does not require fixation once the distal radius fracture has been reduced and stabilised.

Note

Kim JK, Koh YD, Do NH. Should an ulnar styloid fracture be fixed following volar plate fixation of a distal radial fracture? *J Bone Joint Surg Am* 2010; 92: 1-6. **This study included 138 patients, of which 55% had an ulnar styloid fracture. There was no difference in outcomes for these patients compared with those without fracture.**

In patients with instability of the distal radioulnar joint, the ulnar styloid may be fixed with a single K-wire supplemented with figure-of-eight tension-band wiring. The forearm should be immobilised for 6 weeks after fixation.

Femoral neck fracture

Femoral neck fractures predominantly occur in the elderly population and are more common in women. Only 3-5% of femoral neck fractures occur in people younger than 50 years and these are usually due to high-energy trauma.

Anatomy

Normal femoral anteversion is $10\pm7°$, while the neck shaft angle is $130\pm7°$. The tip of the greater trochanter is level with the centre of rotation of the femoral head in the horizontal plane. In a varus hip the centre of the head is lower, while in a valgus hip the centre of the femoral head is higher than the tip of the trochanter. The lesser trochanter is posteromedial on the femoral shaft. The greater trochanter flares posteriorly and in the proximal part.

The lateral epiphyseal artery is the main blood supply to the femoral head. This forms from the retinacular vessels, which run on the surface of the femoral neck deep to the synovial lining. The reticular vessels, in turn, arise from the medial circumflex femoral artery, which runs along the posterior surface of the femoral neck along the intertrochanteric crest. The lateral circumflex femoral artery runs along the base of the neck of the femur anteriorly and gives rise to the anterior retinacular arteries. These mainly supply blood to the neck and contribute little to the supply to the head.

The artery of the ligamentum teres, a branch of the obturator artery, supplies a small part of the femoral head around the fovea.

Diagnosis

The clinical presentation is often typical, with a fall followed by pain in the hip. The leg may be shortened and externally rotated, but this sign is absent in impacted or undisplaced fractures. A full examination is essential to check for other injuries.

Plain radiographs in two planes are the mainstay of diagnosis. Further investigations can be used for fractures not evident on plain radiographs:

- T1-weighted MRI will demonstrate fracture in all cases.
- Fractures can be demonstrated on a bone scan within 72 hours (or sometimes as early as 24 hours).
- A CT scan may show the fracture line. The presence of lipohaemarthrosis on a CT scan is suggestive of fracture.
- Enhanced MRI is very effective for showing AVN at an early stage. A Tc-99m bone scan within 72 hours can predict AVN.

Classification

In 1964, Garden classified femoral neck fractures into four types:

- Incomplete fractures.
- Complete but undisplaced fractures.

- Partially displaced fractures – loss of alignment of the trabeculae in the head and acetabulum.
- Completely displaced fractures – alignment of the trabeculae in the femoral head and acetabulum is restored as there is minimal contact across the fracture site.

Pauwel's 1965 classification is based on the angle between the fracture surface on the femoral shaft fragment and a line perpendicular to the longitudinal axis of the femur. In type I the angle is 30°, in type II it is 30-50° and in type III it is more than 50°.

The importance of this classification lies in the emphasis on biomechanical forces in this area. A fracture with an angle of 30° is subject to predominantly compressive force and is more likely to unite than a fracture with an angle of 70°, which is largely under shear stress.

For practical purposes, types I and II are grouped together as undisplaced fractures and types III and IV are grouped together as displaced fractures.

Management of femoral neck fracture

Femoral neck fracture is an absolute indication for surgical intervention: internal fixation or replacement. Non-operative management is indicated only when the patient is unfit for surgery. Every effort should be made to optimise the medical condition as soon as possible; a prolonged period of recumbency increases the risk of complications.

Ideally, joint medical and orthopaedic teams will assess and manage patients in the perioperative period. Postoperative care in a high-dependency unit helps reduce in-hospital mortality from femoral neck fractures.

Aspiration of the haemarthrosis was proposed to reduce the intra-articular pressure in the capsule. This was thought to improve circulation in the retinacular vessels. However, aspiration has no proven value in restoring vascularity.

Note

Maruenda JI, Barrios C, Gomar-Sancho F. Intracapsular hip pressure after femoral neck fracture. *Clin Orthop Relat Res* 1997; 340: 172-80. **This prospective study with 34 patients found that patients with AVN after 7 years had intracapsular pressures that were lower than their diastolic pressures.**

Permissible delays before surgery

Many patients with a planned hemiarthroplasty have medical complications that must be optimised before surgery. Ideally these patients should be operated upon within 36-48 hours; however, a delay of up to 4 days does not increase mortality.

Note

Moran CG, Wenn RT, Sikand M, Taylor AM. Early mortality after hip fracture: is delay before surgery important? *J Bone Joint Surg Am* 2005; 87: 483-9. **In this prospective observational study of 2,660 patients, mortality was 9% at 30 days, 19% at 90 days and 30% at 12 months. Patients with medical conditions that delayed surgery had a 2.5-times higher risk of mortality. Delaying surgery up to 4 days, however, did not increase mortality.**

For patients with planned reduction and internal fixation, the literature is divided on the need for urgent surgery.

Note

Jain R, Koo M, Kreder HJ, *et al.* Comparison of early and delayed fixation of subcapital hip fractures in patients sixty years of age or less. *J Bone Joint Surg Am* 2002; 84: 1605-12. **This retrospective study compared early (12 hours) versus delayed (>24 hours) fixation in 38 patients. Sixteen percent developed AVN, all of whom were in the delayed treatment group.**

Note

Haidukewych GJ, Rothwell WS, Jacofsky DJ, *et al.* Operative treatment of femoral neck fractures in patients between the ages of fifteen and fifty years. *J Bone Joint Surg Am* 2004; 86: 1711-6. **This retrospective study looked at data from 73 patients. AVN developed in 25% of patients treated within 24 hours and 20% of those who had been treated after 24 hours of diagnosis.**

Fracture reduction

For displaced fractures where internal fixation is intended, a gentle closed reduction is the first step in managing the fracture. The femoral shaft fragment is displaced proximally and rotates externally as a result of the fracture. The reduction is achieved by traction in extension to correct the proximal displacement and internal rotation of the leg to correct the rotational alignment.

Different methods of closed reduction have been described. Reduction can be achieved either with traction in flexion or extension, followed by internal rotation.

Rarely, open reduction is needed. This can be performed with anterior capsulotomy and manipulating the femoral shaft fragment to the head fragment. The procedure is performed on the fracture table and checked with an image intensifier before fixation. Anatomic reduction is desirable.

Screw fixation

Lag screw fixation is undertaken with three or four 6.5mm cancellous screws or 7.3mm cannulated cancellous screws.

The threads of the screws should cross the fracture site. Screws with 16mm threads are preferred to those with 32mm threads.

The screws are inserted in a triangular orientation parallel to each other. The apex of the triangle can be either superior or inferior.

Note

Oakey J, Stover M, Summers H, *et al.* Does screw configuration affect subtrochanteric fracture after femoral neck fixation? *Clin Orthop Relat Res* 2006; 443: 302-6. **An inferior apex is preferable as a superior configuration is associated with a higher risk of subtrochanteric fracture.**

The tips of the screws should be 5-10mm from the subchondral bone. The entry point of screws on the lateral femoral cortex should be above the lesser trochanter. This reduces the risk of subtrochanteric fracture through the screw hole.

Note

Parker MJ, Blundell C. Choice of implant for internal fixation of femoral neck fractures. Meta-analysis of 25 randomised trials including 4,925 patients. *Acta Orthop Scand* 1998; 69: 138-43. **This meta-analysis included 4,925 patients in 25 series. There was no advantage to using side plates. Therefore, cannulated parallel screws are preferred.**

Note

Asnis SE, Wanek-Sgaglione L. Intracapsular fractures of the femoral neck. Results of cannulated screw fixation. *J Bone Joint Surg Am* 1994; 76: 1793-803. **This 8-year follow-up of 141 patients reported that cannulated screws were associated with union in 96% of patients and with AVN in 22%.**

Note

Kauffman JI, Simon JA, Kummer FJ, *et al.* Internal fixation of femoral neck fractures with posterior comminution: a biomechanical study. *J Orthop Trauma* 1999; 13: 155-9. **The authors reported that in non-comminuted fractures, there is no advantage to using four screws over three. In posterior comminution, the use of four screws is considered more stable.**

The spread of screws in the lateral radiograph is related to failure. A wider spread reduces the failure rate (non-union).

Note

Gursamy K, Parker MJ, Rowlands TK. The complications of displaced intracapsular fractures of the hip: the effect of screw positioning and angulation on fracture healing. *J Bone Joint Surg Br* 2005; 87: 632-5. **In this study, reduced spread of screws on the lateral view was associated with a greater risk of non-union.**

Dynamic hip screw

Using a two-hole side plate with a dynamic hip screw is an option for femoral neck fractures. This provides secure fixation and may be advisable in non-adherent patients. It has a higher rate of AVN, but provides better fixation than cannulated screws.

There is a risk of rotational malalignment while inserting the hip screw and a guide wire inserted superior to the hip screw will prevent rotation. Subsequently, the guide wire can be removed or used to insert a lag screw parallel and superior to the dynamic hip screw.

In basicervical fractures, a dynamic hip screw with derotation screw should be used.

Note

Deneka DA, Simonian PT, Stankewich CJ, *et al.* Biomechanical comparison of internal fixation techniques for the treatment of unstable basicervical femoral neck fractures. *J Orthop Trauma* 1997; 11: 337-43. **In this study, dynamic hip screw had a higher load to failure than cannulated screws.**

Hemiarthroplasty

Displaced subcapital fractures in elderly patients (age >80 years) with limited mobility requirements are managed with hemiarthroplasty.

Note

Hui AC, Anderson GH, Choudhry R, *et al.* Internal fixation or hemiarthroplasty for undisplaced fractures of the femoral neck in octogenarians. *J Bone Joint Surg Br* 1994; 76: 891-4. **In this study, internal fixation of minimally displaced or impacted fractures in patients older than 80 years led to a higher rate of secondary surgery.**

Note

Robinson CM, Saran D, Annan IH. Intracapsular hip fractures. Results of management adopting a treatment protocol. *Clin Orthop Relat Res* 1994; (302): 83-91. **This study of 166 patients determined that fixation is preferred in patients younger than 65 years, while a replacement prosthesis is preferred in those older than 80 years. Between 65 and 80 years of age, physiological assessment of the patient is advised to choose the treatment option.**

Note

Leonardsson O, Sernbo I, Carlsson A, *et al.* Long-term follow-up of replacement compared with internal fixation for displaced femoral neck fractures: results at ten years in a randomised study of 450 patients. *J Bone Joint Surg Br* 2010; 92: 406-12. **At 10 years, this randomised study reported a complication rate of 46% with screw fixation versus 9% with hemiarthroplasty. Mortality was 75% at 10 years in both groups.**

The following should be considered:

- Displacement of the fracture.
- The age of the patient.
- Adequacy of reduction achieved.

In patients with chronic renal failure and hyperparathyroidism, a cemented hemireplacement is preferred.

The traditional Austin-Moore hemiarthroplasty (uncemented) or the Thompson hemiarthroplasty (cemented) are used in patients who have a limited activity level or life expectancy. Both procedures are associated with groin pain due to the articulation of the metal head against the acetabular cartilage.

The lack of fixation of the Austin-Moore prosthesis to the femur causes thigh pain.

Cemented versus uncemented

Note

Lo WH, Chen WM, Huang CK, *et al.* Bateman bipolar hemiarthroplasty for displaced intracapsular femoral neck fractures. Uncemented versus cemented. *Clin Orthop Relat Res* 1994; (302): 75-82. **This study reported less subsidence, less thigh pain and a better Harris hip score with cemented versus cementless prostheses.**

Note

Timperley AJ, Whitehouse SL. Mitigating surgical risk in patients undergoing hip arthroplasty for fractures of the proximal femur. *J Bone Joint Surg Br* 2009; 91: 851-4. **In this study, cemented hemiarthroplasty in fracture patients did not increase the risk of mortality. Patients with cemented implants had less pain and a lower revision rate, reoperation rate and risk of death.**

Unipolar versus bipolar

Bipolar hemiarthroplasty has been designed to give better results because of the presence of an additional bearing surface.

Note

Calder SJ, Anderson GH, Harper WM, *et al.* A subjective health indicator for follow-up. A randomised trial after treatment of displaced intracapsular hip fractures. *J Bone Joint Surg Br* 1995; 77: 494-6. **In this randomised controlled trial (RCT) of patients aged 65-79 years with displaced fractures, bipolar prostheses were associated with better scores for pain, mobility and social function.**

Note

Calder SJ, Anderson GH, Jagger C, *et al.* Unipolar or bipolar prosthesis for displaced intracapsular hip fracture in octogenarians: a randomised prospective study. *J Bone Joint Surg Br* 1996; 78: 391-4. **In this RCT of patients older than 80 years, no difference in complication or function was found between unipolar and bipolar hemiarthroplasty.**

Total hip arthroplasty

Total hip arthroplasty is an option for patients with hip arthritis and femoral neck fracture. These patients are unlikely to do well with either fixation or hemiarthroplasty.

Increasingly, total hip replacement is increasingly being used in younger patients with displaced fractures as a definitive treatment. The traditional concerns with hip arthroplasty in patients with femoral neck fractures have focused on a higher dislocation rate.

Note

Blomfeldt R, Törnkvist H, Eriksson K, *et al.* A randomised controlled trial comparing bipolar hemiarthroplasty with total hip replacement for displaced intracapsular fractures of the femoral neck in elderly patients. *J Bone Joint Surg Br* 2007; 89: 160-5. **This study looked at 120 patients with a mean age 80 years and 1-year follow-up. Bipolar hemiarthroplasty and total hip replacement had the same complication rate, but better function was achieved with a total hip replacement.**

Management planning

Undisplaced fractures are managed with cancellous screw fixation or a dynamic hip screw.

Displaced fractures are managed according to age:

- Younger than 65 years – closed reduction/ORIF within 6 hours.
- Older than 80 years – hemiarthroplasty.
- Between 65 and 80 years – fixation or replacement depends on the physiological condition of the patient. Total hip arthroplasty is appropriate in active patients.

Patients with renal failure, neurologic deficit, parkinsonism or hyperparathyroidism have a high failure rate with internal fixation and alternative treatments should be considered.

Complications

Osteonecrosis

The incidence of osteonecrosis is 10-45% after femoral neck fractures. The risk of osteonecrosis depends on the following:

- Initial displacement of the fracture.
- Time gap between injury and reduction.
- Adequacy of reduction (>20° varus/valgus leads to AVN).
- Associated dislocation of the hip.
- Comminution of the posterior part of the neck.

Management options include hemiarthroplasty, total hip replacement, arthrodesis of the hip, valgus osteotomy, core decompression and insufflation of the femoral head with methyl methacrylate. In view of good and reliable long-term results, total hip arthroplasty is often the preferred option for patients with osteonecrosis.

Non-union

The prevalence of non-union has been reported to be 10-30% after 12 months. If the head is viable on MRI scan then valgus osteotomy is an option in young patients. A free vascularised fibular graft can also be considered. If the head is not viable, and in relatively elderly patients, total hip arthroplasty is advisable.

Failure of fixation

This is best managed with total hip arthroplasty.

Infection

Urinary tract infection is present in up to one in four patients undergoing surgery for femoral neck fracture. Treatment is instituted as appropriate but surgery is not delayed unless there is systemic sepsis. Surgical site infection is rare after fixation.

Transfusion requirement

The requirement for transfusion varies with the procedure. The figures quoted are 45% after total hip replacement, 42% after cemented hemiarthroplasty, 29% after uncemented hemiarthroplasty, 19% after a dynamic hip screw and 0% after cannulated screws.

Note

Levi N. Blood transfusion requirements in intracapsular femoral neck fractures. *Injury* 1996; 27: 709-11.

There may be an increased risk of infection in patients receiving a blood transfusion.

Mortality

After femoral neck fracture, the 30-day mortality is 10% and 1-year mortality is 30%.

After cemented hemiarthroplasty, mortality is 20% at 6 months and 28% at 1 year.

The preoperative albumin level has been shown to be an indicator of mortality.

Note

Eiskjaer S, Ostgård SE. Risk factors influencing mortality after bipolar hemiarthroplasty in the treatment of fracture of the femoral neck. *Clin Orthop Relat Res* 1991; 270: 295-300. **The authors reported that risk factors for high mortality include cardiac conditions, pulmonary disease, residence in a nursing home, high serum creatinine and pneumonia.**

Note

Foster MR, Heppenstall RB, Friedenberg ZB, Hozack WJ. A prospective assessment of nutritional status and complications in patients with fractures of the hip. *J Orthop Trauma* 1990; 4: 49-57. **A preoperative albumin level below 3.0g/dL correlated with 70% mortality at 11 months, while levels over 3.0g/dL corresponded to 18% mortality at 11 months.**

Intertrochanteric fracture

Intertrochanteric fractures involve the region of the greater and lesser trochanter of the femur. These are different from femoral neck fractures as the extensive muscle attachments in this area provide good vascularity and hence good healing potential of the fracture, making non-union quite rare. AVN of the femoral head is also rare, with a reported incidence of 1%.

Diagnosis

Clinical features are similar to those of intracapsular fractures of the femoral neck. Presenting patients are usually elderly and this fracture is more common in women. Young patients with this injury have high-energy impacts, in contrast to simple falls in the older age group. The shortening and external rotation may be more marked in patients with intertrochanteric compared with femoral neck fractures.

The bone density bears a relationship to the risk of intertrochanteric fractures. Bone density of less than 0.6g/cm indicates an increased risk of fracture.

The family history is significant, and there is a two-fold increased risk of fracture in women whose mothers sustained a similar injury.

Imaging studies show similar patterns to those for femoral neck fracture. An X-ray in internal rotation may show the undisplaced fractures, which may not otherwise be obvious. A Tc-99m bone scan will be positive after 72 hours. An MRI scan is the most sensitive modality to detect undisplaced fractures.

Classification

The difference between stable and unstable fractures is based on the ability to resist a medial compressive load on physiological loading. Medial comminution or reverse obliquity of the fracture line indicates instability.

Boyd Griffin classification:

- Type I – fracture along the intertrochanteric line.
- Type II – comminuted fracture with the main fracture line along the intertrochanteric line.
- Type III – subtrochanteric fractures with extension just distal to or through the lesser trochanter.
- Type IV – fractures in two planes.

Evans classification:

- Type I – the main fracture line is along the intertrochanteric line. Type I fractures are further classified into those in which stability can be restored by anatomical reduction and those in which it cannot.
- Type II – the main fracture line extends downwards and laterally from the lesser trochanter (also known as reverse oblique fractures).

Other systems of classification include the Jensen-Michaelsen classification and the OTA classification.

Surgical planning

Surgical stabilisation is the standard treatment for intertrochanteric fractures. Non-operative management can be considered only for patients who would be very high risk with surgery. Mortality with non-operative management is around 35%. Shortening and external rotation deformity is the likely outcome.

Only the primary compressive trabeculae can provide sufficient hold for an implant. Anatomic reduction is not necessary, but stable reduction is mandatory. Mild valgus may be desirable. The Dimon-Hughston osteotomy was based on the principle of impaction of the neck into the medullary canal, hence medialising the shaft of the femur to improve stability. The Sarmiento osteotomy describes resection of a lateral wedge so as to reduce the fracture to a more stable valgus position. The osteotomies that have been described are now largely historical and offer no definite benefit over modern fixation devices.

Note

Zuckerman JD, Skovron ML, Koval KJ, et al. Postoperative complications and mortality associated with operative delay in older patients who have a fracture of the hip. *J Bone Joint Surg Am* 1995; 77: 1551-6. **An operation should be performed within 2 days of fracture; delay in operation increases the 1-year mortality.**

Choice of implant

Historical implants used for fixation of these fractures include the Jewett nail plate, which was a fixed-angle, fixed-length device. The development of the sliding screw led to better outcomes as it allowed impaction of the fragments to a stable position with loading, and reduced the rate of implant cutout from the femoral head.

Today, the most commonly used implant for stabilising these fractures is the dynamic hip screw. More recently, intramedullary implants have been developed with a screw into the head of the femur. These are useful for the unstable fractures, reverse oblique fractures and fractures with subtrochanteric extension.

Implant position

Screw placement in the femoral head should not be in the anterior or superior part of the head; central, or slightly posterior and inferior, is acceptable.

The tip-apex distance predicts the risk of cutout of the screw. This distance is the sum of the distance from the tip of the screw to the fovea on the femoral head measured on AP and lateral radiographs. The total distance should be less than 25mm.

Note

Baumgaertner MR, Curtin SL, Lindskog DM, Keggi JM. The value of the tip-apex distance in predicting failure of fixation of peritrochanteric fractures of the hip. *J Bone Joint Surg Am* 1995; 77: 1058-64. **The authors described the tip-apex distance in 198 fractures.**

Note

Baumgaertner MR, Solberg BD. Awareness of tip apex distance reduces failure of fixation of trochanteric fractures of the hip. *J Bone Joint Surg Am* 1997; 79: 969-71. **Awareness of the tip-apex distance reduced the cutout rate from 8% to 0%.**

The sliding hip screw acts as a lateral tension band. A loss of sliding leads to a rigid construct and high failure rate.

Note

Jacobs RR, McClain O, Armstrong HJ. Internal fixation of intertrochanteric hip fractures: a clinical and biomechanical study. *Clin Orthop Relat Res* 1980; 146: 62-70. **Telescoping of the screw within the barrel by 10mm improved strength by 28%, and telescoping by 20mm improved strength by 80%. The average settling of the screw was 5mm in stable fractures and 15mm in unstable fractures.**

Posterior sag does not compromise fixation strength.

Seventy percent of patients need a walking stick 6 months postoperatively compared with 36% preoperatively. First-generation intramedullary nails have a 10° offset at the proximal end. The cutout rate is 3% and the incidence of thigh pain is 17%.

Second-generation nails have 4° angulation at the proximal end and a similar cutout rate to first-generation nails. In shorter nails, where the tip is in the diaphysis, a stress riser may be present, leading to cortical hypertrophy. These nails provide secure fixation and less shortening than a dynamic hip screw.

An intramedullary hip screw buttresses against collapse and shaft medialisation, reducing shortening and blood loss. There is better calcar load sharing.

> **Note**
>
> Hardy DC, Descamps PY, Krallis P, *et al.* Use of an intramedullary hip-screw compared with a compression hip-screw with a plate for intertrochanteric femoral fractures. A prospective, randomized study of one hundred patients. *J Bone Joint Surg Am* 1998; 80: 618-30.

Intramedullary devices that end in the proximal half of the femur are associated with a 3-6% incidence of secondary fracture at the tip of the stem. To avoid this, long intramedullary implants that extend to the distal femur and are locked distally are preferable.

A 95° blade plate or screw device or intramedullary implants are suitable for reverse obliquity fractures.

Calcar-substituting hemiarthroplasty or total replacement arthroplasty is useful for failed fixations. Bone pastes such as calcium phosphate cement can be used to augment fixation.

Most patients are allowed weight bearing to tolerance following surgery.

> **Note**
>
> Koval KJ, Sala DA, Kummer FJ, Zuckerman JD. Postoperative weight-bearing after a fracture of the femoral neck or an intertrochanteric fracture. *J Bone Joint Surg Am* 1998; 80: 352-6. **This study performed gait analysis in 32 patients at 3 months. The patients voluntarily self-protected: 51% were weight bearing at 1 week and 87% at 12 weeks.**

Comparison of proximal femoral nail and gamma nail

> **Note**
>
> Schipper IB, Steyerberg EW, Castelein RM, *et al.* Treatment of unstable trochanteric fractures. Randomised comparison of the gamma nail and the proximal femoral nail. *J Bone Joint Surg Br* 2004; 86: 86-94. **In this multicentre prospective trial, there was more lateral protrusion of the hip screw with the proximal femoral nail compared with the gamma nail. Both nails had similar complication and union rates, and the cutout rate was 7% with both. A second screw in the proximal femoral nail had no benefit. There was no 'knife effect' of two screws in the proximal femoral nail leading to cutout.**

> **Note**
>
> Sadowski C, Lübbeke A, Saudan M, *et al.* Treatment of reverse oblique and transverse intertrochanteric fractures with use of an intramedullary nail or a 95 degrees screw-plate: a prospective, randomized study. *J Bone Joint Surg Am* 2002; 84-A: 372-81. **In patients with a reverse oblique fracture, an intramedullary nail was found to be better than a 95° hip screw. The failure and non-union rate was 36% compared with 5%, respectively.**

The sliding hip screw has been shown to be an effective implant for intertrochanteric fractures involving the lesser trochanter. Fractures of the lesser trochanter disrupt the medial weight-bearing axis and can lead to instability. However, a prospective randomised study has shown no difference in the failure rate of the sliding hip screw and nails.

Note

Barton TM, Gleeson R, Topliss C, et al. A comparison of the long gamma nail with the sliding hip screw for the treatment of AO/OTA 31-A2 fractures of the proximal part of the femur: a prospective randomized trial. *J Bone Joint Surg Am* 2010; 92: 792-8. **The reoperation rate was the same in 210 patients randomised to a long gamma nail or sliding hip screw.**

Reverse oblique fractures and fractures extending into the subtrochanteric area are best managed with intramedullary nailing.

Subtrochanteric fracture

The subtrochanteric area is the segment of the femur at the level of the lesser trochanter and extending 5cm distal to the lesser trochanter. Some fractures may extend proximally to involve the greater trochanter.

Muscle forces are considerable in the subtrochanteric region. The proximal fragment is abducted and externally rotated by the strong abductors. Shortening results from the combined action of the quadriceps, adductors and hamstring muscles.

The subtrochanteric area is a common site for metastasis. The possibility of pathologic fracture should be considered in all subtrochanteric fractures, particularly those with a transverse pattern of fractures.

Classification

Classification is by Russell Taylor:

- Type I – fractures that do not extend into the piriform fossa.
- Type II – fractures extending into the piriform fossa.

Each type is subdivided into two:

- A – the lesser trochanter is intact.
- B – the lesser trochanter is involved.

Management

Subtrochanteric fractures are best managed with internal fixation.

Second-generation nails are preferred for type I fractures. These provide secure fixation in the head of the femur and have good stability. The nails should not be locked in the diaphysis to avoid the risk of a stress fracture at the site of the screw hole. The nails should be long and locked in the distal metaphysis.

Type II fractures are managed with a dynamic hip screw along with bone grafting if needed for medial comminution. The gamma and proximal femoral nails are options, as these are inserted through the greater trochanter instead of the piriform fossa.

Intramedullary implants provide better biomechanical stability compared with extramedullary implants such as the dynamic hip screw.

Complications

- Implant failure – relatively common because of high biomechanical forces in the subtrochanteric area.
- Non-union – if there is no evidence of progression of healing after 6 months, a reamed statically locked intramedullary nail can be inserted.
- Malunion.
- Infection.

Femoral shaft fracture

Historically, femoral shaft fractures were treated by traction in a Thomas splint followed by hip spica. This often resulted in decubitus ulcers, deep vein thrombosis, osteoporosis, muscle wasting, knee stiffness, respiratory complication, shortening and malalignment.

The development of the Küntscher nail was a landmark in the management of these injuries. Gerhard Küntscher also introduced the concept of reaming to allow a larger-diameter nail insertion and improve the contact area between the nail and the bone.

Clinical evaluation

The diagnosis of femoral shaft fracture is usually obvious on clinical examination. Normal Advanced Trauma Life Support (ATLS) protocols should be followed as these are high-energy injuries and associated injuries may be present. Femoral neck fracture may be associated with a femoral shaft fracture and this should be checked before, during and after fracture fixation.

Classification

Classification is by Winquist and Hansen and the AO group. The Winquist classification is based on degree of comminution.

- Type I – minimal or no comminution.
- Type II – at least 50% contact of two major fragments.
- Type III – between 50% and 100% of the circumference of the major fragments is comminuted.
- Type IV – no cortical contact between major fragments.

In the AO classification, the femoral shaft is given the number 32.

- 32A – simple fracture.
- 32B – wedge fracture.
- 32C – complex fracture.

Management

Non-operative treatment in the form of splinting or traction can be used as a temporary measure until internal fixation is performed. The definitive treatment of femoral shaft fractures in adults is by internal fixation. This should be undertaken as soon as the patient's physiologic condition has been stabilised.

> **Note**
>
> Bone LB, Johnson KD, Weigelt J, Scheinberg R. Early versus late stabilization of femoral fractures. A prospective randomised study. *J Bone Joint Surg* 1989; 71: 336-40. **This study found that delays in internal stabilisation of femoral shaft fractures are associated with increased respiratory complications and acute respiratory distress syndrome.**

External fixation

External fixation is an option for patients with severe open fractures or vascular injuries, or for initial stabilisation in haemodynamically unstable patients. Once the vascular repair has been undertaken, or soft tissue cover achieved, external fixation can be converted to an intramedullary nail within 3 weeks without an increased risk of infection.

Ipsilateral femoral neck and shaft fractures

Ipsilateral femoral shaft and neck fractures are generally managed by a cephalomedullary device that enables fixation of both fractures simultaneously using one implant. Plating of the femur fracture and fixation of the femoral neck fracture with screws is an option.

Intramedullary nail

An intramedullary nail is the most common method with which to stabilise femoral shaft fractures. The development of the locking nail expanded the indications for nailing and more comminuted fractures can now be managed. Fractures from the trochanteric to the supracondylar region can be managed with intramedullary nailing.

The first-generation nails were locked proximally and distally, but did not provide fixation into the femoral head. The second-generation nails have a screw or an alternative fixation device inserted into the femoral head, which extends the indications to subtrochanteric and intertrochanteric fractures, and ipsilateral femoral neck and femoral shaft fractures.

A floating knee is a femoral shaft fracture with an ipsilateral tibial fracture. It can be managed with retrograde and tibial nailing. Both procedures are performed through a single incision at the knee.

If the Injury Severity Score is more than 18, early stabilisation is associated with a lower rate of acute respiratory distress syndrome and pulmonary complications.

Note

Winquist RA, Hansen ST Jr, Clawson DK. Closed intramedullary nailing of femoral fractures. A report of five hundred and twenty cases. *J Bone Joint Surg Am* 1984; 66: 529-39. **This study reported 99% union with intramedullary nails.**

Note

Bone LB, Johnson KD, Weigelt J, Scheinberg R. Early versus delayed stabilization of femoral fractures. A prospective randomized study. *J Bone Joint Surg Am* 1989; 71: 336-40. **These authors reported that multiply injured patients had a higher risk of pulmonary complications.**

Note

Brumback RJ, Reilly JP, Poka A, *et al.* Intramedullary nailing of femoral shaft fractures. Part I: Decision-making errors with interlocking fixation. *J Bone Joint Surg Am* 1988; 70: 1441-52. **Static locking was better, as dynamic locking was believed to lead to rotational instability and shortening.**

Intramedullary nailing can be performed on the fracture table using the traction mechanism or on an ordinary radiolucent table with the help of a femoral distractor to achieve reduction. Rare complications with using the fracture table include pudendal, femoral or sciatic nerve palsy, perineal skin damage and occasionally 'well-leg' compartment syndrome.

Retrograde nails

Retrograde nailing is an option in certain situations. The nail is inserted from the intercondylar notch in the distal femur and locked proximally. Indications for retrograde nailing include the following:

- A femur fracture below a total hip replacement.
- A distal femoral fracture above a total knee replacement.
- Obesity that obstructs access to the proximal femur.
- Avoidance of radiation to the proximal femur in pregnant patients.
- Ipsilateral femoral fracture and acetabular fractures so as not to compromise acetabular exposure.
- A contaminated wound around the entry point for antegrade nailing.
- A femur fracture with hip dislocation.
- A femoral fracture with displaced femoral neck fractures requiring closed reduction.

Complications that may result from retrograde nailing include a spread of infection to the knee joint in open fractures, a stiff knee, a 52% decrease in the anterior cruciate ligament blood supply, a 49% decrease in the posterior cruciate ligament blood supply and risk of patellofemoral joint damage if the nail is prominent.

Union rates of 85-95% have been reported.

Reamed versus unreamed

Increased pulmonary complications with reaming in the presence of a chest injury in patients with multiple injuries have been reported by Pape. However, no adverse effect of reaming was detected by Bosse.

Note

Pape HC, Regel G, Dwenger A, *et al.* Influences of different methods of intramedullary femoral nailing on lung function in patients with multiple trauma. *J Trauma* 1993; 35: 709-6. **Reaming was considered to increase the risk of pulmonary complications compared to unreamed nailing.**

Note

Bosse MJ, MacKenzie EJ, Riemer BL, *et al.* Adult respiratory distress syndrome, pneumonia, and mortality following thoracic injury and a femoral fracture treated either with intramedullary nailing with reaming or with a plate. A comparative study. *J Bone Joint Surg Am* 1997; 79: 799-809. **In this study, there was no increase in the risk of acute respiratory distress syndrome after reaming for femoral fractures.**

Some authors have reported similar union rates, although others have found a slower union rate in unreamed versus reamed nails.

Note

Tornetta P 3rd, Tiburzi D. The treatment of femoral shaft fractures using intramedullary interlocked nails with and without intramedullary reaming: a preliminary report. *J Orthop Trauma* 1997; 11: 89-92. **Here, reaming led to faster healing.**

Note

Clatworthy MG, Clark DI, Gray DH, Hardy AE. Reamed versus unreamed femoral nails. A randomised, prospective trial. *J Bone Joint Surg Br* 1998; 80: 485-9. **In this RCT of 45 patients, a union time of 39 weeks was reported with unreamed nails compared with 28 weeks with reamed nails.**

In nail fixation, one distal locking bolt is generally sufficient and the proximal hole should be used. There should be at least 5cm of intact bone between the fracture and the bolt. In comminuted fractures, two bolts are recommended and early weight bearing can be allowed.

Ipsilateral neck and shaft fracture

Options are a nail, plate or retrograde nail combined with screws, or a second-generation nail.

Femur fracture with head injury

Care is taken to avoid intraoperative hypotension and hypoxia in these patients. Intracranial pressure monitoring is advisable.

Complications of femoral fracture

- Infection – the risk is reported to be approximately 1% following internal fixation.
- Delayed union or non-union – options are to dynamise the nail, perform a bone graft or exchange the nail. Exchange nailing is successful in 50% of patients.
- Malunion in the distal third – rotational malalignment is common and averages 16° in some studies.
- Compartment syndrome – rare.
- Neurologic injury – the pudendal and sciatic nerves are at risk due to traction at the time of internal fixation.
- Heterotopic ossification – present in 25% of patients, but routine prophylaxis is not recommended. The extent will depend on muscle damage and reaming. Pulsatile lavage does not reduce the risk.

Note

Giannoudis PV, MacDonald DA, Matthews SJ, *et al.* Nonunion of the femoral diaphysis. The influence of reaming and non-steroidal anti-inflammatory drugs. *J Bone Joint Surg Br* 2000; 82: 655-8. **In this study, NSAIDs were found to delay bone healing in femoral shaft fractures.**

Note

Brown KM, Saunders MM, Kirsch T, et al. Effect of COX-2-specific inhibition on fracture-healing in the rat femur. *J Bone Joint Surg Am* 2004; 86-A: 116-23. **Here, Cox 2 interfered with the healing of femur fractures.**

Distal femoral fracture

The supracondylar area extends from the femoral condyles to up to 5cm above the metaphyseal flare.

Clinical assessment

The clinical assessment follows general principles. The physical examination should assess open injuries, neurological or vascular compromise and other associated injuries.

Imaging

Standard imaging includes AP and lateral views of the knee and femur, along with oblique views to detect fracture extension and configuration. In the lateral view, the lateral condyle appears larger and has a notch in the anterior half, which helps to differentiate it from the medial condyle.

CT scanning, including three-dimensional reconstructions, is very useful for preoperative planning to determine the orientation of fracture lines.

Classification

The fractures are commonly classified based on the comprehensive classification (Table 13.4).

Table 13.4. Comprehensive classification of distal femoral fractures.

Type		Description
A		Extra-articular fractures
	A1	Simple extra-articular fracture
	A2	Metaphyseal wedge fracture
	A3	Extra-articular with complex metaphyseal fracture
B		Partial articular fractures
	B1	Lateral condyle sagittal fracture
	B2	Medial condyle fracture
	B3	Partial articular fracture in the frontal plane
C		Complete articular fractures
	C1	Both condyles fracture
	C2	Simple, complete articular fracture with metaphyseal comminution
	C3	Complete articular fracture with articular comminution

Management

Non-operative management of these injuries carries a poor prognosis and operative stabilisation is recommended.

Fractures with intra-articular extension, fractures above a total knee replacement prosthesis, open injuries and fractures with vascular injury are absolute indications for operative stabilisation.

Treatment options are as follows:

- A 95° fixed-angle condylar screw.
- A 95° fixed-angle blade plate.
- Condylar buttress plate.
- Intramedullary nail – antegrade/retrograde.
- External fixation.
- Less invasive stabilisation system (LISS).

In patients with metaphyseal comminution, the fixation device (LISS or dynamic condylar screw) is used as a bridging implant, without exposure of the metaphysis. This avoids devascularising the fragments and stability is achieved by fixation in the distal and shaft fragments.

Preoperative templating avoids surprises at the time of surgery. The blade or condylar screw should be placed in the middle of the anterior half of the femoral condyle, which will coincide with the axis of the femoral shaft. The distal femur is trapezoid in cross-section, with the posterior aspect being the widest. The blade or the screw will lie anterior to this and hence should be shorter than the widest diameter of the femur seen in the AP view of the image intensifier. A longer screw is likely to impinge on the medial collateral ligament and can be painful.

LISS is based on a locking-screw principle and functions as an internal fixator. It is inserted through a lateral incision and the plate is slid proximally from the femoral condyle to bridge the metaphysis. The screws are locking and proximal screws are unicortical. Fixation into the femoral condyle is through multiple locking screws, which provide stable fixation. Locking plates are now the most commonly used implants for distal femoral fractures.

Knee dislocation

Knee dislocations are high-energy injuries resulting in significant morbidity unless appropriately managed.

Approximately 50% of dislocations can be reduced at the time of presentation. Vascular injuries are present in up to a third of patients with knee dislocation and must be repaired quickly. The amputation rate is 11% with repair within 8 hours, rising to 86% with repair after 8 hours.

One in four patients has neurologic injury and one in five dislocations is an open injury.

There are several types of knee dislocation:

- Anterior.
- Posterior.
- Medial.
- Lateral.
- Rotatory.

Assessment should include the ankle-brachial index. This should be more than 0.9, indicating adequate circulation distal to the knee.

On X-ray, the presence of the lateral capsular sign (avulsion in the intercondylar region) indicates a severe injury.

Management

Non-operative
Non-operative management is indicated if the patient participates in low-demand activities or will be unable to adhere to the postoperative regimen.

Surgery
Surgical repair can be early or delayed. The current trend is towards early reconstruction of all damaged ligaments and the posterior capsule. Early repair may require ligament augmentation or substitution. Posterolateral corner injuries should be treated within 2-3 weeks.

If the knee is unstable after repair, a hinged external fixator can be applied for 6 weeks.

Delayed repair addresses specific instability complications once the patient starts mobilising the knee.

Patellar fracture

Patellar fractures are common. They can be the result of direct or indirect trauma.

Classification

Fractures of the patella can be of several types.

Osteochondral fractures are the result of patellar dislocation, whereby the injury causes a fracture of the medial facet of the patella. The fragment is largely cartilage and partly bone, and is sometimes difficult to visualise on plain radiographs.

The fragments can be replaced and fixed by arthroscopy or mini-arthrotomy. Bioabsorbable screws are useful in these cases. The tear in the medial extensor retinaculum can be repaired to restore stability to the patella.

Transverse fractures are generally the result of indirect trauma in which quadriceps pull results in fracture of the patella. Displaced fractures have an associated tear in the extensor expansion and, if present, will exhibit extensor lag. The gap in the patella is often palpable.

Vertical fractures are due to direct trauma and the extensor mechanism is not disrupted. As the fracture line is parallel to the pull of the quadriceps, the fracture is inherently stable. A step in the articular surface is an indication for ORIF.

Stellate fractures are comminuted fractures due to direct trauma, but the fragments are not displaced and the extensor retinaculum is intact. These can be managed non-operatively.

Comminuted fractures are caused by direct trauma and often need surgical stabilisation.

Management

Undisplaced fractures can be managed non-operatively with an initial hinged brace or cylinder cast immobilisation followed by gradual supervised flexion. Full weight bearing in extension can be allowed from the outset.

Displaced fractures have tears in the extensor reticulum and should be managed surgically. Tension-band wiring of transverse fractures provides adequate fixation and early mobilisation. The presence of more than two fragments can often be dealt with using lag screws to reduce fragments to one another before fixing two main fragments with the tension band.

> **Note**
>
> Weber MJ, Janecki CJ, McLeod P, et al. Efficacy of various forms of fixation of transverse fractures of the patella. *J Bone Joint Surg Am* 1980; 62: 215-20. **A classic article describing the technique of tension-band wiring of the patella.**

Cannulated screws can be used in place of K-wires and the wire loop can be passed through the screws. This is an alternative to tension-band wiring.

Postoperative early motion encourages compression at the fracture site. Weight bearing in extension is allowed as tolerated.

Patellar tendon rupture

Patellar tendon injuries are relatively rare and are usually the result of indirect trauma: flexion of the knee with an actively contracting extensor mechanism. Tendonitis of the patellar tendon or steroid injections in the local area predispose to rupture.

Clinical presentation

Patients exhibit reduced power of knee extension. A gap is usually palpable.

Imaging

Radiographs will reveal patella alta and an ultrasound scan will demonstrate the rupture.

Management

Rupture of the patellar tendon is managed with repair using a Kessler or Krackow suture. The repair is protected with a cerclage wire passed along the superior pole of the patella and through the tibial tubercle. This can be a steel wire or non-absorbable suture, and is tightened with the knee flexed to 90° to maintain the length of the patellar tendon. The steel wire must be removed after 3 months, but cerclage sutures can be left *in situ*.

Quadriceps tendon rupture

Quadriceps tendon rupture commonly occurs within 2cm of the proximal pole of the patella. It is predisposed by steroid injections or diabetes.

Clinical features

Patients have a history of injury followed by pain and an inability to actively extend the knee. In patients with an intact extensor mechanism, active extension may be possible but the power will be diminished.

A gap is often palpable and an ultrasound scan will demonstrate the tear.

Management

Direct repair of the tendon is performed. If there is inadequate tissue on the distal end, repair can be achieved by drill holes in the patella or through suture anchors in the patella.

Postoperative knee flexion should start early if possible, starting from 0 to 30° flexion, and gradually increased so as to achieve unrestricted knee flexion by 6-8 weeks.

Tibial spine fracture

Tibial spine avulsion fractures are injuries of the tibial attachment of the anterior cruciate ligament.

Classification

Classification is by Meyers and McKeever:

- Type I – the anterior edge of the eminence is slightly elevated.
- Type II – greater elevation of the anterior edge of the eminence.
- Type IIIA – the entire eminence is elevated and lies in its bed in the tibia.
- Type IIIB – a displaced eminence with loss of contact with the tibia.

Note

Meyers MH, McKeever FM. Fractures of the intercondylar eminence of the tibia. *J Bone Joint Surg Am* 1970; 52: 1677-84. **Classification of tibial spine fracture.**

A further type IV was added by Zaricznyl, in which the tibial eminence is comminuted.

Clinical presentation

The injury to the knee can be hyperextension, twisting or excess varus or valgus strain. The knee is swollen and painful, with lipohaemarthrosis. Full extension may be blocked.

Imaging

Radiographs of the knee are obtained. A CT scan will help to clearly define the fragment.

Management

The stability of the knee is checked, along with the ability to achieve passive full extension. If full extension is possible, a cast in full extension will reduce the fragment. The anterior horn of the medial or lateral meniscus can block full extension, in which case arthroscopic reduction will be needed.

Fixation of the fragment when there is a block to extension can be achieved by arthroscopic or mini open arthrotomy. Residual cruciate laxity may be noticed postoperatively due to stretching of the ligament prior to bony avulsion at the time of bony injury.

Tibial plateau fracture

Tibial plateau fractures are the result of varus, valgus or axial loading of the knee, which drives the femoral condyle into the proximal tibia. These are high-energy injuries in the young, but relatively low-energy injuries can cause tibial plateau fractures in osteopenic individuals.

Assessing the soft tissue component is an important aspect of management of tibial plateau fractures. This includes local soft tissue, skin cover, open injury and neurovascular assessment. A tilt of more than 5° or articular incongruity of more than 3mm is an indication for surgery.

Imaging

Standard radiographic views, along with oblique films and, if necessary, radiographs of the uninjured contralateral side are obtained. CT scanning is useful for assessment and changes the classification in 10-15% of patients. In addition to plain radiographs, CT scanning with reformats is useful in demonstrating the extent of the fracture and planning fixation. MRI can help to identify an associated torn or trapped meniscus.

Approximately 50% of patients have associated meniscal tears.

Classification

The Schatzker classification is the most commonly used:

- Type I – vertical split fracture of the lateral tibial plateau.
- Type II – split-depression fracture of the lateral tibial plateau. Along with the split, there is depression of the weight-bearing part of the adjacent tibial plateau.
- Type III – pure depression of the articular surface of the lateral tibial plateau.
- Type IV – fracture of the medial tibial plateau.
- Type V – wedge fracture of both the medial and lateral tibial plateaus.
- Type VI – fracture with metaphyseal extension, such that there is no continuity between the metaphysis and diaphysis.

Management

Non-operative management may be appropriate for minimally displaced fractures. A cast is initially required, followed by hinged bracing to allow knee flexion once the fracture is sufficiently healed. Weight bearing is restricted for 6-8 weeks.

Type I fractures are more common in young patients. If undisplaced, these fractures can be managed non-operatively with early mobilisation and avoiding weight bearing. Displaced fractures require reduction and internal fixation. The lateral meniscus is sometimes trapped between the fragments; this can be detected and corrected by arthroscopy.

Type II fractures are managed with open reduction, elevation of the depressed fragment, bone grafting and internal fixation. Early mobilisation limits knee stiffness. These cases can be managed with percutaneous fixation of the split, along with opening a medial cortical window and bone grafting under the depressed fragments. Fractures involving the condyle require buttress plating, but an undisplaced split of the lateral wall can be fixed percutaneously after reduction with pointed clamps applied percutaneously.

A trapped meniscus will interfere with percutaneous reduction and is managed with arthroscopy or limited arthrotomy.

Note

Halzach P, Matter P, Minter J. Arthroscopically assisted treatment of lateral tibial plateau fractures in skiers: use of a cannulated reduction system. *J Orthop Trauma* 1994; 8: 273-81. **This study managed 16 patients with arthroscopy, elevation and autologous bone grafting. All patients except one had good results.**

Type III fractures are common in relatively older patients compared with type I fractures and are related to an osteoporotic proximal tibial bone. If the knee is unstable on examination under anaesthetic then open reduction, elevation of the condyle, bone grafting and internal fixation is performed. Stable fractures can be managed in a hinged brace without weight bearing.

Type IV fractures can be managed non-operatively if undisplaced. Close follow-up is needed to check for any late displacement. Displaced fractures need ORIF.

Type V fractures are often unstable. Internal fixation offers the best chance of anatomic alignment.

Type VI fractures are difficult to manage. The principles of treatment are restoration of the articular surface anatomy and using a bridging implant to connect the epiphysis and diaphysis. Ring fixators have been used in these situations with good results.

Surgical planning

The incisions used for fixation of the fracture are planned so as not to compromise any future reconstructive procedure. Knee replacement surgery is performed through a vertical midline incision and a similar approach is beneficial for access to the fracture. Anatomic reduction of the joint surface is essential and stable fixation will allow early mobilisation.

Protected weight bearing is instituted in the postoperative period and continues for 8-12 weeks. Early movement of the knee is encouraged. For bicondylar fractures, a double-incision technique can be employed: a posteromedial incision is made to manage the coronal split of the medial condyle, while a standard anterolateral approach is taken for the lateral condyle. Any extensile approach to both condyles through one incision, with or without tenotomy of the patellar tendon, is associated with a high rate of wound complications.

Note

Honkonen SE. Degenerative arthritis after tibial plateau fractures. *J Orthop Trauma* 1995; 9: 273-7. **This study followed patients with 131 fractures for 7.6 years. Concurrent meniscectomy increased the rate of degenerative changes from 37% to 74%. Overall, 44% of cases showed evidence of degenerative changes.**

Tibial shaft fracture

In 1964, Nicoll coined the term 'personality of fracture' to describe the differences in outcome based on degree of comminution, periosteal stripping and soft tissue injury.

Blood supply of the tibia

The vascular supply of tibia comes from three sources:

- The nutrient vascular system.
- The periosteal vascular system.
- The epiphyseal metaphyseal system.

The nutrient artery arises from the posterior tibial artery and enters the posterior aspect of the tibia below the soleal line. It divides into an ascending and descending branch. The anterior tibial artery gives rise to most of the periosteal circulation. The nutrient vessels and the periosteal supply comprise the main vascular system involved in the healing of tibial shaft fractures.

Classification

The classification of closed soft tissue injuries in tibial fractures was proposed by Oestern and Tscherne:

- Grade 0 – indirect force, negligible soft tissue injury.
- Grade 1 – superficial contusion or abrasion, simple fracture.
- Grade 2 – deep abrasion, direct trauma and impending compartment syndrome.
- Grade 3 – extensive skin contusion, crushed skin, subcutaneous degloving and compartment syndrome.

Clinical assessment

The following factors influence the choice of treatment method:

- Age of the patient.
- Presence of other injuries, polytrauma.
- Coexisting medical conditions.
- Open or closed fracture.
- Neurovascular conditions.
- Presence of or impending compartment syndrome.
- Fracture comminution.
- Presence or absence of fibular fracture and its level.
- Involvement of the ankle or knee joints.

Imaging

Plain radiographs are taken in two planes, including the knee and the ankle joint. Associated vascular injuries require angiography.

Note

Tornetta P, 3rd. Technical considerations in the surgical management of tibial fractures. *Instr Course Lect* 1997; 46: 271-80. **The central axis of the tibia is lateral to the midline.**

If there is any suspicion of compartment syndrome then compartment pressures should be monitored. Some centres recommend routine continuous compartment pressure monitoring.

Management

The treatment of tibial shaft fractures has changed with the evolution of orthopaedic practice. Non-operative methods – plaster casts, traction and functional bracing – were initially employed. The AO group proposed internal fixation to allow early mobilisation and minimise stiffness.

Non-operative management for selected tibial fractures continues to be used with good results. The ideal indication for non-operative management is a stable closed, isolated, minimally displaced fracture. A long leg cast is applied and weight bearing is limited in the initial stages of treatment, depending on the fracture configuration. Mobilisation is commenced with functional cast bracing after 2-3 weeks, when the fracture becomes 'sticky'.

The acceptable alignment is less than 5° of varus or valgus angulation and less than 10° angulation in the sagittal plane. There should be less than 10° external rotation and less than 10mm shortening. Any degree of internal rotation is not acceptable. Displacement of more than 50% of the shaft diameter is associated with delayed union.

Indications for surgery

- Comminuted fractures.
- Displaced intra-articular fractures.
- Open fractures or severe soft tissue injury.
- Unstable fractures.
- Segmental fractures.
- Bone loss.
- Coexistent injuries to the limb – 'floating knee' fracture of the femur with tibia fracture.
- Polytrauma.
- Neurovascular injury.
- Compartment syndrome.

Comparison of cast treatment and nailing

Stable tibial fractures without significant comminution can be managed by cast immobilisation or intramedullary nailing. Some degree of stiffness of the knee and ankle is seen after prolonged casting.

> **Note**
>
> Bone LB, Sucato D, Stegemann PM, Rohrbacher BJ. Displaced isolated fractures of the tibial shaft treated with either a cast or intramedullary nailing. An outcome analysis of matched pairs of patients. *J Bone Joint Surg Am* 1997; 79: 1336-41. **In this study of 97 closed fractures, the time to healing was 14 weeks with nailing compared with 22 weeks in a cast. The rates of healing were 98% and 90%, respectively. Functional scores for the knee and ankle were better in the group managed with an intramedullary nail.**

Potential complications with a cast include delayed union (19%), non-union (4%), malunion (13-20%) and ankle stiffness.

External fixation

External fixators are reported to be associated with a 20% rate of malunion, 5% non-union and 50% pin-tract infection. External fixation can be used for temporary stabilisation prior to the insertion of a tibial nail in open fractures and polytrauma patients. The safe period for conversion without increasing the risk of infection is 1-2 weeks.

> **Note**
>
> Bhandari M, Zlowodzki M, Tornetta P, 3rd, *et al.* Intramedullary nailing following external fixation in femoral and tibial fractures. *J Orthop Trauma* 2005; 19: 140-4. **In this meta-analysis, external fixation for more than 28 days was associated with a higher risk of infection compared to earlier conversion of external fixation to a nail.**

Ream versus unreamed nails

Reaming the tibial canal is believed to disrupt the endosteal vasculature, but clinical studies comparing reamed and unreamed nails have shown quicker healing with reamed tibial nails.

> **Note**
>
> Blachut PA, O'Brien PJ, Meek RN, Broekhuyse HM. Interlocking intramedullary nailing with and without reaming for the treatment of closed fractures of the tibial shaft. A prospective, randomized study. *J Bone Joint Surg Am* 1997; 79: 640-6. **This RCT included 136 closed tibial fractures. The non-union rate was 4% in the reamed group and 11% in the unreamed group.**

> **Note**
>
> Court-Brown CM, Will E, Christie J, McQueen MM. Reamed or unreamed nailing for closed tibial shaft fractures. A prospective study in Tscherne C1 fractures. *J Bone Joint Surg Br* 1996; 78: 580-3. **This study randomised 50 patients with closed tibial fractures. In the reamed group, the healing time was 15 weeks, screw breakage was 4% and union without further surgery was 100%. In the unreamed group, the average time to healing was 23 weeks, screw breakage was 52% and delayed union occurred in 20% of fractures. There was no difference between the groups in the incidence of compartment syndrome and knee pain.**

Open fracture

Open fractures are increasingly being managed with an intramedullary nail with soft tissue debridement and cover, and the use of external fixators has declined. The current trend is to achieve definitive soft tissue cover within 72 hours along with definitive skeletal stabilisation.

> **Note**
>
> Henley MB, Chapman JR, Agel J, *et al.* Treatment of type II, IIIA, and IIIB open fractures of the tibial shaft: a prospective comparison of unreamed interlocking intramedullary nails and half-pin external fixators. *J Orthop Trauma* 1998; 12: 1-7. **This RCT compared external fixation with an unreamed intramedullary nail in 174 type II and III open fractures. Malalignment was lower in the nail group at 8% versus 21%. Similar infection and healing rates were observed in the two groups.**

No increase in the rate of infection with reaming versus without was found in two studies.

> **Note**
>
> Keating JF, O'Brien PI, Blachut PA, *et al.* Reamed interlocking intramedullary nailing of open fractures of the tibia. *Clin Orthop Relat Res* 1997; 338: 182-91. **Among 112 open fractures, the time to union was 29 weeks for grade I open fractures, 32 weeks for grade II, 34 weeks for grade IIIA and 39 weeks for grade IIIB.**

> **Note**
>
> Court-Brown CM, Keating JF, McQueen MM. Infection after intramedullary nailing of the tibia. Incidence and protocol for management. *J Bone Joint Surg Br* 1992; 74: 770-4. **The incidence of infection was 1.8% in closed and type I fractures, 3.8% in type II, 5.5% in type IIIA and 12.5% in type IIIB open fractures.**

In severe injuries, the decision to amputate is based on muscle damage, vascular damage and plantar sensation.

Intra-articular fracture

Fractures that involve the proximal or distal articular surface of the tibia and extend into the metaphysis are managed with anatomic reduction of the articular surface, followed by stabilisation of the metaphysis. The metaphyseal comminution can be bridged with a locking plate or external ring fixator.

Minimally invasive plate osteosynthesis is the use of a locking plate to bridge the fracture site. The plate is inserted through a proximal incision and passed across the fracture without exposure of the fracture site. The screws are inserted with the help of a jig under image-intensifier control. This technique causes minimal trauma to local tissues and provides a stable fixation, with each locking screw acting as a fixed-angle fixation device.

Complications

- Knee pain – occurs in 10-60% of patients and is more common with the patellar tendon splitting approach. Pain is greater on kneeling and is related to activity.
- Malalignment.
- Non-union – fracture non-union is declared after 9 months. If the fracture is axially stable, dynamisation of the nail can be considered. If not, exchange nailing is the preferred option.
- Compartment syndrome – the prevalence varies from 1-9% in tibial fractures. The

> **Note**
>
> Keating JF, Orfaly R, O'Brien PJ. Knee pain after tibial nailing. *J Orthop Trauma* 1997; 11: 10-3. **In 107 patients with 110 tibial fractures treated by interlocking tibial nailing, removal of the nail brought complete pain relief to 45% of patients, partial relief to 35% and no relief to 20%.**

diagnosis is based on the measurement of compartment pressures; a difference of 30mmHg from the diastolic pressure is used as a cut-off for diagnosis.

- Reflex sympathetic dystrophy.
- Venous thromboembolism.

Tibial plafond (pilon) fracture

Pilon fractures are fractures of the distal tibial metaphysis with intra-articular extension. These comprise 5-10% of all tibial fractures. A fibular fracture is present in 75% of pilon fractures.

The main complications are fracture comminution, soft tissue injury and poor bone quality. The extent of soft tissue injury should be fully recognised even in closed injuries.

CT scans are routinely taken as plain radiographs often underestimate the injury.

Note

Tornetta P, 3rd, Gorup J. Axial computed tomography of pilon fractures. *Clin Orthop Relat Res* 1996; 323: 273-6. **In this study, a CT scan led to change in the treatment plan in 64% of patients.**

Classification

Several classification systems are in use.

Kellam and Waddell:

- Rotational.
- Axial loading.

Ruedi and Allgower:

- Type I – undisplaced cleavage fractures involving the joint surface.
- Type II – displaced cleavage fractures with minimal comminution.

- Type III – metaphyseal and articular comminution.

AO/ASIF (Association for the Study of Internal Fixation):

- 43A – extra-articular.
- 43B – partial articular.
- 43C – intra-articular.

Severe fracture patterns are associated with more complications and poorer outcomes.

Management

Initial management involves assessment of the patient, checking for neurovascular injury, soft tissue injury, swelling and associated injuries.

A CT scan is obtained to determine fracture pattern in the axial plane and plan surgical management.

In comminuted fractures, the surgical plan is to fix the fibula to restore length. Reconstruction of the articular surface is then performed with lag screws. Defects in the metaphysis from bone impaction are bone grafted. A medial or anterolateral buttress plate, or a locking plate, is applied as a neutralisation plate to maintain length.

In 1969, Reudi reported 74% good or excellent results at 4 and 9 years. Out of 75 fractures in this series, only three were open and almost half were low-energy injuries.

Temporary external fixation and delayed ORIF after 2 weeks has good results in 77% of cases. A common trend is to stabilise the skeleton and soft tissue with a spanning external fixator, with or without fixation of the fibular fracture (depending on the initial shortening). Delayed fixation with anatomical reduction of the articular surface and either bridge plating of the metaphysis or hybrid fixator application avoids soft tissue and wound complications.

Note

Patterson MJ, Cole JD. Two-staged delayed open reduction and internal fixation of severe pilon fractures. *J Orthop Trauma* 1999; 13: 85-91. **In this study, 21 consecutive patients were managed by fibular fixation and a medial spanning external fixator initially, followed by removal of the fixator and medial plate after an average of 24 days. Good results were seen in 77%, with no deep infections.**

External fixators can be spanning, hybrid or articulated.

Note

White TO, Guy P, Cooke CJ, Kennedy SA, *et al.* The results of early primary open reduction and internal fixation for treatment of OTA 43.C-type tibial pilon fractures: a cohort study. *J Orthop Trauma* 2010; 24: 757-63. **These investigators treated 95 fractures with ORIF within 24 hours in 70% and within 48 hours in 88%. The risk of deep infection and wound dehiscence was 19% for open fractures and 2.7% for closed fractures.**

Complications

- Wound breakdown – wound-healing problems are experienced by up to 10% of patients. Excess tension on the soft tissues and trauma to the tissues at the time of injury predispose to wound problems.
- Infection – infection is reported in up to a third of patients. Removal of metalwork and extensive debridement may be needed for deep infection. Some patients eventually require amputation.
- Malunion (varus) and non-union – the incidence is between 1% and 5%.

- Post-traumatic arthrosis – ankle fusion is an option for post-traumatic arthritis. Ankle fusion carries a risk of non-union, delayed union, leg-length discrepancy, arthritis in adjoining joints, chronic oedema and pain. Ankle replacement is increasingly being undertaken in post-traumatic arthritis.

Ankle fracture

Classification

Lauge and Hansen classified ankle fractures into five types based on the position of the foot at the time of injury and the direction of the deforming force; for example, 'supination adduction' implies an adduction force on the supinated foot:

- Supination adduction.
- Supination external rotation.
- Pronation abduction.
- Pronation external rotation.
- Pronation dorsiflexion.

Interobserver variability may be high, but the classification explains the injury mechanism. The grading is not a prognostic indicator.

The Danis-Weber classification is based on the level of the fibular fracture:

- Type A – fracture of the lateral malleolus below the level of the plafond.
- Type B – oblique fracture of the lateral malleolus at the level of the syndesmosis. This may be associated with an injury to the anterior tibiofibular ligament.
- Type C – fracture of the fibula proximal to the tibiofibular joint with disruption of the tibiofibular ligament.

Isolated medial malleolus fracture

Undisplaced
Undisplaced fractures are usually treated non-operatively. Fixation may be required for high-demand individuals.

Displaced

Displaced fractures are generally managed with internal fixation. Avulsion of the tip can be treated non-operatively, but fractures near the base of the medial malleolus should be fixed. Tension-band wiring can be used if the fragment is too small for two screws.

Fixation is with two cannulated or partially threaded cancellous screws perpendicular to the fracture plane. In fractures oriented vertically, screws should be horizontal and antiglide screws used to prevent proximal displacement.

Bioabsorbable screws (polyglycolic acid or polylactic acid) have been used. These provide union rates similar to those with metal screws, but there have been reports of a higher local inflammatory response and sterile serous discharge with bioabsorbable screws.

Stress fracture of the medial malleolus may be seen in athletes and presents with tenderness over the medial malleolus. Diagnosis is by radiographs or bone scan and 4-5 months of restricted activity is necessary for healing. Displaced fractures can be treated with internal fixation.

Lateral malleolus fracture

Up to 3mm displacement is acceptable for non-operative management as long as there is no talar shift.

> **Note**
>
> Ramsey PL, Hamilton W. Changes in tibiotalar area of contact caused by lateral talar shift. *J Bone Joint Surg Am* 1976; 58: 356-7. **The authors reported that 1mm of talar shift led to a 42% reduction in the contact area between the tibia and talus.**

Reduction in the tibiotalar contact area increases the peak contact pressure. The deltoid ligament is a prime stabiliser against lateral displacement of the talus. Injury to the deltoid ligament is evidenced by medial tenderness and swelling.

In patients with an isolated lateral malleolus fracture with talar shift, the medial ligament may be interposed in the joint, preventing accurate reduction. The medial aspect should be opened to retrieve the ligament, but primary repair does not appear to offer any significant advantage over simple retrieval of the ligament.

Bimalleolar fracture

Most bimalleolar fractures are managed with fixation of both malleoli. A lateral plate on the fibula can lead to pain over the hardware and only half of patients experience relief with hardware removal.

Posterior plates avoid the problem of palpable hardware, but can cause peroneal tendonitis. A posterior antiglide plate is useful in osteopenic bone where bicortical screws distally achieve better fixation. Screws can be inserted through the plate to compress the fracture site.

Early surgery is recommended before the swelling increases. In the presence of fracture blisters or excess swelling, surgery may have to be delayed for 1-2 weeks. During this time, alignment of the ankle is maintained with a cast or external fixator.

Injury to the syndesmosis

In syndesmotic injuries, the ankle pain is anterior, the squeeze test is positive and there is pain on external rotation of the ankle.

These injuries are caused by external rotation of the talus in the ankle mortise. They can be present in medial malleolus fractures without lateral malleolus fracture or with Danis-Weber type B or C fractures of the lateral malleolus.

Diagnosis is by demonstrating a widened gap between the distal tibia and fibula on radiographs or intraoperative stressing.

A fibular fracture in the mid or distal third with a syndesmotic injury should be fixed along with stabilisation of the syndesmosis.

Fixation can be performed with 3.5mm fully threaded cortical screws from the fibula to the tibia, engaging one tibial cortex. The screw should be 3cm proximal and parallel to the tibial plafond. The direction of the screw is angled 30° anteriorly as the coronal plane of the fibula is posterior to the tibia. Two screws are used in large individuals. An alternative to screws is the tightrope suture.

Routine removal of screws is controversial. Screws left *in situ* are liable to break, but removal before the syndesmosis is healed may cause diastasis. Bioabsorbable screws and tightropes have been used to avoid the issue of implant removal.

> **Note**
>
> Hovis WD, Kaiser BW, Watson JT, Bucholz RW. Treatment of syndesmotic disruptions of the ankle with bioabsorbable screw fixation. *J Bone Joint Surg Am* 2002; 84-A: 26-31. **In this study, 23 patients had a 4.5mm polylevolactic acid screw and were non-weight bearing for 6 weeks postoperatively. There were no significant complications and all patients returned to their preinjury level of work.**

> **Note**
>
> Cottom JM, Hyer CF, Philbin TM, Berlet GC. Treatment of syndesmotic disruptions with the Arthrex Tightrope: a report of 25 cases. *Foot Ankle Int* 2008; 29: 773-80. **Twenty-one patients had a single tightrope and four had two tightropes placed. The mean time to full weight bearing was 5.5 weeks. There was no redisplacement of the syndesmosis at a mean follow-up of 10.8 months.**

Trimalleolar fracture

The fragment is often attached to the distal fibula by the posterior tibiofibular ligament and reduces when the fibular fracture is reduced. Fragments that involve more than 25% of the distal tibial articular surface should be internally fixed. Any amount of posterior subluxation of the talus on the tibia is not acceptable.

In trimalleolar fractures, the fibular fracture should be reduced and held with reduction forceps. The posterior malleolus should then be fixed, ensuring anatomical reduction. The lateral and medial malleoli are fixed after the posterior malleolus. Applying a fibular plate before the posterior malleolus may make reduction difficult. In addition, it obstructs intraoperative imaging of the ankle in the lateral view to assess articular alignment.

Complications of ankle fracture

- Infection.
- Wound problems.
- Malunion.
- Non-union.
- Post-traumatic arthritis.
- Distal tibiofibular synostosis.

Fixation of ankle fractures is associated with a higher rate of non-union, infection and wound-healing problems in patients with diabetes. Prolonged immobilisation is required until fracture healing is satisfactory.

Ankle sprain

The lateral ligament complex around the ankle includes the anterior and posterior talofibular ligaments and the calcaneofibular ligament. The lateral ligament complex provides stability against inversion stress.

Three grades of ankle sprain have been described.

- A stable ankle with ligament stretch.
- A partial tear.
- An unstable ankle.

The clinical signs are as follows:

- Pain over the anterior talofibular ligament – 50% chance of rupture.
- Pain over the calcaneofibular ligament – 70% chance of rupture.
- Pain over the anterior talofibular and calcaneofibular ligaments – 90% chance of rupture.

Management

Management is with proprioception training and acute repair. Acute repair has poor results compared with non-operative management.

> **Note**
>
> Kaikkonen A, Kannus P, Järvinen M. Surgery versus functional treatment in ankle ligament tears. A prospective study. *Clin Orthop Relat Res* 1996; 326: 194-202. In this prospective study, 30 patients were treated with surgery and 30 were managed non-operatively. At 9 months, 60% of the surgically treated patients had excellent or good outcomes while 87% of the non-operatively managed patients had good or excellent outcomes.

Chronic ankle pain/instability

Twenty percent of acute sprains develop chronic instability.

Diagnosis

Clinically, the diagnosis is based on a positive anterior drawer test. Talar tilt stress X-rays will demonstrate the instability.

Management

Management is with direct repair with suture anchors, with or without local tissue augmentation. A success rate of 85% is reported.

The peroneus brevis or plantaris tendon can be used for reconstruction of the lateral ligament complex. Indications for ligament reconstruction are as follows:

- An old injury.
- Failed anatomic repair.
- Insufficient local tissue.
- Osteoarthrosis of the ankle.

Achilles tendon rupture

The most common site for rupture of the Achilles tendon is 2-6cm above insertion. Poor vascularity in this zone contributes to the high rupture rate.

Clinical features

The injury follows an overload and presents with local pain and difficulty walking. A gap is often palpable on examination.

The Thompson test, first described by Simmonds in 1957, is conducted with the patient prone or kneeling on a chair. Squeezing the calf results in plantar flexion at the ankle if the Achilles in intact, and this is compared with the opposite side.

The Matles test is performed with the patient prone and the knees flexed to 90°. The ankle on the side of the rupture will have more dorsiflexion due to loss of the normal tone of the gastrosoleus complex.

In the O'Brien needle test, a needle is inserted into the muscle belly 10cm proximal to the musculotendinous junction. The ankle is plantarflexed and dorsiflexed. Lack of needle movement on movement of the ankle implies tendon rupture.

A sphygmomanometer cuff can be applied over the calf with the foot plantarflexed. Ankle dorsiflexion will elevate the pressure in the cuff if the Achilles tendon is intact. This was described by Copeland.

Imaging

Distortion of the tendon outline may be evident on a lateral radiograph of the ankle. Kager's triangle is the fat pad bounded by the posterior aspect of the tibia, the anterior aspect of the Achilles tendon and the superior aspect of the calcaneum, and can be disrupted in Achilles tendon ruptures.

Ultrasound of the tendon is helpful in diagnosis and for detecting partial ruptures. MRI is rarely needed, but is useful in chronic ruptures.

Management

It is debatable as to whether operative or non-operative management of acute rupture of the Achilles tendon is preferable. Surgery may allow earlier weight bearing with a reduced re-rupture rate, but wound-healing problems and superficial nerve injury are potential risks.

Note

Nistor L. Surgical and non-surgical treatment of Achilles tendon rupture. A prospective randomized study. *J Bone Joint Surg Am* 1981; 63: 394-9. **From a total of 105 patients, 60 were treated with surgery and the rest non-operatively. The re-rupture rates were 4% and 8%, respectively. In the surgery group, 4% of patients experienced deep infection, 20% had superficial nerve complications and 44% had scar adhesions. Plantarflexion strength was similar in the two groups.**

Note

Suchak AA, Bostick GP, Beaupré LA, *et al.* The influence of early weight-bearing compared with non-weight-bearing after surgical repair of the Achilles tendon. *J Bone Joint Surg Am* 2008; 90: 1876-83. **This study randomised 110 patients to weight bearing 2 weeks after repair or non-weight bearing for 6 weeks. Early weight bearing had no detrimental effects and there was no difference between the two groups at 6 months.**

Endoscopic methods have been employed for management and help in checking for adequate apposition of the tendon ends. There is a risk of injury to the sural nerve.

Note

Fortis AP, Dimas A, Lamprakis AA. Repair of Achilles tendon rupture under endoscopic control. *Arthroscopy* 2008; 24: 683-8.

Chronic ruptures of the Achilles tendon are those that remain 6 weeks following the injury. These are managed with open repair if the gap between the two ends is less than 2.5cm. If there is wider separation between the two ends then management options include the following:

- V-Y-plasty of the proximal part of the tendon.
- Turndown flaps of the aponeurosis of the tendon.
- Use of the peroneus brevis, flexor hallucis longus, flexor digitorum longus, free tendon graft or fascia lata strip to bridge the defect.
- Fresh-frozen Achilles allograft.

Talar fracture

Two-thirds of the talus is covered in an articular surface. The bone has no muscle or tendon attachment.

Blood supply to the talus

The blood supply to the talus is demonstrated in Figure 13.3. The artery of the tarsal canal is one of the chief suppliers of blood. It either arises from the posterior tibial artery 1cm proximal to the origin of the medial plantar artery or occurs as a branch of the medial plantar artery.

The contribution from the anterior tibial artery is through the artery of the sinus tarsi. This anastomoses with the artery of the tarsal canal.

Talar neck fracture

Talar neck fractures commonly result from forced dorsiflexion of the ankle, with the anterior margin of the distal tibial articular surface striking the talar neck.

Classification

Hawkins' classification is commonly used:

- Type I – undisplaced fractures of the talar neck.
- Type II – talar neck fracture with subtalar joint subluxation.

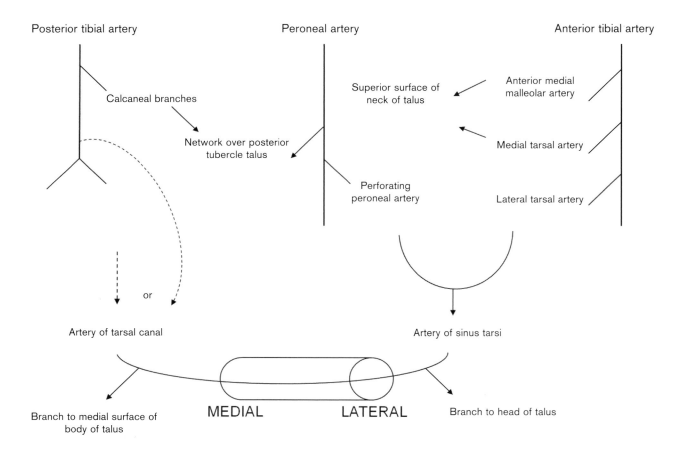

Figure 13.3. Summary of the blood supply to the talus.

- Type III – talar neck fracture with dislocation of the body of the talus from the ankle and subtalar joint.
- Type IV (described by Canale and Kelly) – talar neck fracture with subluxation or dislocation of the talonavicular joint.

> **Note**
>
> Hawkins LG. Fractures of the neck of the talus. *J Bone Joint Surg Am* 1970; 52: 991-1002.

> **Note**
>
> Canale ST, Kelly FB Jr. Fractures of the neck of the talus. Long-term evaluation of seventy-one cases. *J Bone Joint Surg Am* 1978; 60: 143-56.

Management

Undisplaced fractures of the talar neck can be managed non-operatively in a below-knee non-weight-bearing cast, with close follow-up for late displacement.

Displaced fractures require urgent reduction to maintain the blood supply of the talus. A combined dorsomedial and posterolateral approach is used.

A posteroanterior direction of screws is preferred on the grounds of biomechanical stability. Two 4mm screws are adequate. In the presence of gross comminution, compression by screws has to be avoided and plate fixation may be more appropriate. Weight bearing is not permitted for 3 months, but ankle movements may be started.

Complications

- Delayed union or non-union – managed with bone grafting, with or without fixation.

- Malunion – commonly varus malunion of the fracture, which causes hindfoot varus and adduction of the forefoot. Triple arthrodesis is an option to relieve the pain and correct deformity.
- Post-traumatic arthritis of the subtalar and tibiotalar joints is common, occurring in up to 50% of patients.
- AVN – the risk of AVN increases with increasing grade of injury. The presence of subchondral lucency under the talar dome in the AP view of the ankle (Hawkins' sign) 6-8 weeks following the injury indicates an intact blood supply. AVN is managed with tibiocalcaneal or tibiotalar fusion (Blair fusion).

Calcaneal fracture

The os calcis (calcaneum) is a weight-bearing bone. Fractures occur with a fall from a height or high-energy motor vehicle accidents resulting in an axial load. The talus is driven into the calcaneum and splits the bone into two or more parts.

The calcaneum has three facets on the superior surface. The posterior facet articulates with the talus and is separated from the middle and anterior facets by the tarsal canal and sinus tarsi.

The lateral process of the talus is driven into the 'angle of Gissane' on axial loading, resulting in a medial fragment that contains the sustentaculum tali and a lateral fragment.

Classification

On the basis of plain radiographs, there are two main types of intra-articular fractures on a lateral view of the calcaneum: the tongue type and the joint depression type.

In the tongue type of fracture, the fracture line exits through the posterior aspect of the bone. The joint surface is therefore depressed but not directly involved in the fracture. In the joint depression type, there are two primary fracture lines in the coronal plane. These result in the posterior facet being driven down into the cancellous bone. Both fracture lines extend to the superior surface of the calcaneum.

Sanders' classification is used for CT scans. On coronal images, the sustentaculum tali fragment retains its position and the classification is based on displacement and the presence of fracture lines in the lateral fragment:

- Type I – minimal displacement.
- Type II – the posterior facet joint is depressed, but the lateral wall of the calcaneum is intact. This is a three-part fracture.
- Type III – the joint is depressed, along with fracture of the lateral wall. This is known as a four-part fracture.

Clinical features

The local soft tissues should be assessed carefully and a full examination conducted for associated injuries.

Management

Non-operative management is based on elevation, ice and early mobilisation, avoiding weight bearing for 8-12 weeks. Casts are unnecessary for calcaneum fractures.

Surgical treatment is undertaken to restore the alignment of the fragments and correct the widening of the heel. Surgery is delayed for 5-7 days after injury to allow soft tissue revascularisation and resolution of blisters.

The lateral approach is the most common approach to the calcaneum. The fragments are reduced to the sustentaculum tali fragment and the lateral wall is plated.

Primary subtalar arthrodesis is an option for the unreconstructable fracture.

> **Note**
>
> Rammelt S, Grass R, Zawadski T, *et al.* Foot function after subtalar distraction bone-block arthrodesis. A prospective study. *J Bone Joint Surg Br* 2004; 86: 659-68. **The authors looked at distraction bone-block subtalar arthrodesis for malunited calcaneal fractures. Thirty-one patients were recruited, with a mean time from injury to arthrodesis of 36 months. A posterior approach was used, with a distracter applied to restore heel height, tricortical iliac bone graft and restoration of 5° heel valgus. One or two cancellous screws were used. The authors advised that arthrodesis is indicated if loss of calcaneal height is more than 8mm and there is tibiotalar impingement. A total of 5mm height can be restored.**

Malunited calcaneal fracture causes subtalar arthritis, loss of calcaneal height, tibiotalar impingement, increased calcaneal width causing fibulocalcaneal impingement and impingement of the peroneal tendons.

Lisfranc injury

Lisfranc fracture dislocation involves the tarsometatarsal joint. The second metatarsal extends proximal to the other metatarsals and acts as a keystone to stabilise this joint. There are no interosseous ligaments between the first and second metatarsals. The first metatarsal is attached to the medial cuneiform via capsular ligaments. The Lisfranc ligament connects the second metatarsal with the medial cuneiform.

Diagnosis

The mechanism of injury is axial loading of the foot. This is usually seen in high-energy accidents.

The oblique radiograph of the foot should normally show the medial border of the fourth metatarsal aligned with the medial border of the cuboid; the medial border of the second metatarsal aligned with the medial border of middle cuneiform; and the first metatarsal aligned with the medial cuneiform bone. Any loss of alignment should raise the suspicion of a Lisfranc fracture dislocation.

The lateral radiograph should be assessed for any dorsal subluxation of the metatarsals in relation to the tarsal bones. CT scans are helpful to detect occult fractures and confirm alignment of the tarsometatarsal joint.

Management

Undisplaced injuries can be managed non-operatively in a non-weight-bearing short-leg cast for 6-8 weeks.

Displaced fractures require accurate reduction and internal fixation. Open reduction is performed where soft tissue interposition impedes closed reduction. Fixation is achieved by stabilising the first ray to the medial cuneiform with cannulated screws, followed by stabilising the second and third metatarsals with cannulated screws. The fourth and fifth metatarsals are fixed with K-wires for 6 weeks to maintain flexibility.

Weight bearing is not permitted for 6 weeks, and full weight bearing is not permitted for 3 months.

Note

Myerson MS, Fisher RT, Burgess AR, Kenzora JE. Fracture dislocations of the tarsometatarsal joints: end results correlated with pathology and treatment. *Foot Ankle* 1986; 6: 225-42. These authors identified indications for surgery of more than 2mm displacement or a tarsometatarsal angle over 15°.

Note

Calder JD, Whitehouse SL, Saxby TS. Results of isolated Lisfranc injuries and the effect of compensation claims. *J Bone Joint Surg Br* 2004; 86: 527-30. In this study, 13 out of 46 patients with Lisfranc injuries had a poor outcome. Poor outcomes were associated with a delay in diagnosis of more than 6 months and the presence of a compensation claim.

Pelvic ring injuries

Mechanism of injury

Pelvic ring fractures result from high-energy injuries such as motor vehicle accidents, falls and industrial crush injuries. Fractures in the elderly can result from simple falls, where osteoporosis is a contributory factor.

Initial evaluation

- ATLS protocol (Advanced Trauma Life Support) – check airway, breathing, circulation and disability (ABCD) and manage as detailed in ATLS.
- Look for scrotal or labial swelling and wounds on the buttock in open fractures.
- Pain on compression or distraction of the symphysis indicates a pelvic injury.
- Open laceration or skin degloving may be present. Extensive skin degloving is known as a Morel-Lavallée lesion.
- Associated injuries such as urologic, neurologic and head injuries and limb trauma should be assessed.
- Rectal and vaginal examination is mandatory to check for bone-spike penetration into these cavities.

During resuscitation, the following should be checked and corrected:

- Hypotension – a systolic blood pressure below 90mmHg is associated with a 38% mortality rate, compared with 3% in normotensive patients. Ninety percent of pelvic bleeding is venous and from fracture surfaces. Arterial bleeding arises from the internal pudendal, obturator or lateral sacral arteries.

- Hypothermia.
- Acidosis.
- Hypocalcaemia.

A CT scan of the chest and abdomen is obtained to assess any associated injuries.

Imaging

A pelvis AP radiograph is obtained in the emergency department as part of the initial assessment. Approximately 90% of pelvic injuries are diagnosed on an AP view of the pelvis and resuscitation should commence based on this view. Inlet and outlet views are helpful to demonstrate AP and vertical displacement and are taken for decision making and to plan the surgical strategy.

The lateral lumbosacral view may sometimes be needed for suspected lower lumbar or sacral injuries.

Stability

Stability indicates the ability of the pelvis to withstand physiological loading without significant displacement.

Several signs indicate rotational instability:

- Widening of more than 2.5cm of the pubic symphysis.
- An avulsion fracture of the lateral sacrum or ischial spine.
- Widening of the anterior sacroiliac (SI) joint.

Table 13.5. Young's classification of pelvic ring injuries.

Injury	Type	Description
Lateral compression or horizontal fracture of pubic rami	I	Sacral compression on the side of impact
	II	Crescent (iliac wing) fracture on the side of impact
	III	Lateral compression I or II with contralateral anteroposterior compression (open-book) injury
Anteroposterior compression, symphyseal diastasis and/or longitudinal rami fracture	I	Slight widening of the symphysis (<2.5cm) or SI joint Stretched but intact anterior SI, sacrotuberous and sacrospinous ligaments Intact posterior SI ligament
	II	Widened anterior SI joint with symphyseal widening >2.5cm Disrupted anterior SI ligament, sacrotuberous and sacrospinous ligaments Intact posterior SI ligament
	III	Complete SI joint disruption All ligaments disrupted with a widened symphysis or parasymphyseal fractures
Vertical shear	-	Symphyseal diastasis or vertical displacement anteriorly and posteriorly usually through the SI joint, rarely through the iliac wing or sacrum
Combined mechanical	-	Combined injury

SI = sacroiliac

Signs of vertical instability are as follows:

- More than 1cm cephalad migration of a hemipelvis.
- Sacral fractures with a gap (distraction).
- Avulsion of the tip of the L5 transverse process. This is the site of attachment of the iliolumbar ligament.

A CT scan is conducted to detect subtle associated fractures and injuries to the posterior part of the pelvic ring, retroperitoneal haematoma and other organ injuries. Definitive management of the pelvic ring is planned based on the CT scan.

Classification

Young described four types of pelvic ring injuries – lateral compression, AP compression, vertical shear and combined mechanical (Table 13.5).

Note

Burgess AR, Eastridge BJ, Young JW, *et al*. Pelvic ring disruptions: effective classification system and treatment protocols. *J Trauma* 1990; 30: 848-56. **In this study of 210 consecutive patients, classification-system-based protocols reduced mortality and morbidity.**

Table 13.6. Tile's classification of pelvic ring injuries.

Type		Description
A		Stable
	A1	Does not involve the pelvic ring – avulsion of the ischial tuberosity, fracture of the iliac wing
	A2	Stable fracture of the pelvic ring – low-energy injury in elderly patients
	A3	Transverse fracture of the sacrum, fracture of the coccyx
B		Rotationally unstable
	B1	'Open-book' anterior compression – fracture of the pubic rami or pubic diastasis First stage – symphyseal separation <2.5cm; the sacrospinous ligament is intact Second stage – diastasis >2.5cm, rupture of the sacrospinous and anterior sacroiliac ligaments
	B2-1	Lateral compression with ipsilateral fracture
	B2-2	Lateral compression with contralateral fracture (bucket-handle injury)
	B3	As for B2 second stage, but the injury is bilateral
C		Rotationally and vertically unstable Includes vertical shear and anterior compression with posterior ligament injury
	C1	Unilateral fracture of the anterior and posterior ring
	C2	Bilateral injury – one hemipelvis is vertically stable
	C3	Bilateral – both hemipelvises are rotationally and vertically unstable

Tile classification
Tile proposed three types of pelvic ring injuries (Table 13.6).

Classification of sacral fractures
Classification of sacral fractures is by Denis:

- Type I – the fracture line is lateral to the neural foramina.
- Type II – the fracture line is through the foramina.
- Type III – the fracture is medial to the neural foramina.

Crescent fracture
Crescent fracture is a type of lateral compression injury with dislocation of the SI joint and fracture of the posterior iliac wing. These fractures have been subdivided into three types (Day *et al*, 2007):

- Type I – a large crescent fragment with dislocation of less than one-third of the SI joint.
- Type II – an intermediate-size fragment with dislocation of a one- to two-thirds size fragment of the SI joint.
- Type III – a small crescent fragment with dislocation of almost all the SI joint.

> **Note**
>
> Day AC, Kinmont C, Bircher MD, Kumar S. Crescent fracture-dislocation of the sacroiliac joint: a functional classification. *J Bone Joint Surg Br* 2007; 89: 651-8.

Management

The initial management follows ATLS protocols.

Emergency management
A pneumatic antishock garment (PASG) can be used to manage hypovolaemic shock at the scene of injury. The PASG should be released gradually when the patient is in the emergency department. Prolonged use of a PASG runs the risk of compartment syndrome.

In the presence of haemodynamic instability, unstable pelvic injuries are stabilised with a pelvic binder or pelvic wrap. The lower limbs are internally rotated and tied together at the ankles and knees. A custom-made binder or a draw sheet is applied at the level of the greater trochanter to stabilise fractures. This binding technique can be used by paramedics at the scene. Biomechanically, it has been shown to be comparable with anterior external fixation. It is currently the preferred method of initial stabilisation as it is simple, easy to apply and preserves the skin for future definitive surgery.

An anterior pelvic frame can be applied in the operating theatre with two or three pins in the anterior iliac crest. It is indicated in open-book injuries. The C-clamp uses pins placed percutaneously over the region of the SI joints and helps to reduce posterior displacement. The C-clamp is solely an emergency device, while the anterior frame can be used as the definitive treatment in selected cases.

> **Note**
>
> Riemer BL, Butterfield SL, Diamond DL, *et al*. Acute mortality associated with injuries to the pelvic ring: the role of early patient mobilization and external fixation. *J Trauma* 1993; 35: 671-7. **External fixation reduced the mortality rate of hypotensive patients from 41% to 21%.**

The use of CT scanning with contrast helps in the search for bleeding areas. Embolisation of the bleeding artery can be considered as long as the embolisation is from the obturator artery, the superior gluteal artery or another branch of the internal iliac artery. Bleeding from the main trunk of the internal iliac artery, venous bleeding and bleeding from bone surfaces cannot be controlled by embolisation.

Laparotomy and packing of the true pelvis (below the pelvic ring) is also carried out in patients with uncontrolled haemorrhage who are *in extremis*.

Open pelvic fractures still carry a mortality rate of 40-50%. They are managed with aggressive debridement, surgical toilet, skeletal stabilisation and diversion of the bowel and bladder.

Definitive management

Internal fixation of pelvic fractures can be delayed until the patient has been stabilised and other life-threatening associated injuries managed. This often translates to a delay of 5-7 days.

Stable injuries (Tile type A) are managed with early mobilisation and analgesia. Type B and C injuries usually require operative stabilisation.

Rotationally unstable injuries can be managed with the following:

- Anterior external fixator – acceptable as a definitive treatment as long as adequate reduction is achieved and maintained. For definitive management, supra-acetabular pins (low route) are preferred because of a good fixation strength. However, hip joint penetration and injury to the lateral cutaneous nerve are notable complications with this procedure.
- Symphysis pubis plating – a single or double plate across the symphysis. With a Pfannenstiel approach, the plate is placed on the superior and/or anterior aspect.

Vertically unstable injuries require posterior stabilisation in addition to anterior fixation. Posterior fixation can be achieved with the following:

- Iliosacral screws – for SI joint disruptions (percutaneous or open).
- Anterior plating of the SI joint with a retroperitoneal approach.
- Posterior fixation of sacral fractures and the SI joint through an open posterior approach.

For crescent fractures (fracture dislocation of the SI joint), ORIF is recommended.

Outcome

Patients with stable injuries generally do well and experience few long-term complications. Unstable injuries result in poorer outcomes with pain, non-union and malunion. The presence of urogenital and nerve injuries alongside pelvic fracture compromises the outcome.

Acetabular fracture

The reduction achieved at surgery is the single most important factor affecting the outcome of the procedure and relates to the experience of the operating surgeon.

Initial management

Initial management is based on the ATLS protocol. If associated with dislocation of the hip, the hip should be reduced urgently in the emergency department or under image intensifier in the operating theatre. Posterior dislocation may be associated with injury to the sciatic nerve and this must be checked for and documented.

Radiographic evaluation is with an AP view of the pelvis and 45° oblique views (Judet views).

The medial roof arc should also be assessed. A vertical line is drawn through the centre of the acetabulum, with a second line drawn from the centre of the acetabulum to the fracture line crossing the dome of the acetabulum. If the angle between the lines is less than 45° in a displaced fracture, then operative treatment should be considered (Matta). Similarly, anterior and posterior roof arcs can be measured on the Judet views.

On CT scans, the superior 10mm of the acetabular roof corresponds to the 45° roof arc angle. Scans are taken with 3mm intervals. Three-dimensional reconstructions are possible, but the best accuracy is achieved by correlating the plain radiographs with the two-dimensional CT images.

The acetabulum has a horseshoe-shaped articular surface surrounding a non-articular cotyloid fossa. The anterior column is composed of the anterior half of the acetabulum with the iliac crest, iliac spine and pubis, and is represented by the iliopectineal line. The posterior column comprises the posterior half of the acetabulum along with the ischium, ischial spine and posterior part of the ilium and is represented by the ilioischial line. The dome is the roof of the acetabulum. Restoration of the femoral head under the dome is the critical factor in determining the long-term outcome after an acetabular fracture. The neurovascular structures in the pelvis are at risk in acetabular injuries and should be checked.

Corona mortis is a large anastomosis between the external iliac, inferior epigastric and obturator arteries. It can lead to haemorrhage in the ilioinguinal approach.

Classification

Primary fractures:

- Anterior wall.
- Anterior column.
- Posterior wall.
- Posterior column.
- Transverse.

Transverse fractures can be of three types:

- Transtectal – the fracture line is superior to the cotyloid fossa.
- Juxtatectal – at the junction of the cotyloid fossa with the articular surface.
- Infratectal – through the cotyloid fossa.

Complex fractures:

- Posterior column, posterior wall.
- Anterior with posterior hemitransverse.
- Transverse and posterior wall.
- T-fracture.
- Associated both columns.

In associated both-column fracture, the articular fragments of the acetabulum do not maintain any continuity with the SI joint. The obturator oblique view demonstrates the spur sign, which is diagnostic of a both-column injury. This spur is the part of the ilium remaining attached to the SI joint and is seen lateral to the medially displaced acetabulum.

Management

Suprapubic catheters preclude an ilioinguinal approach because of a risk of infection and should be avoided.

Non-operative management

Undisplaced fractures (<2mm displacement) can be managed non-operatively. Traction or non-weight-bearing mobilisation is advised for 8 weeks, with regular radiographic monitoring.

Some comminuted both-column fractures may have 'secondary congruence' in relation to the femoral head and can be managed non-operatively. The comminuted fragments are often displaced medially as a whole and may have gaps, but align themselves in the shape of an acetabulum.

Elderly osteoporotic and medically unfit patients should be considered for non-operative management.

Local soft tissue infection indicates non-operative management. A Morel-Lavallée lesion is localised subcutaneous fat necrosis overlying the pelvis. A surgical approach made through this lesion is associated with a high infection rate.

Internal fixation

Displaced fractures (>2mm displacement, based on the roof arc measurement) should be operated on and fixed internally. Roof arcs should be measured on the AP and Judet views, which will give the anterior, medial and posterior roof arcs.

Posterior wall fractures can lead to hip instability and should be fixed if more than one-third of the posterior wall is fractured.

Displaced fractures through the weight-bearing dome of the acetabulum should be fixed.

Intra-articular fragments are a further indication for internal fixation.

Primary total hip replacement

Primary total hip replacement is indicated by the following:

- Comminuted both-column fracture.
- Unreduced posterior fracture dislocation.

Surgical approaches

Surgery should be performed within 5-7 days.

Standard approaches:

- Kocher-Langenbeck.
- Ilioinguinal.

- Modified Stoppa – a vertical midline incision to expose the inner surface of the ilium.

Extensile approaches:

- Extended ilioinguinal (Letournel and Judet).
- Triradiate approach (Mears and Rubash).
- T-approach.

Management of different fracture patterns

Table 13.7 summarises treatment planning for acetabular fractures.

Table 13.7. Summary of treatment planning for acetabular fractures.

Fracture pattern	Approach	Fixation	Comments
Posterior wall	Kocher-Langenbeck	Lag screw and reconstruction plate	Long-term results depend on marginal impaction, damage to femoral head and screw placement
Posterior column	Kocher-Langenbeck	Lag screw and recon plate	Rotational malalignment must be corrected
Anterior wall	Ilioinguinal or iliofemoral	Buttress plate	May be associated with hip dislocation
Anterior column	Ilioinguinal or iliofemoral	Buttress plate	-
Transverse fractures	Posterior or ilioinguinal	Buttress plate on the exposed column and a lag screw in the other column	Juxta and transtectal fractures should be reduced anatomically
Posterior column and wall	Kocher-Langenbeck	Double plate posteriorly	-
Transverse and posterior wall	Extensile or combined	Based on the fracture pattern	Can be difficult to reduce an anterior fracture through a posterior approach
Transverse and anterior column and posterior hemitransverse fracture	Ilioinguinal or combined	Plate along the pelvic brim	-
Both columns	Combined approach	Based on the fracture pattern	-

Postoperative management

Prophylaxis should be given against thrombosis, heterotopic ossification and infection. Toe-touch bearing is permitted 2 days after surgery and continues for 12 weeks.

Complications of acetabular fractures include the following:

- Mortality (1-2.5%).
- Post-traumatic arthritis:
  - with anatomic reduction, 10% at 1 year;
  - without anatomic reduction, 35% at 1 year.
- AVN (7.5% after posterior dislocation).
- Infection (up to 5%) – there is a higher risk of infection with a Morel-Lavallée lesion if the posterior approach is used and with a suprapubic catheter if the ilioinguinal approach is used.
- Sciatic nerve injury – can be present in 10% of patients with acetabular fractures as part of the injury. The sciatic nerve is also at risk with the posterior approach (risk of injury is 2-6%).
- Heterotopic ossification – present in 50% of patients undergoing the posterior (Kocher-Langenbeck) or combined approach. The risk is lower with the ilioinguinal approach. Prophylaxis is with indomethacin (preferred; 25mg three times a day for 6 weeks) or radiation.
- Thromboembolism – present in 50% of patients. If proximal deep vein thrombosis is detected then an inferior vena cava filter should be considered. Filters should also be used in high-risk patients. Preoperative prophylaxis is

with low-molecular-weight heparin, followed postoperatively by warfarin for 6 weeks.

Total hip replacement for post-traumatic arthritis following acetabular fracture

The results of total hip replacement for post-traumatic arthritis are often not as good as primary total hip replacement for osteoarthritis. Complications include retained hardware, scarring, heterotopic ossification and early loosening.

Note

Berry DJ, Halasy M. Uncemented acetabular components for arthritis after acetabular fracture. *Clin Orthop Relat Res* 2002; 405: 164-7. This study included 34 hips in 33 patients, with a 10-year follow-up. The mean patient age at surgery was 49 years. Nine patients underwent revision for osteolysis, loosening, poly wear or dislocation.

Fracture in children

Hip fracture

Hip fractures in children are relatively rare compared with other childhood injuries.

Classification
The classification was proposed by Delbet (Table 13.8).

Table 13.8. Delbet's classification of femoral neck fractures in children.

Type	Description	Risk of avascular necrosis (%)
I	Epiphyseal separation with or without dislocation of the femoral head from the acetabulum	~100
II	Transcervical fractures	50
III	Basal neck fractures	25
IV	Intertrochanteric fractures	10

Blood supply to the femoral head

From birth to the age of 4 years, the metaphyseal vessels arising from the medial and lateral circumflex femoral arteries are the major supply to the femoral head, along with the artery along the ligamentum teres. By the age of 4 years, the physis is more developed and the retinacular vessels become the major supply. These arise from the medial circumflex femoral artery.

Management

Type I fractures are treated with anatomic reduction (either closed or open) and stabilisation with a pin or screws. These must cross the epiphyseal plate in order to stabilise the fracture and smooth pins should be used in children to minimise growth impairment at the physis. Type I injuries are associated with dislocation of the capital physis in 50% of children. This carries an almost 100% rate of AVN of the capital physis.

Type II and III fractures can be treated non-operatively with a cast in young children if they are undisplaced or if anatomic reduction can be achieved. ORIF can be performed but crossing the physis is avoided if possible.

Type IV injuries have a low risk of AVN and are treated either in a spica or by internal fixation with a screw with a side plate (paediatric hip screws).

Complications

AVN is a complication related to initial displacement and a time lag between injury and reduction. The risk of AVN is highest with type I and lowest with type IV fractures.

Coxa vara can result from growth arrest at the physis, with relative overgrowth of the trochanteric physis. Malreduction\or loss of alignment can also lead to coxa vara. Subtrochanteric valgus osteotomy is an option if the neck shaft angle is less than 110°.

Physeal growth arrest can be caused by damage at the time of injury or threaded pins crossing the physis.

Non-union is possible in patients where anatomic reduction is not achieved.

Chondrolysis is a rare complication.

Hip dislocation

Hip dislocation is a rare injury in children. It is generally related to high-energy trauma. The diagnosis is evident on radiographs or cross-sectional imaging.

Management is directed towards concentric reduction, either with closed manipulation or open reduction.

Femoral shaft fracture

Femoral shaft fractures can occur from simple falls or high-energy injuries. Non-accidental injury accounts for almost half of femoral shaft fractures in infants.

Management

Femoral shaft fractures can be managed with various methods depending on the age of the child, and the management must be individualised according to the clinical situation. The options include spica application, traction followed by spica, external fixation, flexible intramedullary nails and a dynamic compression plate. In general, children younger than 5 years can be managed in a spica cast. Beyond this age, flexible intramedullary nails are preferred. Antegrade femoral nailing is an option in skeletally mature patients.

Indications for surgery in young children include open fractures, multiple injuries, an associated head injury, neurovascular injury and floating knee (ipsilateral femoral and tibial fracture). Surgery is also indicated in situations where it is difficult to maintain reduction by closed methods.

Spica

The early application of spica is an option in children younger than 5 years. Children older than 5 years can be difficult to manage at home in a spica cast. It can be difficult to maintain reduction with spica and there is a possibility of shortening.

Traction

Traction used to be a common method of treatment, but the long period of hospitalisation required has diminished its role in modern orthopaedics. Traction is usually applied for 2-4 weeks and is followed by spica cast application. It can be used on its own as a definitive treatment method.

External fixation

External fixation is an effective method in children. It is easy to apply, minimally invasive and provides adequate stabilisation. Conversely, external fixation it associated with pin-site infections, the inconvenience of a frame, knee stiffness and refracture after frame removal.

Flexible intramedullary nails

Flexible intramedullary nails are increasingly being used for femoral shaft fractures because of their minimally invasive nature and ability to maintain reduction effectively. They are generally inserted retrograde and the entry point is proximal to the distal femoral physis. The nails can be bent into a C- or S-shape to provide three-point fixation across the fracture.

Weight bearing is restricted until a callus is seen on the radiographs, but some stable fracture patterns can be progressed on weight bearing at an earlier point.

Antegrade femoral nailing is avoided in skeletally immature children because of the risk of AVN from direct damage to the blood supply and coxa valga via damage to the trochanteric growth plate.

Dynamic compression plate

Plating of the femur provides a stable construct. Plating is associated with a relatively bigger scar and more blood loss. The risks are plate breakage and fracture through a screw hole after plate removal.

Complications

Leg-length discrepancy may occur due to malreduction and shortening of the injured limb. The shortening is compensated for by overgrowth of the femur following fracture. This may be up to 1cm.

Supracondylar femoral fracture

These fractures are difficult to reduce and stabilise non-operatively because the pull of the gastrocnemius tends to flex the knee and produce angulation at the fracture site. Cross-pins or screws can be used.

Distal femoral physeal fracture

These injuries can be seen in newborns, and are caused by pulling on the leg during delivery in a breech presentation. In older children, physeal separation is associated with high-energy trauma.

Undisplaced injuries can be managed with cast immobilisation. Displaced fractures require reduction and can be stabilised with smooth pins crossing the physis or by screw fixation into the metaphyseal fragment.

Physeal injuries can lead to growth arrest with consequent angular deformity or limb-length discrepancy. The injury should be followed up to skeletal maturity.

Patellar fracture

Patellar fractures in children present and are managed in a similar manner to adult patellar fractures. A sleeve fracture of the patella is through unossified cartilage, and the radiographs may give a false appearance of a small fragment.

Patellar dislocations are common in children. Most dislocations or subluxations of the patella reduce spontaneously and present as a painful knee. Tenderness along the medial border of the patella and apprehension on lateral subluxation indicate a possible patellar dislocation.

Acute patellar dislocations are managed with reduction and 1-2 weeks of immobilisation. Once the pain settles, quadriceps exercises can be started. Quadriceps setting exercises are started initially, followed by closed-chain exercises.

A significant number of patients with acute patellar dislocation have an osteochondral fracture involving the patellar surface or the lateral femoral condyle.

Tibial tubercle fracture

Avulsion injuries of the tibial tubercle are classified into three types:

- Type I – avulsion of a small fragment of the tuberosity.
- Type II – avulsion extending to the proximal tibial physis.
- Type III – avulsion of the tuberosity extending to the proximal tibial articular surface.

Displaced fractures are managed with ORIF by screws. Arrest of physeal growth can lead to a recurvatum deformity in the growing child.

Tibial fracture

Proximal tibial epiphyseal injuries can be Salter Harris type I or II. The close proximity of the arteries posteriorly means there is a risk of vascular injury.

Displaced fractures are managed with closed reduction and percutaneous pins. Open reduction is rarely needed. The physis should not be crossed with threaded pins. Growth arrest leading to deformity occurs in one in four patients and follow-up is advisable.

Fractures of the proximal tibial metaphysis are prone to late valgus deformity. These injuries should therefore be followed up. If a deformity becomes evident, surgery to correct it should be delayed for 3 years as some deformities will spontaneously correct.

A toddler's fracture is an undisplaced oblique fracture of the distal tibia seen in infants and is the result of a low-energy trauma. A short-leg walking cast for 3 weeks is sufficient.

Tibial diaphyseal fractures in older children are managed with closed reduction and long leg cast application. Surgical options for open fractures, irreducible fractures and unstable fractures are external fixation, flexible intramedullary nails and plate fixation.

Triplane fracture

Triplane fractures are fractures of the distal tibia in the skeletally immature patient, involving the distal tibial growth plate. The fracture plane is sagittal in the epiphysis, horizontal through the growth plate and coronal through the posterior distal tibial metaphysis.

Triplane fractures are Salter Harris type IV injuries. They are often minimally displaced and can be managed in a cast with close monitoring for displacement. Displaced fractures require internal stabilisation with one or two screws. A CT scan will show the displaced fragments.

There is a potential for growth arrest with these injuries.

Seymour lesion

A Seymour lesion is an injury of the physis of the distal phalanx associated with injury to the skin and nail fold. The physeal plate is proximal in the phalanx and is close to the nail fold. Displacement of this physis leads to an open injury.

Humeral shaft fracture

In neonates, fractures of the proximal end of the humerus involving the growth plate are usually Salter Harris type I injuries. The growth plate is susceptible to injury. Older children have type II or III injuries. The vast majority are managed with non-operative methods due to good remodelling and quick healing.

Humeral shaft fractures are rare in children and non-operative measures such as a cast or brace with sling are adequate for immobilisation. Operative intervention is rarely needed.

Supracondylar humerus fracture

Supracondylar humerus fracture is a common elbow injury in children. It is sustained as a result of a fall on an outstretched hand. Rarely, it may be due to a direct fall onto the elbow.

Demographics

The most common age of presentation is 4-7 years, as this is a period of rapid metaphyseal remodelling. Most are hyperextension injuries. It is more common in boys.

Classification

Classification is by Gartland:

- Type I – undisplaced fractures.
- Type II – fractures with angulation but an intact posterior cortex.
- Type III – complete fracture with displacement. These can be flexion- or extension-type injuries.

Clinical assessment

These fractures can be associated with neurovascular injury and a thorough assessment is vital.

There is often significant local swelling and tenderness. Open fractures require urgent debridement and K-wire stabilisation. In some closed fractures, the proximal fragment may be buttonholed through the brachialis and can pucker the skin on the anterior aspect of the elbow.

The nerves should be assessed and recorded. The anterior interosseous nerve is the most common nerve involved in this injury. The distal circulation is assessed, noting both the capillary refill time and the radial and ulnar pulses. Flexing the elbow can obstruct distal circulation; if this occurs, the arm should be splinted in a semi-flexed position until reduction and stabilisation can be performed.

Imaging

Baumann's angle is the angle between the longitudinal axis of the humerus and a line drawn along the axis of the capitellar physis. The normal angle is 70-78°.

On the lateral view, a line drawn along the anterior cortex of the humerus should intersect the middle one-third of the capitellum.

Radiographs are helpful to classify the injury, assess displacement and look for associated injuries.

Management

No vascular compromise

Undisplaced (type I) injuries can be managed in a plaster splint.

Type II injuries require manipulation and splint application to restore alignment.

Type III injuries are managed with closed reduction and percutaneous pin fixation. Open reduction is sometimes required if there is soft tissue interposition or if the brachialis is impaled by the fragment.

One pin is inserted from the medial epicondyle to engage the opposite cortex and the other is inserted from the lateral condyle. Two diverging pins from the lateral side are acceptable, but will not be as mechanically stable as cross-pins.

The timing of surgery has been a matter of some debate. It is advisable to undertake reduction before the local soft tissue swelling progresses to the extent of compromising circulation.

> **Note**
>
> Sibinski M, Sharma H, Bennet GC. Early versus delayed treatment of extension type-3 supracondylar fractures of the humerus in children. *J Bone Joint Surg Br* 2006; 88: 380-1. **In this study of 77 children, 43 children were pinned within 12 hours and the rest were managed more than 12 hours after the injury. There was no difference in outcome between the two groups.**

Note

Walmsley PJ, Kelly MB, Robb JE, et al. Delay increases the need for open reduction of type-III supracondylar fractures of the humerus. *J Bone Joint Surg Br* 2006; 88: 528-30. **In this retrospective study of 171 children, 126 were managed within 8 hours and 45 were managed after 8 hours. Those in the delayed group were more likely to require open reduction.**

Note

Leet AI, Frisancho J, Ebramzadeh E. Delayed treatment of type 3 supracondylar humerus fractures in children. *J Pediatr Orthop* 2002; 22: 203-7. **In this study of 158 patients, there was no increase in operative time, closed reduction and complications with delays in surgery of up to 21 hours.**

Olecranon pin insertion and traction is an option for the management of supracondylar fractures. It requires a hospital stay and is hence not a favoured method. Traction can be applied in a brace, which allows earlier discharge from hospital but has a relatively higher complication rate.

Note

Matsuzaki K, Nakatani N, Harada M, Tamaki T. Treatment of supracondylar fracture of the humerus in children by skeletal traction in a brace. *J Bone Joint Surg Br* 2004; 86: 232-8. **This study of 193 patients with supracondylar fracture, including 15 radial nerve injuries and 14 median nerve injuries, investigated bracing with skeletal traction using an olecranon pin. Four children (2%) developed cubitus varus and one child had restricted flexion. Lateral and posterior displacement was not significant.**

Vascular compromise

Fractures with vascular compromise should be reduced as an emergency. In most cases, the distal circulation is impaired because of tenting of the artery over the fracture site and will be restored immediately or within a few minutes of reduction.

If the circulation is still impaired, exploration of the brachial artery is undertaken by a vascular surgeon. Intimal tears are managed with a vein graft and lacerations in the artery can be repaired directly or with a graft.

In many patients, the collateral circulation may be adequate to maintain perfusion.

Management of the 'pink pulseless hand' following supracondylar fracture has been somewhat controversial. Recent evidence from vascular surgery units advocates exploration of the 'pink pulseless hand' to avoid the risk of ischaemia.

Note

Blakey CM, Biant LC, Birch R. Ischaemia and the pink, pulseless hand complicating supracondylar fractures of the humerus in childhood: long-term follow-up. *J Bone Joint Surg Br* 2009; 91: 1487-92. **This study followed 26 children. A poor outcome was noted in children where the vessels were not explored despite a pink hand.**

Nerve injuries in association with supracondylar fractures

Nerve injuries are usually neurapraxias and recover with time. If there is no recovery after 4-6 months, then nerve conduction studies are undertaken and neurolysis considered.

Complications of supracondylar fractures:

- Nerve and vascular injury.
- Malunion.
- Elbow stiffness.
- Myositis ossificans.

The risk of malunion is minimised with pin fixation. Cubitus valgus is better tolerated, but can lead to stretching of the ulnar nerve. Cubitus varus is cosmetically disabling and a supracondylar dome or lateral closing wedge osteotomy is required for correction.

Separation of the distal humeral physis

This injury is seen in neonates and young children. The cartilaginous capitellum is not visible on radiographs and the appearance may be of elbow dislocation. Elbow dislocations are extremely rare in neonates. Ultrasound is diagnostic and demonstrates the capitellum.

Treatment is with closed reduction and splintage in flexion.

Lateral humeral condyle fracture

Lateral condyle fractures mainly involve the cartilaginous end of the distal humerus. There is little soft tissue cover to enable reduction and these fractures are likely to lose alignment if not internally stabilised.

Because these are intra-articular injuries there is a high rate of non-union. Fractures that are displaced more than 2mm should be reduced and fixed.

Classification
Classification is by Milch:

- Type I – Salter Harris type IV injury involving the capitellum. The lateral part of the trochlear ridge remains attached to the humerus.
- Type II – Salter Harris type II injury involving the capitellum and the lateral part of the trochlear ridge.

Management
Undisplaced fractures can be immobilised in a cast and followed up closely to ensure there is no displacement.

Displaced fractures should be reduced (either closed or open) and stabilised with two smooth pins. Kocher's approach is used for exposure. The blood supply is from the posterior aspect and the soft tissues on this side should be protected. An anterior arthrotomy can be established to confirm the reduction.

The pins are removed at 4-6 weeks.

Complications
Complications include non-union, malunion and their consequences. Non-union is managed with bone grafting and fixation *in situ*. Cubitus varus is possible in patients with malunion and can cause ulnar nerve palsy. Elbow stiffness may result from anatomic repositioning and fixation *in situ* should be considered.

Anterior transposition of the ulnar nerve will relieve stretch on the nerve.

Medial epicondyle fracture

These are avulsion injuries from a valgus force to the elbow. The fragment is separated and may become trapped within the elbow joint if the elbow was dislocated at the time of injury.

In most patients, displaced fractures are managed by resting the arm in a sling. Fibrous union can be expected and functional limitation is minimal. Fixation of the fragment is indicated for high-demand patients and those with associated elbow dislocation. A single screw is adequate to achieve compression at the fracture site.

Radial head dislocation

Radial head dislocations in children may be congenital or traumatic.

Congenital dislocations have the appearance of a rounded radial head lacking concavity on the proximal aspect, relative overgrowth of the radius and a hypoplastic capitellum. Congenital dislocations have a poor outcome if reduction is attempted.

Traumatic dislocation can occur as an isolated injury or in association with ulnar fracture (known as the Monteggia injury).

Imaging

The longitudinal axis of the radius should be co-linear with the capitellum in all views of the elbow. Any loss of alignment indicates incongruence of the radiocapitellar joint.

Management

If diagnosed early, within 3-4 weeks, radial head dislocations can be reduced by closed manipulation.

If diagnosed late, open reduction is required. The annular ligament is reconstructed using strips of the triceps fascia passed through tunnels in the proximal ulna to maintain concentric reduction of the radial head. Many different techniques have been described. Bell Tawse used a strip from the central part of triceps fascia, while Lloyd-Roberts and Bucknill used the lateral part of the fascia. The harvested strip is left attached to the ulna at the distal end.

> **Note**
>
> Lloyd-Roberts GC, Bucknill TM. Anterior dislocation of the radial head in children: aetiology, natural history and management. *J Bone Joint Surg Br* 1977; 59-B: 402-7.

> **Note**
>
> Bell Tawse AJ. The treatment of malunited anterior Monteggia fractures in children. *J Bone Joint Surg Br* 1965; 47: 718-23.

Radial neck fracture

Radial neck fractures are the result of a valgus force on the elbow. There is good remodelling potential at this site in children and up to 30° of angulation can be accepted. Fractures angulated by more than 30° are managed with closed reduction and splintage.

If the angulation is more than 50°, a percutaneous pin can be used to physically push the fragment into alignment while applying a varus force to distract the joint. The blunt end of a Steinmann pin or a 3.2mm guide wire is useful for this purpose. An option is to pass a flexible nail with a bent tip retrograde in the medullary canal of the radius and lever the fragment back into alignment with the tip of the nail. This is known as the Metaizeau technique. Most fractures are stable after reduction and can be splinted for 2-3 weeks followed by immobilisation. A K-wire can be used across the fracture site to transfix the fragment, but a transcapitellar wire should be avoided because of risk of breakage.

Open reduction is an option where closed reduction fails, but carries a high risk of damage to the growth plate.

Monteggia fracture

A Monteggia fracture dislocation is a fracture of the ulna with dislocation of the radial head.

Classification

Classification is by Bado:

- Type I – anterior dislocation of the radial head.
- Type II – posterior dislocation of the radial head.
- Type III – lateral dislocation of the radial head.
- Type IV – dislocation of the radial head with fracture of both the radius and ulna.

Management

Acute injuries are managed with closed reduction of the radial head and immobilisation. Inability to achieve congruent reduction indicates an infolded annular ligament or button-holing of the radial head through the joint capsule; open reduction is needed. Ulnar fractures can be fixed internally for stability.

Injuries diagnosed late require either open reduction of the radial head or techniques to reconstruct the annular ligament. Ulnar corrective osteotomy can be combined with the procedure.

Radius and ulna diaphyseal fracture

Fractures of the radius and ulna are the most common long-bone fractures in childhood. Accurate reduction is important to minimise loss of pronation and supination. The remodelling potential depends on the age of the patient, the extent of the deformity and the distance of the fracture from the physis.

Malrotation of the fragment translates into a similar loss of range of rotation. Rotational deformities do not remodel, but angulation in the plane of movement will improve with time in the growing child.

The proximal and distal radioulnar joints should be visualised on radiographs and checked for any dislocation or subluxation.

Management

Greenstick fractures are managed non-operatively with manipulation and a long-arm plaster cast. Undisplaced fractures are also managed non-operatively.

Displaced fractures of both the radius and ulna can be unstable and anatomic reduction is important to restore function. Options for internal fixation are intramedullary titanium elastic nails or plate fixation.

Plate fixation provides anatomic rigid fixation with rotational control, but leaves longer scars. Intramedullary nails can be inserted with minimal access and are effective in maintaining reduction but provide limited rotational control. Nails often require removal.

> **Note**
>
> Myers GJ, Gibbons PJ, Glithero PR. Nancy nailing of diaphyseal forearm fractures. Single bone fixation for fractures of both bones. *J Bone Joint Surg Br* 2004; 86: 581-4. **Twenty-five patients underwent single-bone intramedullary fixation for fractures of both forearm bones. There was no difference in function if one or both bones were fixed. A cast was required after single-bone stabilisation.**

> **Note**
>
> Bhaskar AR, Roberts JA. Treatment of unstable fractures of the forearm in children. Is plating of a single bone adequate? *J Bone Joint Surg Br* 2001; 83: 253-8. **Twenty patients underwent plating of both bones while 12 underwent plating of the ulna only. There was no difference in function or alignment between the two groups.**

Distal radius fracture

Fractures of the distal radial metaphysis not involving the growth plate are managed in a cast if minimally displaced. Fractures with an initial angulation of more than 30° and displacement of more than 50% are at high risk of malalignment. These fractures can be stabilised with one or two K-wires passed percutaneously to transfix the fracture.

Fractures of the distal radius at the level of the growth plate are very common. Most of these can be reduced by manipulation and maintained in a cast. There is some risk of growth arrest following these injuries. A single smooth pin inserted from the radial styloid crossing the physeal plate is used to stabilise unstable fractures.

Galeazzi fracture is a fracture of the distal third of the radius along with disruption of the distal radioulnar joint. It is managed with anatomic reduction and internal fixation of the radius. A Galeazzi equivalent is a distal radius fracture with separation of the distal ulnar physis.

Cervical spine injuries

Cervical spine injuries have a bimodal incidence. Up to 30% of such injuries occur in young men.

Mechanism

Cervical spine injuries are often the result of road traffic accidents or falls. Penetrating injuries and sports injuries also account for a small percentage. Cervical spine injury must be suspected in patients who cannot be adequately assessed because of head injury or impaired consciousness.

Vertebral artery injury occurs in about 20% of patients, with a higher risk in flexion distraction or flexion compression injuries. In 17% of patients there is reconstitution of the blood flow. Bilateral injuries can lead to delayed cortical blindness and recurrent quadriparesis.

Assessment

General:

- Head injury, pupillary size, Glasgow Coma Scale.
- Facial lacerations or fractures.
- Cerebrospinal fluid otorrhoea or rhinorrhoea.
- Spinal shock.
- Urinary incontinence or retention.

Spine:

- Localised tenderness.
- Gaps in the spinous processes.

Neurologic:

- Careful assessment to detect an incomplete injury.

Sensory:

- Assess pin-prick sensation, light touch using a cotton ball and perianal sensation: 0 is absent, 1 is impaired, 2 is normal and NT is not testable.
- Proprioception is an important posterior column sensation.

Motor:

- Assessed in 10 paired myotomes from rostral to caudal.

In addition, the following should be assessed:

- Diaphragmatic function using fluoroscopy.
- Abdominal reflexes and Beevor's sign.
- Bulbocavernosus reflex for spinal shock.
- Babinski reflex.
- Tone.
- Imaging.

Imaging

The cervical spine should be immobilised at the scene of the accident. X-rays are obtained in the resuscitation room and should include the AP, lateral (including the C7-T1 junction) and odontoid peg views. Cervical spine radiographs miss 20-25% of spinal injuries, but these can be identified with a CT scan of the cervical spine. A CT scan should be obtained in all patients with a suspected or radiographically detected cervical spine injury. MRI is useful in patients with neurological deficit.

The presence of a cervical spine injury should prompt a search for an associated second injury in the spine, the incidence of which is about 10%.

The four alignment lines should be identified on the lateral radiograph: along the anterior borders of the cervical vertebrae; along the anterior extent of the spinal canal; along the posterior margin of the canal; and along the tips of the spinous processes. Any step of more than 3mm or an increase in the soft tissue outline anterior to the vertebral bodies raises suspicion of a cervical spine injury. Unilateral facet dislocation produces a step in the vertebral alignment of less than 25% of the vertebral width. A step of 25-50% indicates bilateral facet dislocation.

Another indicator is the atlantodens interval, which is the space between the posterior border of the anterior arch of the atlas and the anterior margin of the odontoid process. The atlantodens interval should be less than 3mm in adults and less than 5mm in children.

On the open-mouth odontoid-peg view, the distance between the odontoid and the lateral mass of the atlas should be equal on both sides, with the lateral margin of the mass in line with the lateral margin of the C2 body.

Management

The goal of management is to stabilise the spine, prevent the progression of neurological deficit and allow early rehabilitation.

The indications for surgical stabilisation are progressive neurological deficit, associated injuries and spinal instability.

Thoracolumbar spine fracture

Holdsworth proposed the two-column concept of spinal stability. The posterior longitudinal ligament

Table 13.9. Denis classification of thoracolumbar spine fracture.

Injury	Type	Description
Compression fracture	A	Failure of the superior and inferior end plates
	B	Failure of the superior end plate
	C	Failure of the inferior end plate
	D	Failure of the central body
Burst fracture	A	Failure of the superior and inferior end plates
	B	Failure of the superior end plate
	C	Failure of the inferior end plate
	D	Axial loading and rotational injury
	E	Axial loading and lateral flexion injury
Flexion distraction (chance)	-	Horizontal avulsion injuries with the axis of rotation anterior to the anterior longitudinal ligament
Fracture dislocations	A	Slice fracture with rotational shear through the body
	B	Same as A, but through the disc anteriorly
	C	Translational shear injury, failure of facet joint, superior body translated anteriorly
	D	Same as C The neural arch is fractured and remains posteriorly as a floating lamina
	E	Anteroposterior translation with disruption of the ligaments
	F	Rotation and anterior translation of the superior body on the inferior body

complex is the chief determinant of stability. If this is disrupted then the spine is unstable. Stable fractures include anterior wedge fractures, burst fractures and extension injuries. Unstable injuries are shear injuries and fracture dislocations. Denis proposed the three-column concept of spine stability. The anterior column includes the anterior half of the vertebral body and the anterior longitudinal ligament. The middle column includes the posterior half of the vertebral body and the posterior longitudinal ligament. The posterior column includes the posterior arch.

The transition zone is from T11 to L1. It is the junction of the immobile kyphotic thoracic spine and the mobile lordotic lumbar spine. Sixty percent of thoracolumbar spine fractures occur in this area.

Thoracolumbar spine fractures have been classified by Denis (Table 13.9).

Compression fracture

In a compression fracture the anterior column fails under compression, the middle column remains intact and the posterior column remains intact or fails under tension. These injuries commonly occur between T11 and L2. On plain X-rays, measure Cobb's angle and the percentage loss of vertebral height.

If the posterior vertebral angle is more than 100° then this is a burst fracture (see next). There will be interpedicular widening on the AP view and posterior cortical disruption.

Kummell's disease is delayed progression of kyphotic deformity. It is characterised by worsening back pain and osteonecrosis of the vertebral body (post-traumatic). Patients may have neurological deficit.

Burst fracture

Burst fractures involve failure of the anterior and middle column in axial load. They commonly occur between T11 and L2. On X-rays, measure Cobb's angle, the percentage loss of vertebral height and interpedicular widening.

Signs of instability:

- Progressive kyphosis.
- Progressive neurologic deficit.
- Substantial posterior column injury.
- More than 50% loss of vertebral height with kyphosis.

Indications for surgery are as follows:

- Kyphosis of more than 20-30°.
- Subluxation of the posterior facets.
- An increase in the interspinous process distance.
- Loss of more than 50% of vertebral height.

Short-segment pedicle screws have a high failure rate if anterior stabilisation is not achieved and should be removed after 18 months.

An isolated anterior approach can be used if surgery is delayed for more than 2 weeks or if there is compression by the thecal sac.

Flexion distraction injury

The anterior column fails under tension or compression, the middle column fails under tension and the posterior column fails under tension. MRI and CT with sagittal reconstructions should be obtained.

Associated intra-abdominal injuries occur in 45% of patients, and 10-15% experience neurologic deficit.

In view of the good healing potential of bone, patients with no neurological deficit can be managed with a hyperextension cast or total-contact thoracolumbosacral orthosis for 3 months.

Fracture dislocation

All three columns are disrupted. Horizontal translation or rotation will be evident on radiographs.

Management is with multisegment posterior instrumentation. Stabilisation of two levels above and below the fracture is recommended.

Spinal cord injury

Grading

A commonly used grading systems is that of Frankel (Table 13.10).

Grade	Frankel
Table 13.10. Spinal cord injury grading.	
A	No motor or sensory function
B	Sensory function only, no motor function
C	Motor function is useless
D	Motor function is useful
E	Normal motor and sensory function

Emergency management

A full neurological examination is carried out. It is important to rule out spinal shock by checking the bulbocavernosus reflex.

Sacral sparing may be the only indication that the injury is incomplete. In complete injuries, 80% of patients regain function in one root above the injury level while 20% regain two roots.

The National Acute Spinal Cord Injury Study determined a benefit with methylprednisolone infusion (30mg/kg over 1 hour and then 5.4mg/kg/hour) for patients with an acute spinal cord injury:

- Continue for 24 hours if started within 3 hours.
- Continue for 48 hours if started within 8 hours.

There is, however, some controversy relating to the efficacy of steroids. Many centres do not use steroids as a standard of care, but do include them as a management option.

> **Note**
>
> Bracken MB, Shepard MJ, Collins WF, *et al.* A randomized, controlled trial of methylprednisolone or naloxone in the treatment of acute spinal-cord injury. Results of the Second National Acute Spinal Cord Injury Study. *N Engl J Med* 1990; 322: 1405-11. In this study, 162 patients with an acute spinal cord injury were given methylprednisolone, 154 were given naloxone and 171 were given placebo. A benefit was seen with methylprednisolone in patients with complete and incomplete lesions.

> **Note**
>
> Hugenholtz H, Cass DE, Dvorak MF, *et al.* High-dose methylprednisolone for acute closed spinal cord injury – only a treatment option. *Can J Neurol Sci* 2002; 29: 227-5. This systematic review concluded that the evidence to support the use of methylprednisolone is weak (level I to II-1).

Imaging

- X-ray of the entire spine.
- CT to determine the ratio of the transverse diameter of the canal to the AP diameter – a wide transverse diameter indicates interpedicular widening.
- MRI if there is any neurological deficit to assess cord damage and epidural haematoma.

Management

Assess stability:

- Extent of damage to the posterior column.
- Extent of collapse.
- Extent of kyphosis.

The posterior column provides the greatest resistance to progressive kyphosis.

The neutral-zone theory of Panjabi describes a continuum between stability, hypermobility and frank instability.

Indications for surgery are as follows:

- Progressive neurologic deficit.
- Major neurological deficit with canal compromise.
- Progressive kyphosis.
- Substantial rotational or translational malalignment.
- Soft tissue chance fracture.

Surgical approaches

The indications for an anterior approach are as follows:

- Injury to the posterior column.
- Incomplete neurologic deficit in flexion injury with canal compromise.
- Secondary decompression following posterior stabilisation.
- Significant anterior spinal instability.

An anterior approach provides direct decompression, but there is no difference in neurologic outcome.

- For T4-T9 injuries – right transthoracic approach.
- For T10-L1 injuries – thoracoabdominal approach with subphrenic extension.
- For T12-L5 injuries – subpleural retroperitoneal approach.
- For T2-T4 injuries – lateral extrapleural parascapular approach or extension of a cervical spine approach with partial manubriectomy and partial excision of the medial third of the clavicle. Sternal splitting may be needed.

In the posterior approach, instrumentation should be two or three levels above and two levels below. The distraction restores vertebral height and partial canal clearance is achieved by ligamentotaxis. Canal clearance of 40-75% is possible in acute injuries.

Posterior short-segment fusion (one level above and below) is associated with a high rate of proximal screw pullout if there is anterior column compromise. This technique is not commonly used.

In the 'rod long, fuse short' technique, rods are removed after 1 year. However, arthritis develops in unfused segments. Progressive kyphosis after rod removal and late back pain are other complications, and this technique is therefore not commonly used.

For fracture dislocations, fixation can be performed from the back initially with anterior reconstruction performed if needed. The fixation must extend three levels up and two or three levels below.

The extent of canal compromise has been correlated with neurological deficit in some studies, but this is not universally accepted. Any remaining canal compromise decreases by 50% with remodelling over the 12 months following the injury.

An anterior approach is used to reduce canal impingement; a posterior approach with ligamentotaxis may also reduce canal impingement. Sharpey's fibres help with reduction in the posterior approach. Indirect reduction should be performed within 3 days of injury and is less effective in the presence of more than 67% canal compromise due to annular ligament disruption.

A 'flat back' after posterior instrumentation was a problem with the initial instrumentation systems, but square terminal-rod hook constructs allow sagittal contouring.

At the thoracolumbar junction, short-segment pedicle screw constructs have a high failure rate without anterior stabilisation.

Posterolateral decompression

Posterolateral decompression allows access to the anterior thecal sac either through or lateral to the pedicle. Bone anterior to the retropulsed fragments is removed through curettes and pituitaries. This should only be performed in the lower lumbar spine below the conus.

Potential complications include neurologic damage, inadequate decompression and poor visualisation for grafting.

Complications of surgery

- Neurologic deterioration (1%) caused by overdistraction, overcompression, malreduction or an instrument in the spinal canal.
- Instrumentation failure.
- Pseudarthrosis (2-8%).
- Delayed vascular erosion caused by metal-vessel contact in anterior instrumentation.
- Retrograde ejaculation caused by damage to autonomic nervous system (4%).
- Injury to the great vessels.
- Infection.

Surgery does not improve the chances of neurologic recovery. Animal studies, however, have shown better results with early decompression.

Kyphosis is not related to back pain and functional impairment. Damage to the discovertebral complex and posterior facet joints may be responsible for back pain.

Sacral fracture

Anatomy

The S1 nerve root has the foraminal exit area, and the root occupies one-third of the area of the foramen. The S4 nerve root has the largest foraminal exit area, with the root occupying one-sixth of the area.

The anterior rami of S2-S5 conduct parasympathetic impulses for sexual, bladder and bowel function.

Evaluation

Bruising, tenderness, swelling and posterior sacral osseous prominence may be evident with sacral fracture, but 30% of cases are missed on the initial presentation.

A Morel-Lavallée lesion is indicated by degloving of the lumbosacral fascia and a subcutaneous fluid mass.

The examination should assess spontaneous and maximum anal sphincter contraction, light touch and pin-prick along the perianal S2-S5 dermatomes, and bulbocavernosus and cremasteric reflexes.

Assessment

Imaging should include an X-ray of the pelvis: AP, inlet and outlet views.

X-ray signs include the following:

- Fracture of the L5 transverse process – present in 51% of patients.
- A paradoxical inlet view of the sacrum seen on the AP view – 92% of patients.
- 'Stepladder sign' – anterior sacral foraminal disruption.

CT, MRI, bone scan and single-photon emission CT can help to define the injury.

Perineal somatosensory evoked potentials and anal sphincter electromyography can assess neurological deficit from spinal injuries.

Classification

Denis proposed the three-zone classification:

- Zone 1 – the fracture line is lateral to the neural foramen.
- Zone 2 – the fracture involves the neural foramina.
- Zone 3 – the fracture extends to the spinal canal.

Zone 3 is further subdivided based on the pattern of fracture lines into H-type, U-type, lambda fracture and the T-fracture.

Management

Many sacral injuries are managed non-operatively, but the indications for surgery are being more clearly defined with an improved understanding of these injuries and their prognosis.

Indications for surgery include open injuries, fractures with neurological compromise and unstable fractures with progressive displacement.

Fixation of the sacrum can be achieved anteriorly or posteriorly. Percutaneously placed SI screws, plate fixation posteriorly, lumbar pedicle screws with iliac screw fixation and anterior plates are options for stabilising sacral injuries.

Open fracture

An open fracture is a combined bone and soft tissue injury where the fracture haematoma communicates with the exterior through the skin or with a mucous membrane.

The management recommendations for open fractures were published in 2009 through a joint effort of the British Orthopaedic Association and the British Association of Plastic, Reconstructive and Aesthetic Surgeons.

Classification

The Gustilo-Anderson system is most commonly used for classifying open fractures. It is applicable after initial wound debridement:

- Type I – wound of less than 1cm, clean, minimal contamination, minimal soft tissue injury.
- Type II – wound of more than 1cm, moderate contamination, some soft tissue damage, moderate comminution of bone.
- Type III – wound of more than 10cm, high contamination, comminuted fracture:
  - IIIA – severe soft tissue injury, bone cover possible;
  - IIIB – loss of bone coverage, requires soft tissue procedure;
  - IIIC – loss of bone coverage, vascular injury requiring repair.

> **Note**
>
> Gustilo RB, Anderson JT. Prevention of infection in the treatment of one thousand and twenty-five open fractures of the long bones: retrospective and prospective analyses. *J Bone Joint Surg Am* 1976; 58: 453-8. **Classification system for open fractures.**

> **Note**
>
> Brumback RJ, Jones AL. Interobserver agreement in the classification of open fractures of the tibia. The results of a survey of two hundred and forty-five orthopaedic surgeons. *J Bone Joint Surg Am* 1994; 76: 1162-6. **Gustilo and Anderson classification had intraobserver agreement of 60%.**

The Mangled Extremity Severity Score (MESS) of Johansen (1990) is also used (Table 13.11).

Principles of management

Open fractures should be managed at specialist centres with experienced plastic surgical and orthopaedic teams working together. These centres should have appropriate facilities for the required procedures, including theatre space and intensive care, microbiology, prosthetic and rehabilitation support.

The initial management is performed as an emergency following the ATLS guidelines. Resuscitation of the patient is the priority.

Broad-spectrum antibiotic prophylaxis (co-amoxiclav 1.2g every 8 hours or cefuroxime 1.5g every 8 hours) should be administered as soon as possible. Clindamycin is given to patients who are allergic to penicillin.

Table 13.11. The Mangled Extremity Severity Score.

Criteria	Description	Score
A. Skeletal soft tissue injury	Low energy (stab or simple fracture)	1
	Medium energy (open or multiple fractures, dislocation)	2
	High energy (close-range gunshot, crush injury)	3
	Very high energy (as above plus gross contamination)	4
B. Limb ischaemia*	Pulse reduced or absent, normal perfusion	1
	Pulseless, paraesthesia, diminished capillary refill	2
	Cool, paralysed, insensate, numb	3
C. Shock	Systolic blood pressure always >90mmHg	0
	Transiently hypotensive	1
	Persistent hypotension	2
D. Age	<30 years	0
	30-50 years	1
	>50 years	2

* The ischaemia score is doubled if the ischaemia time is >6 hours.

The patient's tetanus vaccination status should be ascertained and prophylaxis administered as appropriate.

A picture of the wound should be taken for the patient's records and to inform the multidisciplinary team. No irrigation or exploration is performed in the emergency department. Haemorrhage is controlled with direct pressure. Significant arterial bleeding requires vascular surgery support. The wound is dressed with a sterile dressing soaked in saline and the extremity is splinted. Appropriate radiographs are requested, making sure to include other injured areas.

The patient is moved to the operating suite as soon as possible for wound debridement and operative management of the fracture. Plastic surgeons should be involved at an early stage and vascular surgeons may be consulted for major vascular injuries.

Urgent surgical exploration is needed for patients with gross contamination, multiple injuries, compartment syndrome or an ischaemic limb.

Management in the operating room

Thorough debridement and washout of the wound with normal saline is the key to a good outcome. All dead, devitalised tissue is excised, with the obvious exception of neurovascular structures. Small wounds are surgically extended to gain access and perform adequate debridement. An assessment is made regarding skin loss.

Bone debridement may be required. A bleeding bone is the best indicator of viability, hence a tourniquet should not be inflated for this part of the procedure. Loose fragments of bone and non-viable ends should be removed. Articular surface fragments are fixed back with rigid fixation. Pulse lavage is not recommended.

Bones can be stabilised at the time of debridement if there is no bone loss. In patients with bone loss, spanning external fixators or ring fixators are used. Internal fixation is performed when soft tissue cover can be achieved, which should be within 3 days (preferably) and usually within 7 days. Free flaps should be applied within 7 days.

Recombinant human bone morphogenetic protein has recently been used in the management of open fractures. It reduces the risk of secondary interventions and quickens fracture and wound healing. Patients undergoing this treatment have been found to have less hardware failure and a lower risk of infection.

> **Note**
>
> Govender S, Csimma C, Genant HK, *et al.* Recombinant human bone morphogenetic protein-2 for treatment of open tibial fractures: a prospective, controlled, randomized study of four hundred and fifty patients. *J Bone Joint Surg Am* 2002; 84: 2123-34.

If no skin loss

- Following debridement, the fracture is managed with stable internal fixation.
- The wound is left open and surgical extensions, if any, are sutured.
- A second look is planned after 48-72 hours, depending on the degree of contamination.
- At this second look, a healthy and granulating wound can be sutured or covered with a skin graft or myocutaneous flap.

- Infected wounds are managed with further debridement, with follow-up after a further 48 hours.

If skin loss

Thorough debridement and internal fixation is the first step. Once the fracture has been stabilised the skin can be covered with a flap, either at the same time as the initial debridement or as a staged procedure after 48-72 hours, depending on the degree of contamination and adequacy of debridement. A vacuum-foam dressing is applied until definitive surgery can be performed.

Evidence for the management of open fracture

Antibiotics in open fractures

> **Note**
>
> Gosselin RA, Roberts I, Gillespie WJ. Antibiotics for preventing infection in open limb fractures. *Cochrane Database Syst Rev* 2004; 1: CD003764. **This review determined that antibiotics reduce the risk of infection by 59%.**

Pulse lavage is not recommended for washout

> **Note**
>
> Hassinger SM, Harding G, Wongworawat MD. High-pressure pulsatile lavage propagates bacteria into soft tissue. *Clin Orthop Relat Res* 2005; 439: 27-31.

Reamed or unreamed nailing in open fractures

> **Note**
>
> Keating JF, O'Brien PJ, Blachut PA, *et al*. Locking intramedullary nailing with and without reaming for open fractures of the tibial shaft. A prospective, randomized study. *J Bone Joint Surg Am* 1997; 79: 334-41. This study found no difference in the non-union, function or infection rates with or without reaming in 88 open tibial fractures. Patients with reamed nails had lower rates of screw breakage.

Chapter 14 Nerve injuries and neuromuscular disorders

Nerve injury

The spinal nerves are formed by union of the dorsal (sensory) and ventral (motor) roots. These nerves supply dermatomes and myotomes, respectively, as segmental nerves or through the formation of a plexus – as in the limbs.

There are 31 spinal nerves: eight cervical, 12 thoracic, five lumbar, five sacral and one coccygeal. There are also 14 sympathetic nerves, which exit with the 12 thoracic and the first two lumbar nerves.

Nerve degeneration and regeneration

Injury to an axon results in Wallerian degeneration in the stump distal to the injury. The production of axoplasmic calcium is increased, and the axoplasm and cytoskeleton are broken down. The debris is cleared within 4 weeks. Schwann cells start dividing within 3 days and form cytoplasmic processes. The cells line the empty endoneurial tubes forming bands known as Büngner's bands, which act as channels for the regenerating axons. Macrophages remove myelin by phagocytosis and stimulate Schwann cells to secrete nerve growth factor.

Proximal to the injury, retrograde or primary degeneration ensues. This extends only to the first node of Ranvier. This process is similar to Wallerian degeneration.

The axonal cell body swells and undergoes chromatolysis. The nucleus migrates to the periphery of the cell.

Axonal growth starts within 24 hours of injury, and continues at a pace of 1-2mm/day. Establishing a link with the regenerating axon distally leads to progression of healing and fibre maturation. The presence of intact tubes (endoneurium) guides the axons along the tract. Neurites that fail to make a distal connection die off or form neuromas.

Classification of nerve injuries

The first widely used classification of nerve injuries was proposed by Seddon in 1943. Three groups were described:

- Neurapraxia – physiological disruption of the nerve, potentially with localised disruption of the myelin sheath. Recovery is complete after this type of nerve injury.
- Axonotmesis – the axon is disrupted and there is distal Wallerian degeneration. The endoneurium and the Schwann cell are preserved and good functional recovery is possible.
- Neurotmesis – severance of the endoneurial tube and the Schwann cell, and disruption of axons. The perineurium and the epineurium are also disrupted. Recovery is variable and nerve repair is indicated to restore continuity.

In 1951, Sunderland proposed a more detailed and useful classification, dividing the nerve injuries into five groups (Table 14.1).

Table 14.1. The Sunderland classification of nerve injuries.

Grade	Description
I	Disruption of myelin; physiological dysfunction
II	Disruption of myelin and axon
III	Disruption of myelin, axon and endoneurium
IV	Disruption of myelin, axon, endoneurium and perineurium
V	Disruption of myelin, axon, endoneurium, perineurium and epineurium

Grade I nerve injury is equivalent to neurapraxia in the Seddon classification. The axon is intact, there is no Wallerian degeneration and recovery is complete. The first modality to recover is sympathetic function, followed by pain and temperature. Proprioception and motor function are the first to be affected and the last to recover.

Tinel's sign (paraesthesia in the distribution of the nerve on percussion at the site of injury) is present in all injuries where there is anatomical damage (grades 2-5). Tinel's sign is progressive in grades 2 and 3, where there is some continuity of the nerve and spontaneous recovery, and not progressive in grade 4 and 5, unless nerve repair is undertaken.

In grade 2 nerve injury, disruption of the axon leads to Wallerian degeneration, but the intact endoneurial tube helps in near-complete recovery. Neuron death in proximal injuries is the cause of some loss of function in this type. Tinel's sign is present and advances distally and the 'motor march' is evident. This means proximal muscles regain function earlier than distal muscles, as regeneration progresses distally in the nerve.

Disruption of the endoneurium in grade 3 injuries causes disorganisation of axonal growth and some loss of function is expected.

The epineurium is intact in grade 4 nerve injury. Tinel's sign is present at the site of injury, but does not progress unless the nerve is repaired successfully.

Grade 5 injuries carry little hope of recovery without surgical repair and functional loss is complete without treatment.

A sixth degree is described by McKinnon, where a part of the nerve is transected and the remaining part suffers an injury of varying degree. This can result in a neuroma-in-continuity.

Evaluation of nerve injury

The first step in diagnosis is to take a detailed history and conduct a physical examination. The history will explain the mechanism of nerve injury, associated injuries, coexisting medical conditions and degree of neurologic involvement. In longstanding nerve injury, evidence of recovery is an important factor with prognostic implications.

Metabolic disorders, collagen diseases and malignancies can cause nerve dysfunction and should be elicited in the history.

The examination of each nerve elicits sensibility in the autonomous distribution, and examination of specific muscles innervated by the nerve. Injuries to the muscle may cause loss of sensation, and this should be differentiated from paralysis due to nerve injury.

Motor deficit indicates a lower motor neuron lesion with atonic paralysis. The grading of muscle strength is shown in Table 14.2.

Table 14.2. Grading of muscle strength.

Grade	Description
0	Complete paralysis
1	Muscle flicker
2	Muscle contraction with gravity eliminated
3	Muscle contraction against gravity
4	Muscle contraction against gravity and resistance
5	Normal muscle contraction

Because of overlap of sensory distribution between cutaneous nerves, the autonomous area of any particular nerve is examined to determine loss of sensory innervation. This is the zone supplied solely by the nerve.

Surrounding the autonomous zone is the intermediate zone, which is the generally accepted anatomical distribution of the nerve. The intermediate area will demonstrate some loss of sensation in the event of a nerve injury.

The maximal zone is beyond the intermediate zone, and indicates the entire distribution of the nerve. If the surrounding nerves are blocked and the nerve is stimulated, the area where sensations are perceived is known as the maximal area.

In addition to sensory and motor deficit, autonomic loss results in loss of sweating in the distribution of the nerve. Sweat droplets can be observed with an ophthalmoscope or checked with the iodine starch test. The presence of sweating indicates continuity of autonomic innervation.

Tinel's sign is elicited by percussion along the course of the nerve from distal to proximal, and checking for tingling in the distribution of the nerve. The presence of Tinel's sign indicates axonal regeneration, while distal advancement of Tinel's sign indicates progression of axonal regeneration along the course of the nerve. Sunderland grade 2 and 3 injuries are characterised by a progressive Tinel's sign, as are grade 4 and 5 injuries after repair. Tinel's sign is present and does not progress along the nerve if repair is not undertaken in grades 4 and 5. Grade 1 injuries do not exhibit Tinel's sign as there is no axonal injury or regeneration.

Another feature of a nerve injury is a lack of skin wrinkling in water. Changes in cutaneous circulation cause vasodilation for 2-3 weeks, followed by vasoconstriction.

Nerve recovery

Nerve recovery following injury follows a specific sequence. Pain and temperature sensation are the first to recover, followed by touch and the perception of 30Hz vibration, moving touch, constant touch, 256Hz vibration and finally stereognosis. Perception of touch is determined with Semmes Weinstein monofilaments.

A grading system for sensory recovery has been proposed by the British Medical Research Society (Table 14.3), while motor recovery is graded by the Medical Research Council. Recovery is tested in the autonomous area of the nerve.

Table 14.3. Grading of recovery from the British Medical Research Society and Medical Research Council.

Sensory recovery		Motor recovery	
Grade	Description	Grade	Description
S0	Absence of sensibility in the area	M0	No contraction
S1	Recovery of deep cutaneous pain	M1	Perceptible contraction in proximal muscles
S2	Partial recovery of superficial cutaneous pain and touch	M2	Perceptible contraction in proximal and distal muscles
S3	Recovery of superficial cutaneous pain and touch; absence of over-response	M3	Power against resistance in proximal and distal muscle groups
S4	Recovery of two-point discrimination	M4	Synergistic and independent movements possible
S5	Complete recovery	M5	Complete recovery

Investigations

Electromyography

Electromyography studies are helpful in evaluating nerve injuries. A needle electrode is inserted into the muscle. Normal muscle does not show any activity at rest. In denervated muscle, fibrillation potentials on needle insertion appear on an electromyogram at 8-14 days and spontaneous potentials are evident after 2-4 weeks. Fibrillations persist until reinnervation or muscle atrophy.

Polyphasic motor unit potentials on voluntary activity are a sign of reinnervation.

Nerve conduction studies

Nerve conduction studies involve placing an electrode on the skin overlying the nerve and measuring the response from the muscle. The distance between the stimulating and recording electrode is divided by the time between stimulus and response, giving the velocity of conduction.

For motor nerves, the muscle is stimulated through the nerve. The response time is noted. The stimulating electrode is moved closer to the distal end and again the response time is noted. The ratio of the distance between the two points of stimulation and the difference in latency time gives the conduction velocity between these two points.

In the event of significant axonal injury, Wallerian degeneration in the distal segment will impair the amplitude of evoked potentials within 5-10 days. The presence of normal conductivity in the distal segment 10 days following injury indicates a good prognosis.

Somatosensory evoked potential

The somatosensory evoked potential is checked by stimulation of the sensory nerve and measuring potentials on the scalp. It is useful for spinal cord monitoring during spinal surgery.

Management of nerve injuries

The initial management of nerve injuries follows Advanced Trauma Life Support guidelines and patient resuscitation.

In open injuries, wound management is undertaken and primary repair of the nerve is preferable if possible. Primary repair is accomplished within a few hours of injury.

If there is a delay in achieving repair because of medical reasons, associated injuries or lack of skilled personnel, repair can be accomplished within 7 days and wound management is carried out as standard practice. Repair within 7 days is known as delayed primary repair. Beyond 7 days, repair is classified as secondary repair.

Closed nerve injuries are observed for signs of recovery while maintaining the range of motion of joints and preventing contractures.

Nerve palsy that develops following the manipulation of a fracture should be explored to rule out entrapment.

Nerve repair

Nerve repair is undertaken as soon as possible after a diagnosis of nerve injury, and with the availability of expertise and equipment.

The surgery is performed under general or regional anaesthesia with tourniquet control. Magnification with loupes or an operating microscope is essential. The preparation of the extremity should allow for the incision to be extended to gain exposure if required. A nerve stimulator is helpful to determine the need for neurolysis of a neuroma-in-continuity.

In patients undergoing secondary repair, the orientation of the two nerve ends may be difficult and the arrangement of the fascicles is matched on either side.

The technique for nerve repair can be epineurial or fascicular. There is no proven advantage of one over the other. In epineurial repair, the epineurium of one end is sutured to the corresponding epineurium of the other end.

Fascicular repair involves repair of the perineurium. It potentially provides more accurate repair as long as the fascicles are matched. The presence of suture material within the substance of the nerve may interfere with regeneration and inaccurate matching of fascicles leads to a poor result.

Fascicle matching can be conducted with intra-operative nerve stimulation, which requires the patient's cooperation. Immunohistochemical identification can be performed in the first few days after nerve injury. This technique relies on detecting acetylcholinesterase in motor axons and carbonic anhydrase in sensory axons. It requires excision of some nerve tissue from the two ends and some processing time, but does not depend on patient cooperation.

Nerve grafting is helpful in patients with a significant gap. Commonly used donor nerves are the sural nerve and the medial and lateral cutaneous nerves of the forearm (Table 14.4).

Nerve tubes or axonal guidance channels have been used to guide the regenerating axons across a gap. These are arteries or veins from the patient used as a conduit, or synthetic materials such as collagen or silicon. The use of such channels is still developing.

Results of nerve repair

The following factors influence the results of nerve repair:

- Age – older patients have worse outcomes following nerve repair.
- Tension on the repair site – the gap between nerve ends determines the tension of the repair. Prior to repair, the nerve has to be resected to the level of undamaged funiculi. Extensive nerve damage may require more resection and with more resection, the arrangement of the funiculi within the nerve changes between the two ends, making repair less successful. The gap can be minimised by nerve mobilisation or transposition, positioning the joint to relieve tension on the nerve or, in rare events, shortening the bone or nerve grafting.
- Timing of repair – early repair is associated with better outcomes. However, repair should be undertaken only when adequate facilities and

Table 14.4. Donor nerves for nerve grafting.

Nerve	Length of graft obtained (cm)	Anatomy
Sural nerve	30-40	Adjacent to the short saphenous vein
Medial cutaneous nerve of the forearm	18-20	Adjacent to the basilic vein
		Minimal scar problems
		The anterior branch or both the anterior and posterior branches can be used
Lateral cutaneous nerve of the forearm	8	Along the ulnar border of the brachioradialis
		Leaves a prominent scar
Nerves supplying the third web space	24	Useful for median nerve injury
		Expendable nerves
Dorsal cutaneous branch of the ulnar nerve	Variable	For ulnar nerve injury
Terminal branches of the anterior interosseous nerve	Variable	To reconstruct digital nerves
		No sensory or motor morbidity

expertise are available and the patient has been resuscitated and stabilised.

- Level of injury – proximal injuries have a less favourable outcome compared with distal injuries.
- Quality of repair – the quality is determined by the condition of the nerve ends, repair without tension, preservation of the blood supply and accurate apposition of the fascicles.
- Experience of the surgeon – experience directly correlates with outcomes.

Neuroma-in-continuity

In neuroma-in-continuity, the neuroma is dissected and the damaged nerve fascicles identified.

A simpler technique is to use a nerve stimulator proximal and distal to the injury site to identify the electrically silent sensory and motor fibres, and then use a nerve graft to reconstruct them. This avoids dissection of the neuroma and reduces the risk of injury to the lesser injured fibres.

Complex regional pain syndrome

Complex regional pain syndrome is an abnormal sympathetic response in a limb following an injury. Patients suffer pain, stiffness, discolouration, increased sweating and osteoporosis. Other terms used to describe this or similar conditions include reflex sympathetic dystrophy, causalgia and Sudeck's dystrophy.

In the initial stage there is swelling, redness, increased sweating and increased local temperature. The pain is out of proportion to what is expected following the injury. After about 2 months these features are replaced by reduced sweating and stiffness. In the late stage, atrophic changes persist.

Two types of complex regional pain syndrome have been described:

- Type I occurs after an injury.
- Type II occurs in association with a peripheral nerve lesion.

Treatment is with physical therapy, with or without sympathetic blocks. Stellate ganglion blocks have been reported as effective in upper limbs and surgical sympathectomy can be considered for patients in whom blocks have transient efficacy.

Entrapment neuropathies

Pronator teres syndrome

Pronator teres syndrome describes compression neuropathy of the median nerve along its course in the anterior aspect of the elbow joint. The nerve can be compressed by the lacertus fibrosus, pronator teres or fibrous origin of the flexor digitorum superficialis.

Abnormal anatomy, repeated activity or trauma can predispose to this condition.

Patients typically complain of aching in the forearm after activity. Depending on the muscle involved in compression, pain can be reproduced by resisted pronation (indicates the pronator teres), resisted flexion and supination (indicates the lacertus fibrosus) or flexion of the fingers (indicates the flexor digitorum superficialis band).

Nerve conduction studies can aid diagnosis and treatment is through avoidance of activity or surgical release.

Anterior interosseous syndrome

Anterior interosseous syndrome describes compression of the anterior interosseous branch of the median nerve under the pronator teres.

The presenting features are aching in the forearm and a weak pinch. Patients are unable to touch the tips of their index finger and thumb together due to a weak flexor pollicis longus and flexor digitorum profundus (FDP). Weakness of the pronator quadratus is evident by weak pronation in extension.

Release of the deep head of the pronator teres alleviates the symptoms.

Cubital tunnel syndrome

Entrapment of the ulnar nerve at the elbow can be caused by medial epicondyle fractures, bony spurs or entrapment under the origin of the flexor carpi ulnaris muscle.

The sensory component is reduced sensation in the ulnar aspect of the hand. Signs of ulnar motor deficit are wasting of the interossei (evident in the first dorsal interosseous), wasting of the flexor carpi ulnaris and the ulnar part of the FDP, weak adduction of the thumb (Froment's sign) and weak abduction of the little finger (Wartenberg's sign). Tinel's sign may be positive and ulnar clawing may be present. Ulnar clawing is absent if the ulnar half of the FDP is weak – for instance, in a high lesion. An ulnar nerve injury near the elbow (high lesion) denervates the ulnar half of the FDP; hence, the degree of clawing is less.

Nerve conduction studies are helpful and release of the ulnar nerve is performed within the tunnel without anterior transposition.

Ulnar tunnel syndrome

Ulnar tunnel syndrome describes compression of the ulnar nerve in Guyon's canal. Guyon's canal lies in the ulnar side of the carpal tunnel on the collar side of the wrist. It contains the ulnar nerve and artery.

Guyon's canal is formed between the pisiform and the hook of hamate. The floor is the transverse carpal ligament and the roof is the volar carpal ligament. The nerve can be compressed by ganglions, fractures of the hook of hamate, lipomas or arthritis of the pisotriquetral joint.

Clinically, the sensory branch of the ulnar nerve is spared and the ulnar clawing is marked because FDP innervation is intact. Phalen's and Tinel's signs may be positive.

Splinting can help to relieve symptoms. Surgical treatment is decompression of the nerve or excision of the hook of hamate.

Posterior interosseous nerve

The posterior interosseous branch of the radial nerve can be compressed along its course by the origin or distal border of the supinator muscle, the origin of the extensor carpi radialis brevis or the arcade of Frohse. Other potential causes are elbow dislocation, dislocation or excision of the radial head or rheumatoid arthritis of the elbow.

Symptoms are related to motor deficit and aching in the posterior compartment of the forearm. Clinical signs are weak wrist extension and radial deviation of the wrist on extension. The extensor carpi radialis longus deviates the wrist to the radial side on extension and escapes denervation because it is supplied by the radial nerve above the level of the supinator.

Surgical decompression of the nerve is recommended.

Radial tunnel syndrome

Compression of the posterior interosseous nerve can cause aching in the extensor compartment of the forearm. The symptoms are worse after activity. Characteristically, there is no motor deficit. Patients have tenderness over the extensor mechanism about 5cm distal to the lateral epicondyle and pain over the origin of the extensor carpi radialis brevis on resisted extension of the middle finger.

The site of tenderness and nerve conduction studies help differentiate this condition from tennis elbow.

Surgical release is recommended when non-operative measures fail.

Wartenberg syndrome

Wartenberg syndrome describes neuritis of the superficial sensory branch of the radial nerve. Patients do not have motor deficit and local steroid injection may help to resolve symptoms. Surgical release may be required.

Brachial plexus injury

The brachial plexus is predominantly formed from five nerve roots – from the fifth cervical to first thoracic spinal nerves. The fourth cervical or the second dorsal root may contribute.

Injuries to the brachial plexus are usually traction injuries from motor vehicle accidents; motorbike accidents account for a significant percentage of cases. Distraction of the head away from the shoulder stretches the upper roots, while violent abduction of the arm leads to traction injury to the lower roots.

Classification

Brachial plexus lesions are classified by Leffert into five types:

- Supraclavicular (75% of all injuries).
- Infraclavicular.
- Post-anaesthetic.
- Radiation injury.
- Obstetric palsy.

Supraclavicular lesions are further divided into supraganglionic (where the roots are avulsed from the cord) or infraganglionic (where the injury is at the level of the root or the trunks).

In postganglionic (infraganglionic) injuries, patients have associated sensory loss. These injuries may be amenable to repair.

Evaluation

A local examination is performed for swelling and bruising, and a detailed neurological examination of sensory and motor loss is performed to document the injury. Tinel's sign, if detectable, should be documented to monitor progress.

A cutaneous axon reflex response differentiates preganglionic from postganglionic palsy. A scratch on the skin with histamine results in an axonal wheal-and-flare formation if nerve innervation is intact. In preganglionic injury, the flare is present and the wheal is absent. In postganglionic injury, the wheal and vasodilation are present but the flare is absent.

The long thoracic nerve and the dorsal scapular nerve arise from the roots. Dysfunction of these nerves indicates an injury that is proximal to their origin.

A feature of lower preganglionic injury is Horner's syndrome. Patients with Horner's syndrome have ipsilateral ptosis (drooping of the upper eyelid), miosis (pupillary constriction), anhydrosis (loss of sweating on the side of the face) and enophthalmos (sunken eye).

Specific injury patterns

- Erb's palsy – involves trauma to the C5, C6 and C7 roots. It is characterised by shoulder adduction and internal rotation, elbow extension and forearm pronation. Sensory loss corresponds to the roots involved. Obstetric palsy often has an Erb's pattern.
- Klumpke's palsy – involves trauma to the C8 and T1 roots. The wrist and finger flexors are weak.

Imaging

A plain radiograph of the cervical spine will detect any fracture/subluxation. A high diaphragm on a chest radiograph indicates phrenic nerve palsy.

A magnetic resonance scan or computed tomography myelogram assesses root avulsions.

Nerve conduction studies and electromyography are important to diagnose specific injury patterns. These are undertaken 3-4 weeks following the injury.

Management

Brachial plexus injuries often involve high-energy impact, and there may be associated injuries to the spinal cord or vessels of the upper limbs. These should be assessed and managed based on Advanced Trauma Life Support protocols.

The techniques for dealing with brachial plexus injury are direct repair, nerve grafting or neurotisation. Direct suture repair can be augmented with fibrin sealants to achieve a stronger repair. Nerve grafting follows standard techniques. The use of vascularised nerve grafts has not shown significant benefit over that of non-vascular nerve grafts.

Root avulsions cannot be repaired. In this situation, local nerves can be diverted to help the patient achieve some function. The spinal accessory nerve is used for shoulder abduction and intercostal nerves are used to gain elbow flexion.

The order of priorities when restoring function is elbow flexion, shoulder stabilisation, hand sensation, wrist extension, finger flexion and intrinsic function.

Shoulder abduction can be restored by transfer of the trapezius to the deltoid. The latissimus dorsi can be transferred posteriorly to function as an external rotator of the shoulder. Shoulder fusion is an option for stabilising the shoulder.

The pectoralis minor is used for elbow flexion via the biceps.

Neurotisation involves transferring a functioning motor nerve to the denervated muscle. A nerve that supplies a synergistic muscle will be able to restore function more quickly to a denervated muscle and hence avoid muscle atrophy. For instance, the ulnar nerve fibres in the upper arm can be transferred to the musculocutaneous nerve to restore elbow flexion (Oberlin procedure). Many other intraplexal or extraplexal transfers have been described, based on whether the donor nerve is part of the brachial plexus.

Recovery from brachial plexus injury can take 18 months or more.

Neuromuscular disorders

The diagnosis of neuromuscular disorders begins with an accurate history, family history and clinical examination. Measurement of serum creatinine phosphokinase and aldolase levels is helpful. Nerve conduction studies, electromyography and nerve and muscle biopsies are further tests that will help to establish a diagnosis.

Creatinine phosphokinase levels are checked. A muscle biopsy is performed, with tissue obtained from involved but functioning muscle at the musculotendinous junction and sent for both light and electron microscopy. A nerve biopsy is conducted at the sural nerve.

In myopathy, the amplitude and duration of muscle action potential is reduced, while the frequency is increased on electromyography testing. In neuropathy, the changes are reversed: the frequency is reduced, while the amplitude and duration are increased. Myotonic dystrophy is characterised by a 'dive-bomber' sound on needle insertion into the muscle. This indicates a reduced frequency, duration and amplitude of action potentials.

Nerve conduction studies are normal in muscle diseases, but will be affected in neuropathies.

Duchenne muscular dystrophy

Duchenne muscular dystrophy (DMD) is inherited as a sex-linked recessive trait. Approximately 70% of patients have a family history, and the remaining cases occur as a result of spontaneous mutation. DMD is far more common in men, but can occur in women with Turner syndrome. The site of the mutation is the Xp21 region of the X chromosome.

Mutation in the dystrophin gene, located on the short arm of the X chromosome, leads to the synthesis of an unstable protein that is rapidly degraded. As a result, the muscle fibres are replaced by fat and fibrous tissue.

Clinically, children with DMD meet their milestones within the first year, but walking is often delayed. Children tend to walk on their toes and have frequent falls. The disease becomes more apparent around the ages of 3-6 years.

The calf muscles feel enlarged and firm due to fatty and fibrous infiltration (pseudohypertrophy). The tibialis posterior muscle retains strength till later stages, while other muscles lose power; this causes an equinovarus deformity of the foot.

The gait is a wide-based, circumduction gait and there is increased lumbar lordosis.

The Gower test is performed by asking children to stand from a squatting position. Children will use their arms to support themselves when standing up from a squatting position because of proximal muscle (gluteal) weakness in the lower limbs.

The Meryon test indicates a lack of shoulder stability when children are lifted with one arm around the chest. If the shoulder muscles have normal strength, children will contract their shoulder muscles to increase stability. Affected children are unable to do this.

Sinus tachycardia and right ventricle hypertrophy may be present. Most patients are wheelchair bound by 12 years and survival beyond 20 years is unusual.

The diagnosis is supported by elevated creatinine phosphokinase levels (>100 times normal) and DNA analysis. Muscle biopsy and dystrophin testing are diagnostic.

Creatinine phosphokinase levels are highly elevated in patients with DMD and can be 200 times normal in children with DMD in the first year of life. The levels decline later as muscle tissue is replaced with fibrous tissue. Creatinine phosphokinase levels are also elevated in women carrying the DMD gene and are an important diagnostic tool. The levels rise after activity, and this rise is higher in women who carry the DMD gene than in those who do not.

Management

The principal aim of treatment is to keep children mobile for as long as possible. Surgical intervention is indicated when mobility declines due to contractures.

Flexion and abduction contractures of the hip, flexion contractures of the knee and equinovarus contractures of the foot are seen. These are addressed by multiple-level tenotomies and bracing.

It is easier to maintain mobility with early interventions than to restore mobility after it has declined due to contractures. Walking should be resumed immediately after surgery. A little equinus is helpful for ambulation and should not be fully corrected. Transfer of the tibialis posterior anteriorly is an option to avoid progression of equinovarus deformity.

Scoliosis is a major problem. Spinal deformity should be addressed in the early stages before significant pulmonary and cardiac compromise arise. Posterior dorsolumbar fusion is performed with instrumentation and facet joint fusion at all levels. The fusion can be extended to the pelvis to avoid pelvic obliquity progressing.

Becker's muscular dystrophy

Becker's dystrophy is a milder form of DMD. The underlying process is similar to DMD, except that there is some intracellular dystrophin. The level of functional dystrophin determines the severity of the disease.

The incidence is one in 30,000 male births and transmission is sex-linked recessive. The symptoms and signs present around the age of 7 years and survival into the fourth or fifth decade of life is common.

Treatment is aimed at correcting contractures and maintaining mobility.

Emery-Dreifuss muscular dystrophy

Emery-Dreifuss muscular dystrophy is a sex-linked recessive disorder. The presentation is in the second decade of life with equinus of the ankle, flexion contracture of the elbow, extension contracture of the neck and tightness of the lumbar paravertebral muscles.

Cardiac abnormalities are often seen and may be asymptomatic. These should be actively investigated and treated. There is a high incidence of sudden cardiac death due to these abnormalities.

Management requires correction of Achilles contractures and stretching for neck and back contractures.

Facioscapulohumeral muscular dystrophy

Facioscapulohumeral muscular dystrophy is an autosomal dominant condition with weakness of the facial and shoulder muscles.

Weakness of the facial muscles means that patients are unable to whistle, purse their lips or wrinkle their brow. Shoulder muscle weakness causes a winged scapula and weak shoulder abduction.

The responsible gene is located on chromosome 4. Early childhood onset is associated with marked symptoms and the child is confined to a wheelchair by the age of 8-9 years. Onset in the teenage age or later has a more gradual course. Eventually, patients develop muscle weakness in the lower extremities.

Scapulothoracic fusion is an option to stabilise the shoulder joint.

Myotonic dystrophy

Myotonic dystrophy is an autosomal dominant condition characterised by muscle weakness and an inability of muscle to relax after contraction. Transmission can be autosomal recessive.

Patients have a tent-shaped mouth, dull expression, temporal baldness, hyperostosis of the skull, gonadal atrophy, dysphasia and dysarthria. Hip dysplasia, scoliosis and clubfoot may be associated with myotonic dystrophy. Clubfoot deformities are often resistant to treatment and talectomy may be needed. Cardiac abnormalities may be present, along with compromised respiratory function.

Charcot-Marie-Tooth disease

Charcot-Marie-Tooth disease (CMTD; also known as peroneal muscle atrophy) is an autosomal dominant (chromosome 17) neuromuscular disorder causing progressive muscle atrophy and loss of proprioception. Inheritance can be X-linked or autosomal recessive.

Onset of CMTD is usually within the first two decades of life. Patients present clinically with foot weakness, metatarsal pain, clawing of the toes and high-arched feet. Balance is impaired and spinal ataxia may be present. The foot deformity progresses to cavovarus.

The rigidity of the foot deformity is assessed by the Coleman Block test. A detailed neurological examination is conducted for muscle strength and sensory impairment. Patients may have acetabular dysplasia and scoliosis and these should be specifically examined.

Radiographs of the foot are obtained in a weight-bearing position to document the degree of forefoot adduction and cavus.

Treatment of the cavovarus deformity should be instituted early, before the deformity is fixed. Soft tissue releases may be combined with metatarsal osteotomy in the early stages, while fixed deformities require triple arthrodesis.

Tendon transfers are an option where the deformity is not fixed.

For claw toes, the Jones procedure can be performed. This involves transfer of the long toe extensors to the metatarsal necks and fusion of the interphalangeal joints. Hibbs procedure involves transfer of the toe extensors to the middle cuneiform in patients with weak ankle dorsiflexion. The tibialis posterior can be transferred anteriorly to augment weak ankle dorsiflexors.

Variants of Charcot-Marie-Tooth disease
Variants of CMTD are summarised in Table 14.5.

Table 14.5. Variants of Charcot-Marie-Tooth disease (CMTD).

Variant	Inheritance	Age of onset	Features
Roussy Levy syndrome	Autosomal dominant	Infancy	CMTD features with static hand tremor
Dejerine-Sottas syndrome	Autosomal recessive or dominant	Infancy	Pes cavus, sensory loss in all four limbs, clubfoot, scoliosis
Refsum disease	Autosomal recessive	Childhood or puberty	Hypertrophic neuropathy, ataxia, areflexia, retinitis pigmentosa, distal sensory and motor loss in hands and feet
Neuronal CMTD	Autosomal dominant	Middle age	Mainly affects the ankle and foot muscles

CMTD is discussed in more detail in Chapter 5.

Spinal muscle atrophy

Spinal muscle atrophy is an autosomal recessive (chromosome 5) degeneration of the anterior horn cells. It results in progressive weakness and areflexia, but sensory function is preserved.

Three different types of spinal muscle atrophy are recognised, based on the age of onset:

- Type I, acute infantile – severe generalised weakness in infants aged less than 6 months, leading to respiratory failure.
- Type II, chronic infantile – begins within the first year of life, but tends to remain static over many years.
- Type III, juvenile – gradual onset in childhood and a progressive course.

The infantile form is known as Werdnig-Hoffman disease, while the juvenile form is Kugelberg-Welander disease.

As the primary abnormality is in the anterior horn cell the muscles show denervation, but nerve conduction studies are normal. A fine tremor and fasciculation of the tongue may be apparent. Weakness is predominantly of the proximal muscles. Serum creatinine phosphokinase levels are normal.

Evans, Drennan and Russman proposed a classification based on function:

- Type I – never able to sit independently and does not have head control.
- Type II – has head control and can sit, but cannot walk.
- Type III – has limited walking using bracing.
- Type IV – can walk and run before onset of weakness.

Patients with the acute infantile form have a poor prognosis and limited survival. Juvenile disease can lead to joint contractures and coxa valga. Hip instability should be managed with corrective proximal femoral osteotomy. Scoliosis is a disabling feature in the juvenile form and is managed by bracing or posterior fusion. Compromise of respiratory function is a significant risk factor.

Friedreich's ataxia

Friedreich's ataxia is an autosomal recessive condition (chromosome 9) resulting in spinocerebellar degeneration. Onset is in childhood or puberty. The clinical triad is ataxia, areflexia and a positive Babinski reflex. Mobility declines and most patients are unable to walk by their teenage years. Associated features are cardiomyopathy, pes cavus and scoliosis. Areflexia manifests as loss of ankle and knee deep-tendon reflexes.

Surgical intervention is needed for foot deformities. These are managed with tenotomies of the long toe flexors and Achilles tendon, or by triple arthrodesis for correction of the cavovarus deformity. Scoliosis can be managed non-operatively in the case of mild curves and by posterior instrumentation and fusion for severe curves.

Chapter 15 Imaging

Musculoskeletal imaging

A number of imaging modalities are available for musculoskeletal disorders. Each modality has a specific role in management. Multimodality imaging is often required in the diagnostic process.

Plain film (X-ray)

Plain films are the mainstay of imaging in various orthopaedic disorders, particularly trauma. They offer a quick and easy way of obtaining the necessary information in orthopaedic patients. The main drawback is the radiation dose, although this is often minimal when imaging the extremities or in comparison with computed tomography (CT). Plain films are also used in postoperative follow-up to assess healing and look for complications.

Computed tomography

CT, which relies on ionising radiation, is a popular imaging modality. It has benefited tremendously from advances in computer software and the development of smaller slice thicknesses. It is now possible to post-process the data in a multitude of ways, the most common of which is multiplanar reformatting. This refers to the reconstruction of data in any desirable plane, most often the sagittal and coronal planes. Curved reformats are also possible and are used, for example, in patients with scoliosis for imaging of the spine.

Some software packages enable three-dimensional (3D) reconstruction of images, including volume rendering and surface reconstructions (Figure 15.1). Such programs are particularly useful for giving surgeons a 3D overview of complex fractures and complex spinal abnormalities. It is also possible to 'ghost-out' structures to make fracture lines more clearly visible.

CT has higher spatial resolution than magnetic resonance imaging (MRI). However, it offers relatively poor contrast resolution and is inferior to MRI for evaluating soft tissues. CT is a much quicker scan than MRI and is therefore less susceptible to artefacts in patients who are unable to keep still. In addition, it allows faster turnover of patients.

Due to high-quality imaging, CT scans are increasingly used in the diagnostic work-up, especially in trauma patients. Furthermore, metallic artefacts from implants can be significantly reduced with the newer CT machines and software packages, allowing much greater visualisation and interpretation of the pathology. CT is also used to aid biopsy of deep-seated lesions and in performing joint injections, such as for the sacroiliac and thoracic facet joints. The major drawback of CT is its reliance on ionising radiation.

Common applications of CT in musculoskeletal disorders are as follows:

- Trauma, especially fractures of the spine, pelvis, tibial plateau, ankle, calcaneum and midfoot.

- Postoperative evaluation to assess complications, state of bone fusion, periprosthetic fractures and prosthesis failure.
- Assessment of some bone lesions, such as osteoid osteoma.
- Deep-seated soft tissue lesion biopsy or bone biopsy.
- Guided injections.

Magnetic resonance imaging

The use of MRI has rapidly grown in clinical practice. MRI provides high-contrast images and may reveal pathology that is invisible on plain films.

An MRI scan is acquired by placing the patient in a strong magnetic field, which aligns the nuclei of elements with odd atomic numbers in the body along the magnetic field. The nuclei affected most is hydrogen. This becomes the steady state in the magnetic field, and a radiofrequency (RF) pulse is then applied in this steady state. After the RF pulse is switched off, the steady state returns to equilibrium with the release of energy in the form of an RF signal, which is detected with the receiver coil.

The above-described spin echo technique gives T1- and T2-weighted images, depending on the time of application of the RF pulse (TR, repetition time) and the timing of signal acquisition (TE, echo time). Different tissues in the body have different T1 and T2 relaxation times: liquids have long T1 and T2 times, while fat has low T1 and T2 values. Varying the TE and TR times can vary the T1 or T2 weighting of images.

Field strength indicates the strength of the magnet. In clinical practice, commonly used MR scanners have field strengths of 1-1.5 Tesla, which allows a shorter imaging time and thinner slices than older scanners. In addition, 3 Tesla scanners are becoming more common in clinical practice. Low-field-strength magnets of 0.3 Tesla have an open configuration and are convenient for imaging claustrophobic patients and extremities such as the elbow and wrist.

MRI is usually performed in at least two and possibly three orthogonal planes.

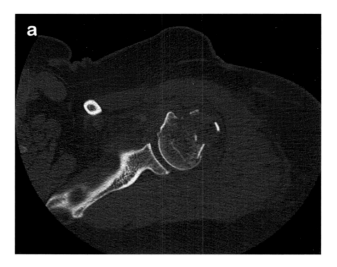

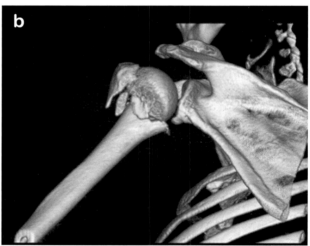

Figure 15.1. (a) An axial computed tomography scan of the left shoulder, demonstrating a comminuted humeral neck fracture. (b) A volume-rendered three-dimensional reconstruction of the same humeral neck fracture.

Commonly used sequences in clinical practice

The commonly used sequences in daily practice are T1, T2, proton density and STIR (short tau inversion recovery).

T1

Short TE and TR times give a T1-weighted sequence, where water returns a low signal and fat returns a high signal. This is a rapidly acquired sequence that provides excellent anatomical detail.

Fat, sub-acute haemorrhages and proteinaceous fluids are bright, while fluid is dark. T1-weighted images are generally considered good for looking at bone marrow. However, they are not as good for detecting bone or soft tissue oedema. T1 imaging following gadolinium administration (see later) is often used as a problem-solving tool.

T2

Long TE and TR times give a T2-weighted image that is excellent for demonstrating pathological conditions such as oedema, inflammation, infection and tumour (all associated with increased water content). One way to remember this is with the mnemonic 'World War 2' – water is white on T2.

Proton density

Proton-density sequences use a short TE and long TR. This sequence is a mix of T1 and T2, with contrast intermediate between T1- and T2-weighted images. This sequence is used in the assessment of menisci and other structures as part of routine knee protocols. It is often used with fat suppression.

STIR

A STIR sequence is a specialised spin echo sequence that suppresses the fat from the image, making fluid-containing lesions more conspicuous. This is a very sensitive technique to detect soft tissue and marrow pathology.

T2* (gradient echo T2)

This is a faster T2 sequence with bright fluid, as in the usual spin echo T2 sequence. It is particularly good for imaging the ligaments, articular cartilage and fibrocartilage. The advantage of this sequence is that very thin sections can be obtained, which are useful for 3D volume reconstruction. However, this sequence is degraded significantly by metal because of susceptibility artefacts.

Fast-spin echo

This is an accelerated method of acquiring T2 and proton-density images and is generally referred to as a 'fast' or 'turbo' technique. Fat remains bright on fast or turbo T2 and therefore fat-saturated sequences are often used. This sequence also reduces artefacts from metal prostheses and should be employed if previous instrumentation is present.

Gadolinium

Gadolinium administration is used to differentiate between cystic and solid masses, and viable and necrotic tissue, among other uses. T1-weighted sequencing with fat suppression is usually used when gadolinium is administered, making the pathology stand out.

MR arthroscopy

MR arthrography involves MR scanning subsequent to the intra-articular injection of gadolinium, clearly demonstrating intra-articular structures. This technique is especially useful in assessing the glenoid and acetabular labrum in the context of shoulder instability and femoroacetabular impingement. MR arthrography is also useful in the characterisation of hyaline cartilage and osteochondral defects.

Contraindications to MRI

The following objects are contraindicated within the MRI scanning room: intracerebral aneurysm clips, cardiac pacemakers, defibrillators, biostimulators, internal hearing aids and metallic orbital foreign bodies.

Relative contraindications are first trimester pregnancy, middle-ear prosthesis and penile prosthesis. Orthopaedic implants including prosthetic joints, screws, plates and rods can be scanned, but steel implants cause artefacts. Titanium devices produce significantly less artefacts. Metallic external fixators should not be scanned.

Common applications

Common applications of MRI in musculoskeletal disorders are as follows:

- Spine pathology – back pain, sciatica.
- Knee joint evaluation – meniscus and cruciate ligament tears (Figure 15.2), hyaline cartilage defects.
- Shoulder joint evaluation – rotator cuff tear, anterior or posterior dislocation.

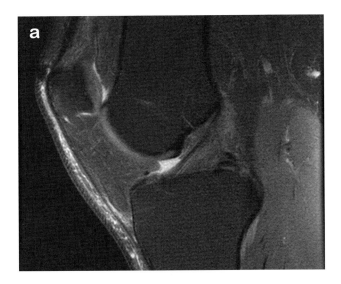

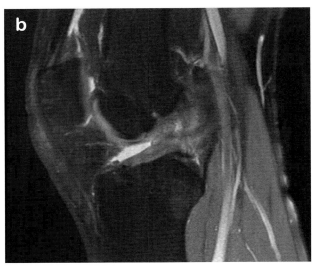

Figure 15.2. Fat-suppressed sagittal proton-density image of the knee demonstrating (a) a normal and (b) ruptured anterior cruciate ligament.

- Wrist – triangular fibrocartilage complex and intrinsic ligament tears.
- Soft tissues and bone neoplasms – to characterise and define the extent of lesions.
- Avascular necrosis.
- Osteomyelitis (including discitis).
- Arthritis.
- Bone marrow pathology.

Ultrasound

Musculoskeletal ultrasound (US) imaging is a rapidly expanding modality. Compared with MRI, US is less expensive and more patient friendly, avoiding the claustrophobia sometimes seen during MR examinations. Its real-time and dynamic nature can direct examiners towards the symptomatic area, allowing them to focus on the relevant area. The dynamic capability allows examiners to observe pathologic movements in tendons, bursae or joints with continuous patient feedback.

However, US images are often difficult to interpret. MR and US are often used as complementary imaging modalities to help interpretation. Another limitation of US is its dependence on body habitus; it is not particularly useful in obese patients because of poor beam penetration of high-frequency probes. US is also an operator-dependent technique and often demonstrates spurious pathologies where none exists.

US offers advantages over CT when used for interventions, because it does not use ionising radiation or contrast. US guidance decreases the inaccuracy rate of blind injections into the knee or shoulder joint, which can approach 30% in some instances.

Common applications

US is commonly used to evaluate tendon pathology, especially the rotator cuff tendons. Many studies have been performed on this subject and sensitivity can approach 100% for full-thickness tears, with much lower sensitivity for partial-thickness tears. The Achilles tendon is another well-defined structure imaged with diagnostic US. Dynamic US imaging allows small tendon tears to become more apparent. This technique can also be used to detect biceps, peroneal or posterior tibial tendon subluxations.

Diagnostic US can also be used for imaging ligaments such as the ulnar collateral ligament of the elbow, the anterior talofibular and calcaneofibular ligaments of the ankle, and the medial and lateral collateral ligaments of the knee. When combined with stress imaging, US is a particularly useful modality to identify medial collateral ligament tears. It is not good for detecting intra-articular knee pathology such as meniscal or cruciate ligaments, for which MRI is superior.

US is also an excellent imaging modality for detecting small joint effusions and to guide interventions such as joint aspiration. Doppler US can detect increased blood flow in the synovium and active synovitis of inflammatory or infectious aetiology. Labral tears of the shoulder and hip are best diagnosed with MRI, but diagnostic US can be used if the defect extends to the peripheral margin of the joint and if it is associated with ganglion formation. The portability, ease of use and high spatial resolution of US make it an excellent tool for imaging muscular injuries and superficial nerves.

Common applications of US in musculoskeletal disorders are as follows:

- Shoulder – rotator cuff pathology.
- Assessment of soft tissue lumps and bumps.
- Tendinosis or tenosynovitis, especially around the ankle and wrist (Figure 15.3).
- Infection – assessment of joint effusion, soft tissue collection.
- To perform guided injections.
- To perform guided biopsy or drainage.

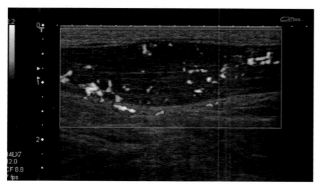

Figure 15.3. An ultrasound image demonstrates Achilles tendinosis.

Radioisotope bone scan

Radioisotope bone scanning involves the use of radiopharmaceuticals, the most common of which is Technetium-99m (Tc-99m) attached to diphosphonate. This is incorporated into the surface of calcium hydroxyapatite crystals of the bone to produce insoluble calcium phosphate complexes.

An isotope bone scan thus provides 'functional' imaging, as the complexes accumulate in areas with increased blood flow or increased bone turnover. Osteoblastic lesions are indicated by increased bone turnover, while lytic lesions are usually visible due to the surrounding rim of reactive bone. Bone uptake is demonstrated on whole-body views and spot views of the region of interest acquired 2-4 hours after injection (delayed phase). In a three-phase bone scan, images are obtained not only in the delayed phase (showing osteoblastic activity), but also in the 'blood flow' and 'blood pool' phases. The three-phase bone scan is commonly used to investigate bone infection, trauma and reflex sympathetic dystrophy. The first (blood flow) phase involves a dynamic flow study, with images obtained every 2-3 seconds for 30 seconds following injection. Imaging in this phase indicates the vascularity of the lesion. The second phase (blood pool) is obtained at 5 minutes, and reflects extracellular fluid uptake within the bone due to changes in capillary permeability.

A positive bone scan in all three phases can suggest an acute lesion of less than 4 weeks with an increased blood flow, whereas a scan positive in only delayed images suggests an abnormality with increased osteoblastic activity.

SPECT and SPECT/CT

Conventional planar imaging provides a two-dimensional projection of a 3D source of activity. Single-photon emission CT (SPECT), which involves taking projection images at many angles in a tomographic fashion, is able to remove the activity from overlying or underlying tissues, which would otherwise obscure the image at the required depth of interest. This results in improved visualisation. SPECT is particularly useful for accurately visualising the posterior elements of vertebrae.

Hybrid imaging combines the functional images obtained with an isotope scan with the anatomical information obtained from CT, so overcoming the drawbacks of both modalities. SPECT with CT correlation, for example, may be useful in assessing anterior knee pain, and can demonstrate patellofemoral osteoarthritic change, patellar enthesopathy or osteochondral bone bruising.

Common causes

Common causes of 'hot spots' on a bone scan are as follows:

- Trauma and stress fractures.
- Previous arthroplasty – can be positive for up to 3 years.
- Malignant tumours and metastasis.
- Arthritis.
- Infections – osteomyelitis.
- Paget's disease.
- Fibrous dysplasia.
- Benign tumours.
- Bone infarction.
- Soft tissue uptake due to an infection, inflammation or tumour.

Common applications

In patients with bone tumours, bone scanning is used to stage disease (i.e., look for metastasis; Figure 15.4), assess areas of bone pain with negative radiographs, determine response to treatment, assess the ribs and sternum (which are difficult to assess with plain radiographs) and detect other sites of involvement.

The term 'superscan' indicates widespread skeletal disease. This results in diffuse and uniform increased isotope uptake in the skeleton, rather than localised hot spots, and can give a false impression of normal skeletal uptake. The kidneys and bladder, which are normally visualised in bone scans due to isotope

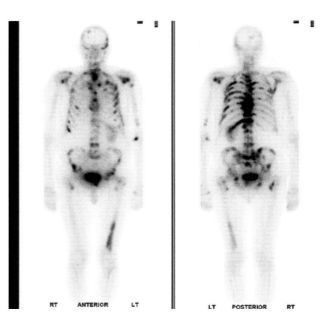

RT   ANTERIOR   LT   LT   POSTERIOR   RT

Figure 15.4. Whole body planar bone scan (in delayed phase) demonstrates widespread bony metastasis in a patient with prostate cancer.

excretion, are not well visualised in a superscan. This is commonly termed 'absent kidney sign'.

Positron emission tomography

Positron emission tomography (PET) is another form of highly sensitive metabolic imaging in nuclear medicine. It depends on the detection of gamma rays emitted indirectly by a positron-emitting radionuclide (tracer). The most commonly used tracer is [18F]-2-fluoro-2-deoxy-D-glucose (FDG). FDG, as a glucose analogue, is taken up by high-glucose-using cells such as brain, heart and cancer cells. Malignant cells concentrate this tracer and retain it until radioactive decay. As a result FDG-PET can be used for the diagnosis, staging and monitoring of cancers.

Common indications for PET imaging include the following:

- Head and neck malignancies for detection of the primary lesion.
- Differentiating scar tissue from recurrent disease.
- Monitoring response to treatment.

Chapter 16 Clinical examination

Shoulder

History

The history elicits the following:

- Age.
- Handedness.
- Occupation and leisure activities.
- Pain.
- Instability.
- Stiffness.
- Weakness.
- Catching or locking.
- Any associated medical problems.

Pain

- Localised or diffuse.
- Night pain is present in frozen shoulder, cuff tears, glenohumeral arthritis, infection and tumours.
- Sudden severe pain may point to resolving calcific tendonitis or acute brachial neuritis (Parsonage Turner syndrome).
- A painful arc in 60-120° abduction indicates impingement. A painful arc in terminal abduction indicates acromioclavicular joint (ACJ) disease.

Instability

- Traumatic or atraumatic.
- Details of the first episode – mechanism of injury, treatment.
- Frequency and ease of instability.
- Voluntary subluxation or dislocation.

- Degree of functional limitation is assessed.
- Generalised laxity.
- Family history.

Weakness

- Rotator cuff problems – sudden trauma or gradual attrition.
- Brachial plexus injury – violent trauma, penetrating injury.
- Entrapment of suprascapular nerve – causes diffuse posterolateral shoulder pain, weak abduction and external rotation (ER).
- Axillary nerve injury.
- Facioscapulohumeral muscular dystrophy – family history of shoulder weakness starting in early childhood, facial weakness, unable to hold arms in abduction.

Stiffness

- Frozen shoulder – common in the middle aged, women and those with diabetes.
- Longstanding glenohumeral arthritis.
- Rheumatoid.
- Chronic dislocation.
- Synovial chondromatosis.
- Tumour.

Examination

Inspection

- From the front – symmetry, contour, prominence of clavicle, ACJ, deformity, deltoid wasting, scars, level of anterior axillary fold. Biceps – pop-eye appearance.

- From the side – contour, swelling.
- From the back – scapulae – shape, position, webbed skin at base of neck, winging of the scapula, wasting of supraspinatus, infraspinatus. To see winging, ask patients to elevate their arms and push against a wall.
- From above (seated patient) – swelling, clavicle.

Palpation
- Temperature.
- Tenderness over:
  - glenohumeral joint;
  - ACJ;
  - clavicle;
  - coracoid – inflammatory arthritis and frozen, tender inferior and lateral to coracoid;
  - scapula;
  - bicipital groove;
  - axilla;
  - posterior joint line – in osteoarthritis.
- Rupture of biceps tendon, pectoralis tendon.
- General hyperlaxity.

Movements
- Abduction – 170°.
- Adduction.
- Forward elevation.
- ER – can the patient reach on top of the head or behind the head with the elbow forwards and backwards? Normal rotation is around 50-70°.
- Internal rotation (IR) – the level of spinous process that the patient can reach up behind the back; normally, between T5 and T10 is recorded.
- Extension.
- Scapulohumeral rhythm – observed from behind.

Impingement
- Anterior or lateral pain, night pain.
- Painful arc 60-120° of abduction, relieved by local anaesthetic.
- Neer test – forward elevation.
- Hawkins' test – flexion to 90° and IR causes pain.
- Injection of local anaesthetic in the subacromial space relieves pain in impingement.

Tests for anterior and posterior instability
Tests for anterior and posterior instability are shown in Table 16.1.

Tests for rotator cuff muscles
- Supraspinatus:
  - Jobe test – in 60° abduction, 30° forward flexion and pronation. Resisted abduction is painful;
  - empty-can test – in 90° abduction, 30° forward flexion and full IR. Resisted abduction is painful;
  - full-can test – in 90° abduction, 30° forward flexion and 45° ER. Resisted abduction is less painful.
- Subscapularis – IR:
  - lift-off test – ask the patient to lift the arm away from the back against resistance and to maintain this position;
  - Napoleon sign or belly-press test – ask the patient to push into the abdomen and bring the elbows anterior to the coronal plane. If the elbow falls back, the test is positive;
  - hug test – ask the patient to place the palm over the contralateral posterior axillary fold and apply IR force against resistance. The pectoralis major is neutralised due to IR. It is possible to do this test even if the shoulder is stiff.
- Infraspinatus:
  - ER with the arm by the side;
  - passively perform full ER and ask the patient to hold the arm in that position;
  - if there is weakness, the arm will fall into IR (drop sign);
  - ER lag sign – the patient sits with the examiner standing behind. Passively abduct to 20° and full ER at the shoulder, with the elbow at 90°. Ask the patient to hold this position.
- Teres minor – weakness of ER in 70° abduction.

Other shoulder muscles
- Serratus anterior – pushing against a wall from the affected arm makes the medial border of the scapula more prominent. This is known as winging of the scapula.
- Deltoid – 90° abduction against resistance to test the power of the deltoid.

Table 16.1. Summary of shoulder tests for instability.

Test	Patient position	Procedure	Inference
Anterior instability			
Drawer	Sitting	Stand behind patient	Anterior instability
		Push head in centre of glenoid	
		Push forwards and backwards	
		Normally – slight anterior translation is possible, as well as about half of head diameter posterior translation	
Sulcus	Sitting or standing	Pull hand down in ER	Sulcus below acromion – inferior instability
Fulcrum	Supine, 90° abduction	Extend and externally rotate arm (apprehension test)	Anterior instability
		Push back on head – more ER possible (relocation test)	
		Push head anteriorly – less ER possible (augmentation test)	
Crank or apprehension test	Sitting	90° abduction, ER causes apprehension	Anterior instability
		Test in 45° abduction – for middle glenohumeral ligament	
Posterior instability			
Jerk test	Sitting	IR, flex to 90°, axially load humerus and move arm horizontally	Jerk indicates posterior instability
Push-pull	Supine	90° abduction, 30° flexion	Apprehension indicates posterior instability
		Pull wrist up and push proximal humerus down	

ER = external rotation; IR = internal rotation

- Biceps:
  - Yergason test – arm by the side and elbow to 90°. The patient starts in full pronation and is asked to supinate against resistance. Pain in the bicipital groove suggests bicipital tendonitis;
  - Speed test – the elbow is flexed to 30° with supination and the patient is asked to flex against resistance.

Acromioclavicular joint pathology

- Tenderness on full abduction.
- Pain over the ACJ when the arm is adducted across the midline in 90° flexion in full pronation.
- O'Brien test – adduct arm, forward elevate to 90° and thumbs up – resisted forward flexion elicits pain.
- Injection of local anaesthetic in the ACJ relieves pain.

Tests for superior labrum anterior posterior lesions

- Speed test – flexed 90°, supination – resisted forward flexion.
- Cross arm adduction in full supination.
- Abduction to 90°, supination – resisted abduction.
- Crank test – abduct to 160°, axial load, IR and ER – causes pain. Can also be performed in 90° abduction.

Examination for associated conditions

- Cervical spine movements – flex-extend, lateral rotation 80°, lateral flexion 40°.
- Neurological examination.
- Vascular assessment – Adson's test, Roos sign.
- Elbow – see next.

Elbow

History

- Age.
- Dominance.
- Occupation.
- Antecedent trauma.
- Sporting activities.
- Pain – nature, location, severity, associated with movement, radiation.
- Movements.
- Instability.
- Crepitus.
- Cervical spine symptoms.
- Previous problems.
- Other joint problems.

- Family history – haemophilia.
- General health.

Examination

Inspection
- Posture.
- Scars.
- Swelling.
- Rheumatoid nodules.
- Deformity.
- Carrying angle.

Palpation
- Lateral supracondylar ridge:
  - lateral epicondyle;
  - common extensor origin;
  - lateral collateral ligament (LCL);
  - tenderness over extensor carpi radialis brevis;
  - capitellar joint line – osteochondral fracture;
  - sulcus between the radial head and capitellum;
  - radial head – orientation to the capitellum, crepitus, movements.
- Anterior:
  - medial to lateral – brachioradialis, biceps, brachial artery, median nerve;
  - myositis ossificans;
  - rupture of biceps.
- Medial epicondyle:
  - common flexors;
  - tenderness over pronator teres – pronator syndrome;
  - ulnar nerve – check for Tinel's sign at the point of entry into the flexor carpi ulnaris.
- Posterior:
  - tip of the olecranon;
  - relationship of the three bony landmarks;
  - triceps tendon;
  - olecranon fossa – loose body;
  - olecranon bursa.

Movements
- Carrying angle in full extension.
- Flexion extension, 0-140°, active and passive.

- Supination and pronation – 85° from the mid prone position.

Power
- Flexion in 90°.
- Extension in 90°.
- Pronation.
- Supination.

Special tests
- Lateral epicondylitis:
  - resisted wrist extension causes pain locally (lateral epicondyle area);
  - resisted middle-finger extension causes pain locally;
  - passive volar flexion of the wrist with the elbow extended and pronated elicits pain locally;
  - weak pinch grip between the thumb and middle finger;
  - local anaesthetic injection can help the diagnosis.
- Medial epicondylitis:
  - tenderness at the medial epicondyle;
  - pain on resisted wrist flexion;
  - passive extension of the wrist and elbow causes pain;
  - clenching the fist causes pain;
  - local anaesthetic injection helps to relieve the symptoms.
- Pronator syndrome:
  - causes diffuse forearm pain; sensory median nerve changes may be present;
  - Tinel's sign is positive at the elbow for the median nerve;
  - resisted pronation for 60 seconds reproduces pain;
  - resisted elbow flexion and supination reproduces pain;
  - resisted middle finger flexion at the proximal interphalangeal joint (PIPJ) reproduces pain.
- Impingement:
  - impingement can be present in the posterior or anterior compartment of the elbow;
  - osteophytic changes at the tip of the olecranon suggest posterior impingement;
  - pain may occur on hyperextension in the fully extended elbow;
  - anterior impingement is caused by osteophytes on the coronoid or radial head.
- Varus instability – this is checked in a 30° flexed elbow, with full IR at the shoulder. Varus stress is applied and the gap between the capitellum and the radial head is assessed.
- Valgus instability – flex the elbow to 30°, hold the patient's forearm between the arm and the trunk and apply valgus force. The milking test was described by O'Brien – fully flex the elbow, hold the thumb so that the forearm is fully supinated and apply valgus force to the elbow.
- Posterolateral rotatory instability (LCL damage) – a lateral pivot shift test is performed in the supine position, with the shoulder and elbow flexed to 90°. A valgus and axial force is applied to the elbow and the elbow is slowly extended. This causes apprehension and at 40°, the ulna reduces with a clunk. The clunk may not always be evident, but the test is positive if the patient feels apprehension.
- Posterolateral rotatory drawer test – the elbow is flexed to 90° and supinated. Anteroposterior translation force is applied and instability assessed. The test is repeated in 30° flexion.
- Apprehension test – reluctance to fully extend the elbow while rising from a chair using the arms to push up, or reluctance in doing push-ups.

Wrist

History

- Pain.
- Weakness.
- Swelling.
- Injury.
- Clunk.

Examination

Inspection
- Alignment of the forearm and hand – any deformities:
  - radial malalignment;
  - evidence of rheumatoid disease;

- Madelung deformity.
- Swelling:
  - in snuff box, De Quervain's tenosynovitis in the first dorsal compartment;
  - ganglion;
  - carpal boss – over second and third carpometacarpal joints (CMCJs);
  - extensor digitorum brevis manus – extra muscle.
- Scars – ask the patient to supinate and examine for swelling and scars.

Palpation
- De Quervain's – pain and swelling over the first dorsal compartment. Wet leather sign – crepitus in the local area.
- Wartenberg's neuralgia – pain and tenderness over the cutaneous branch of the radial nerve.
- Intersection syndrome – tenderness between the first and second compartments.

Movements
- Flexion/extension.
- Radial and ulnar deviation (in pronation).
- Pronation and supination.

Neurologic and vascular examination
- Motor and sensory.
- Allen's test.

Assess shoulder, elbow and cervical spine
Shoulder, elbow and spine problems can give rise to symptoms in the hand. These areas should be assessed as part of the hand examination.

Special tests
- De Quervain's – Finkelstein test – adduction of the thumb and ulnar deviation of the wrist causes pain.
- Scapholunate instability:
  - Kirk Watson – the examiner places his/her fingers dorsally over the scapholunate ligament and a thumb on the scaphoid tubercle on the volar aspect. Pressure is applied on the tubercle and the wrist is moved from ulnar to radial deviation. The scaphoid subluxes dorsally as the thumb prevents it from flexing. This test is positive in approximately 36% of normal individuals;
  - scaphoid thrust test – in the same position as Kirk Watson, pressure is applied to the scaphoid tubercle in slight radial deviation and dorsal dislocation of the scaphoid is palpated;
  - scaphoid lift – the lunate is stabilised and the scaphoid is lifted volarly and dorsally.
- Midcarpal instability:
  - radiocarpal and midcarpal drawer test – the examiner holds the forearm with one hand and the metacarpals with the other hand. Distraction and then a volar and dorsal translating force is applied. Then the distal hand is moved proximally to the proximal carpal row and the test is repeated. This is not a very specific test;
  - midcarpal shift test – the forearm is stabilised. The examiner places a thumb over the capitate dorsally and pushes down, along with ulnar deviation of the wrist. If a clunk is felt as the wrist ulnar deviates, the test is positive;
  - pivot shift pattern – the elbow is placed on a firm surface and with the forearm fully supinated. Pressure is applied on the dorsoulnar aspect of the carpus and the wrist is ulnar deviated. A normal wrist goes into less supination as the capitate engages the lunate.
- Lunotriquetral instability:
  - Reagan ballottement test – the lunate is fixed between the thumb and index finger of one hand, and the triquetrum is held between the thumb and index finger of the other hand and displaced dorsally and volarly. Pain indicates a positive test;
  - shear test – the examiner places a thumb on the dorsum of the lunate and pushes the pisiform from the volar side. Pain on pressing indicates lunotriquetral instability;
  - compression test – the examiner presses over the ulnar snuff box between the extensor carpi ulnaris and the flexor carpi ulnaris distal to the ulnar styloid. This loads the triquetrohamate and triquetrolunate joints, eliciting pain.
- Pisotriquetral arthritis – grind test – the pisiform is compressed in a radial and ulnar direction between the thumb and index finger. Pain in the local area is a positive test.

- Ulnar wrist pain – ulnocarpal stress test – an axial load is applied to the wrist while supporting the forearm. Pain on the ulnar side of the wrist indicates ulnar side pathology. This is useful as a general screening test.
- Distal radioulnar joint:
  - compression test – pain on supination and pronation while compressing the distal radioulnar joint indicates distal radioulnar joint pathology;
  - piano key test – the forearm is stabilised and pressure applied over the distal ulna. Increased excursion indicates dorsal subluxation (instability);
  - radioulnar drawer test – the radius is stabilised, and the ulna is held between the thumb and index finger and moved dorsally and volarly. Comparison is made with the other side;
  - dimple sign – longitudinal traction is applied across the wrist while pushing down on the dorsal aspect of the ulna. The appearance of a dimple at the level of the distal radioulnar joint indicates volar subluxation.
- Extensor carpi ulnaris subluxation – in the supinated and ulnar deviated forearm, dorsiflexion can cause pain and subluxation of the tendon.
- Hamate fracture – patients have tenderness over the hook of hamate. Pain is increased with resisted flexion of the ring and little finger with the wrist in ulnar deviation.

Hand

History

- Age.
- Dominance.
- Occupation and leisure activities.
- Nature of injury.
- Associated medical conditions – diabetes, gout, arthritis, systemic diseases.
- Pain – night pain indicates deep infection.
- Swelling.
- Weakness.
- Numbness.

- Deformity.
- Instability.
- Snapping tendons – extensor tendons (due to disruption of the sagittal bands of the metacarpophalangeal joint [MCPJ]).
- Stiffness.
- Loss of dexterity.
- Cold intolerance.
- Congenital malformations.

Examination

Inspection and palpation
- Posture – position of wrist, MCPJ, PIPJ.
- Tremor.
- Size.
- Swelling – infection, ganglion, giant-cell tumour of tendon sheath.
- Colour – vascular lesions, sympathetic dystrophy.
- Nails – clubbing, splinter haemorrhages, subungual haematoma, mucous cysts, glomus tumour.
- Skin creases.
- Deformity.
- Muscle wasting – first dorsal interosseous, thenar.
- Sensation – biro test, water immersion test.
- Crepitus.
- Thrill.

Movements
- MCPJ, 0-90°.
- PIPJ, 0-110°.
- Distal interphalangeal joint (DIPJ), 0-90°.

Metacarpophalangeal joint
- Range of motion, ulnar shift, subluxation.
- Extensor digiti quinti sign – full flexion of the little finger MCPJ indicates an intact extensor digiti quinti.
- Rupture of the extensor digiti of the ring and little fingers is known as a Vaughn-Jackson lesion.
- Rupture of the extensor pollicis longus over Lister's tubercle.

Table 16.2. The Leddy classification of flexor digitorum profundus avulsion.	
Type	**Description**
I	The end of the tendon retracts into the palm
II	The end of the tendon retracts to the level of the proximal interphalangeal joint
III	A bony fragment is held in distal pulley proximal to the distal interphalangeal joint

Flexor tendon injury

- History of injury.
- The flexor digitorum superficialis (FDS) and flexor digitorum profundus (FDP) are tested separately. FDPs to the middle, ring and little finger have a common muscle belly.
- The Leddy classification of FDP avulsion is shown in Table 16.2.

Trigger finger/thumb

- Neonates have triggering of the thumb and fixed flexion of the interphalangeal joint (IPJ).
- There may be a palpable nodule at the level of the A1 pulley.
- Trigger finger/thumb is more common in people with diabetes and rheumatoid disease.
- Adults have pain and tenderness at the base of the finger at the A1 pulley.
- If triggering is at the level of the FDS chiasma, pain is felt at the level of the PIPJ.

Osteoarthritis

- Pain, stiffness and deformity of the PIPJ or the first CMCJ.
- Loss of grip strength.
- Heberden's nodes, stiffness and Bouchard's nodes over the PIPJ.
- Grind test for the first CMCJ – rotate the base of the first metacarpal against the trapezium.
- Thumb CMCJ arthritis – adduction and hyperextension deformity of the MCPJ.

Rheumatoid hand

History
- Drug treatment.
- Cervical spine symptoms.
- Temporomandibular joint arthritis.

Examination
- Cervical spine, shoulder and elbow movements.

Hand examination
- Inspection – dorsal and volar aspects.
- Skin.
- Deformities.
- Nails – splinter haemorrhages and vasculitis at the fingertips.
- Scars from previous surgeries.
- Function.
- Grip – tripod, pinch and key grips.
- Opposition.

Flexor tenosynovitis

- Fullness over the wrist or along the tendon sheath.
- Stiffness.
- Crepitus at the wrist or A1 pulley.
- Triggering.
- Flexor pollicis longus rupture over the scaphoid osteophytes – Mannerfelt lesion.
- Carpal tunnel syndrome.

Table 16.3. The Nalebuff classification of swan-neck deformities.

Type	Description
I	All joints are mobile
II	Intrinsic tightness
	Bunnell test (reduced PIPJ flexion with the MCPJ extended)
III	Limited PIPJ flexion in all positions of the MCPJ
IV	A stiff PIPJ with articular disruption

MCPJ = metacarpophalangeal joint; PIPJ = proximal interphalangeal joint

Swan-neck deformity

The Nalebuff classification of swan-neck deformities is shown in Table 16.3.

Boutonnière deformity

- Stage I – a correctable extensor lag at the PIPJ; limited DIPJ flexion.
- Stage II – the PIPJ is flexed 30-40°. DIPJ flexion is restricted on passive correction of PIPJ flexion.
- Stage III – fixed PIPJ flexion and articular damage.

Thumb deformities

- Type I – Boutonnière deformity. A flexed MCPJ and extended IPJ.
- Type II – type I with subluxation of the CMCJ.
- Type III – swan-neck deformity. An adducted CMCJ, extended MCPJ and flexed IPJ.
- Type IV – laxity of the ulnar collateral ligament and an adducted first metacarpal joint.
- Type IV – an extended MCPJ and flexed IPJ. No adduction.

Psoriatic arthritis

- Extension contractures.
- Nail pitting.
- Arthritis mutilans leading to flail digits.

Dupuytren's

History
- Feet.
- Nodules.
- Diabetes, cirrhosis, epilepsy.
- Previous surgery.

Examination
- Record the flexion contractures.
- Investigate whether the hand can be laid flat on the table.
- Perform Allen's test on digits to check for vascular insufficiency.
- Look for Garrod's pads on the knuckles and on the dorsum of the PIPJ.

Radial club hand

- This may be associated with TAR (thrombocytopenia with absent radius) syndrome, Fanconi syndrome and Holt-Oram syndrome.

- Movements of shoulder and elbow are recorded.

Syndactyly

- Family history.
- Poland syndrome, Apert syndrome.
- Syndactyly can be complete/incomplete, simple/complex.

Spine

History

- Pain:
  - mechanical – worse with activity and better with rest;
  - onset, duration and course;
  - aggravating and relieving factors;
  - radiation;
  - site, severity;
  - night pain;
  - relation to coughing;
  - effect on lifestyle.
- Neurologic symptoms – bladder or bowel symptoms.
- Loss of weight, fever, change in bowel or bladder habits.
- Deformity.
- Duration, progression, previous treatments.
- Impact on social life.
- Physical development – menarche, recent growth spurt.
- Other illnesses:
  - ankylosing spondylitis – stiffness, fatigue, rare in those of Afro-Caribbean descent;
  - spinal dysraphism/neoplasm – change in gait, bladder or bowel function.
- Medical, social, family history.
- Congenital defects in small children, perinatal history.

Examination in standing

- Gait

- Asymmetry:
  - torticollis;
  - asymmetric shoulders;
  - prominent scapula;
  - waist asymmetry;
  - pelvic obliquity;
  - thoracic hypokyphosis.
- Spinal movements:
  - flexion – Schober's test – a horizontal line is drawn at the lumbosacral junction and a perpendicular line is drawn in the midline 5cm below and 10cm above this line. The vertical line should increase by at least 6cm in length on forward bending;
  - chest expansion – should be at least 5cm, measured just under the axilla.
- Trunk rotation:
  - 20% of adolescents have trunk asymmetry on forward flexion, but only 2% have scoliosis. An asymmetric spine on forward flexion indicates a spinal tumour or infection, or a herniated disc;
  - measure the angle of trunk rotation with a scoliometer. If the angle is more than 7°, an X-ray evaluation is recommended.
- Foot – cavus foot, asymmetric foot size, progressive foot deformity, Gower sign.

Examination in sitting

- Cervical spine:
  - torticollis;
  - range of motion;
  - tenderness;
  - a short neck, low hairline and decreased range of motion are signs of Klippel-Feil syndrome;
  - 13% of patients with a cleft lip have a spinal deformity, generally spina bifida or vertebral hypoplasia;
  - Goldenhar syndrome is indicated by epibulbar dermoid, a preauricular tag, hemivertebra and block vertebra.
- Check power of upper limbs.
- Sitting straight leg raise (SLR).

Supine and prone

- Examine the hips, knees and ankles. A Thomas test is performed for hip flexion.
- Examine the sacroiliac joint with the FABER (flexion, abduction and external rotation) test.
- SLR:
  - to rule out hip disease;
  - a restricted SLR without pain indicates hamstring tightness due to myostatic contracture or spasticity;
  - tight hamstrings are also seen in Scheuermann's kyphosis and spondylolysis;
  - a reduced SLR with pain indicates nerve root inflammation.
- Lasegue test – pain on dorsiflexing the foot during a SLR.
- A contralateral SLR is specific for nerve root compression on the painful side.
- Popliteal angle measurement helps to confirm suspected tension signs. The angle between the femur and the tibia with the hip flexed to 90° is checked. More than 50° is abnormal.
- A femoral stretch test is performed in the prone or lateral position. The thigh is extended with the knee flexed. Anterolateral thigh pain indicates involvement of L2, L3 or L4 dermatomes.
- A prone hyperextension test is performed to see if the hyperkyphosis is correctable. The patient is asked to raise his/her head and shoulder up.
- Neurologic examination.
- Peripheral pulses.
- Galeazzi test to compare the length of the femur on each side.
- A reverse Galeazzi test is performed in the prone position with the knees flexed to 90°. The relative height of the foot indicates the discrepancy in the length of the tibia.

Adult spine

Additional points in adults

- Occupation.
- Social activities.
- Sports.
- Time off work.
- Legal proceedings.
- Unsteady gait.
- Neck and arm pain.
- Back pain radiating to the legs.
- Leg pain after walking indicates claudication, and is often relieved by forward flexion.

Examination

Inspection
- Swelling.
- Scars.
- Deformity.
- Forward-bend test to see rib hump.
- Kyphosis – cervicothoracic kyphosis is seen in ankylosing spondylitis. Thoracic kyphosis is seen in Scheuermann's disease and multiple wedge fractures.
- Lumbar lordosis – lost in degenerative disease and increased in spondylolisthesis.
- Shoulder asymmetry and pelvic tilt.
- Gait – an antalgic gait indicates lumbar radiculopathy, while a broad-based gait indicates cervical myelopathy.

Palpation
- Along spine.
- Abdominal examination.
- Rectal examination.

Movements
- Cervical – flexion, extension, rotation and lateral flexion.
- Thoracic – rotation. Not a very useful test.
- Lumbar – Schober's test.

Cervical spine – special tests

Spurling's manoeuvre is performed to investigate cervical radiculopathy due to disc herniation. The neck is hyperextended, flexed laterally and rotated to the side of the suspected lesion. Reproduction of symptoms suggests cervical radiculopathy.

The shoulder abduction relief test is positive if symptoms are relieved with abduction of the ipsilateral shoulder.

Lhermitte's sign is pain or paraesthesia in a lower limb on flexion of the neck.

Thoracic outlet syndrome

Thoracic outlet syndrome is characterised by pain and paraesthesia in the arm on overhead activity.

In Adson's test, the head is extended and rotated to the affected side. The radial pulse is obliterated on deep inspiration.

In the Roos test, the shoulder is abducted to 90° and the elbows flexed to 90°. The shoulder is braced back and the patient asked to extend and flex the fingers. Reproduction of pain is a positive test.

Lumbar spine

- SLR:
  - nature of pain reproduced;
  - Lasegue sign – pain on dorsiflexion of the foot.
- Bow string test – flex the hip to 45° and the knee to 45°, and press in the popliteal fossa over the nerve. A positive test indicates sciatic nerve tension.
- Ask the patient to sit up with the knees extended. This is an alternative way to examine the supine SLR.
- Flip test – the knees are flexed over the edge of a couch and gradually extended, one knee at a time. This may produce symptoms similar to the SLR.
- Cross-over sign – indicates disc protrusion in the 'axilla' of the nerve root instead of in the more common 'over the shoulder' of the nerve root.
- Femoral stretch test – in a prone position, the knee is flexed to 90° and the foot lifted, leading to extension of the hip. A positive test indicates neuropathy of L2, L3 or L4 nerve roots.

Hips

History

- Pain:
  - groin or thigh;
  - radiation;
  - constant pain indicates infection.
- Stiffness – difficulty in trimming toe nails.
- Childhood problems.
- Previous surgeries.

Examination

Inspection on standing

- From the front – pelvic tilt, muscle wasting, rotational deformity.
- From the side – lumbar lordosis, surgical scars.
- From the back – Scoliosis, gluteal wasting, scars.
- Shortening – use wooden blocks to measure discrepancies.
- Trendelenburg test – the patient should stand for 30 seconds. The test is positive in myelomeningocele, spinal cord lesions, superior gluteal nerve injury, fractures of the neck of the femur, hip dislocation and coxa vara.

Gait

- Pain.
- Stiffness.
- Shortening.
- Gluteal insufficiency.
- Using walking aids.

In an antalgic gait, the patient has a short stance and leans to the affected side.

In a short-leg gait, the centre of gravity shifts to the short side in stance. In addition, the centre of gravity drops.

In a Trendelenburg gait, the patient drops his/her pelvis on the opposite side, and lurches to the same side.

In a gluteus maximus gait, there is forward thrust of the pelvis and backward thrust of the trunk.

Examination in supine position

- Lumbar lordosis.
- Level of the anterior superior iliac spine.
- Swelling.
- Tenderness.
- Scars.
- Deformity.
- Shortening – in full extension – true and apparent.
- Galeazzi sign.
- Special tests to measure shortening.
- Bryant's triangle.
- Nelaton's line – from the ischial tuberosity to the anterior superior iliac spine. The tip of the greater trochanter normally lies below this line.
- Schoemaker's line – this is a line from the greater trochanter to the anterior superior iliac spine projected onto the abdomen from both sides. The lines should normally meet in the midline above the umbilicus.

Palpation

- Tenderness.
- Temperature.

Movements

- Thomas test – to measure fixed flexion deformity.
- Extension – measured in the prone position.
- Abduction – in extension and flexion. Abduction in flexion is the first to be lost in osteoarthritis.
- Adduction.
- IR, ER in extension and 90° flexion.
- Anteversion – patients with high anteversion have increased IR. To assess anteversion, the patient is prone with IR at the hips (feet apart). As the feet are brought back to neutral, the angle of the tibia with the vertical is measured at the point where the greater trochanter is in true lateral. This is the angle of anteversion.

Measurement

- True shortening.
- Apparent shortening.
- Muscle wasting.

Special tests

- Rectus femoris test – Ely's test. This is performed in the prone position, with the knees flexed. The ipsilateral hip will rise if there is contracture of the rectus femoris.
- Iliotibial band (ITB) – Ober test. This is tested in the lateral position, with the affected hip up. The hip is extended and abducted. If there is a contracture, adduction is restricted.
- Labral tears:
  - supine, flexed, adducted and IR causes pain;
  - supine at the edge of a table, extension and ER of leg causes pain.

Knees

History

- Injury.
- Locking – true or pseudo locking.
- Effusion.
- Localised swelling – duration, pain and variation in size. If constant or increasing in size, consider neoplasia.
- Pain – severity, rest pain, walking distance, stairs and walking aids. Constant pain indicates a tumour or infection.
- Stiffness.
- Giving way – true instability.
- Lifestyle.

Examination

Inspection in supine position

- Swelling.
- Redness.
- Surgical scars.
- Obvious deformity.
- Muscle wasting.
- Varus/valgus – put feet together and measure intermalleolar distance.
- Leg-length discrepancy.

Inspection in standing position

- Varus/valgus.
- Recurvatum/fixed flexion.
- Foot – excess pronation.

- Limb-length discrepancy.
- Scars on the back of the knee.

Gait
- Ligamentous instability can lead to thrust while walking.

Sitting
- Extensor lag.
- Patellar tracking.

Palpation
- Local temperature.
- Tenderness along the medial and lateral joint line.
  - tender on femoral attachment of the medial collateral ligament;
  - 'figure of four' test to see LCL tenderness.
- Patellar tendon.
- Posterior palpation.
- Fluid in the knee joint, patellar tap.
- Retropatellar tenderness – Clarke's test.
- Apprehension on pushing the patella laterally.

Movements
- Hyperextension.
- SLR and extensor lag.
- Flexion – both knees together.

Meniscal lesions

McMurray's test – in the supine position, the knee is flexed and the examiner places an index finger and thumb on the medial and lateral joint line. The other hand applies axial load and rotation in varying flexion. Pain on the medial joint line in ER indicates medial meniscus pathology, while pain on the lateral joint line in IR indicates lateral meniscal pathology.

Patellofemoral joint

- Assess rotation of the leg and foot position.
- Assess patella position, size and height.
- Observe tracking.
- Palpate the retinaculum for tenderness.
- Assess medial and lateral movement of the patella for laxity of the retinaculum.

- Patellar apprehension test.

Instability

- Varus/valgus – instability is checked in 30° flexion to relax the posterior capsule and cruciate ligaments. Increased laxity on valgus stress indicates medial collateral ligament laxity, while increased laxity on varus stress indicates lateral collateral ligament laxity.
- Lachman test – checked with the knee in 15-30° flexion and with a thumb on the anteromedial joint margin. Anterior subluxation of the tibia is compared with the contralateral side and the firmness of the 'end point' is assessed. In anterior cruciate ligament (ACL) injury, there is increased anterior translation of the tibia and the end point is soft.
- Drawer test.
- Posterior sagging of the tibia – the patient flexes both hips and both knees to 90°. Normally, the tibial plateau is 1cm anterior to the femoral condyle. A comparison is made with the contralateral side.
- Quadriceps active test – the patient's position is as for assessment of posterior sag. Contraction of the quadriceps causes anterior movement of the tibia, indicating posterior cruciate ligament (PCL) injury.
- Pivot shift – a valgus force and IR is applied to the knee, and the knee is flexed from an extended position. If the tibia reduces back on flexing around 20-30°, this indicates ACL deficiency. The prerequisites for a pivot shift test are an intact medial collateral ligament, intact ITB and the knee not locked (full extension possible). The ITB passes posteriorly as the knee flexes, causing the tibia to reduce in flexion. Instability is increased if the hip is abducted as this relaxes the ITB.
- For minor ACL instability – an alternative method for examination is for the patient to take a lateral position with the affected side up. The pelvis is rolled back 30° and the medial border of the foot placed on a table with the knee extended – this internally rotates the tibia on the femur. The examiner places both thumbs on either side posteriorly and both index fingers

anteriorly on the joint margin and pushes into flexion. At the starting position, the tibia is subluxed anteriorly and reduces at 30° due to tension in the ITB. A positive test indicates ACL deficiency.

- Houston test/toe lift-off test – both great toes are held together and gently lifted off the bed with the knee extended. Increased ER of the tibia and recurvatum indicates PCL, posterolateral corner or LCL injury.
- Rotary drawer test – an anterior drawer that is increased in 30° ER and decreased in 15° IR indicates anteromedial instability. An anterior drawer that is increased in 15° ER and decreased in 30° IR indicates anterolateral instability.
- Jerk test – flex to 90°, valgus, IR and extend the knee. In patients with ACL deficiency, relocation occurs at 30°.
- Posterolateral corner injury:
  - ask the patient to walk and look for varus thrust;
  - reverse pivot shift – the lateral tibial plateau reduces from a posterior subluxed position. Valgus, ER stress and flex-extend knee and the tibia reduces. This indicates injury to the PCL, LCL or arcuate complex;
  - dial test in the prone position;
  - ER increased at 30° flexion – posterolateral corner injury;
  - ER increased at 90° flexion – posterolateral corner plus PCL injury.

A summary of knee ligament tests is shown in Table 16.4.

For patients with knee arthritis

History
- Severity of pain, rest pain.
- Functional level – walking distance, stair climbing, walking aids.
- Impact on lifestyle, ability to use public transport.
- Previous surgical procedures, steroid injections.

Examination
- Gait – check for ligamentous laxity, thrust.
- Scars.
- Deformity and limb alignment.
- Vascularity of feet.
- Hindfoot and forefoot deformities.
- Tenderness – joint line or retropatellar.

Table 16.4. Summary of knee ligament tests.

Ligament	Tests
Anterior cruciate ligament	Anterior drawer, Lachman test, pivot shift, lateral position test
Anteromedial instability	Increased anterior drawer in 30° external rotation
Anterolateral instability	Increased anterior drawer in 15° internal rotation
Posterolateral corner	Increased external rotation in 30° flexion
Posterior cruciate ligament	Reverse pivot shift
Posterior cruciate ligament, posterolateral corner	Increased external rotation in 90° flexion
	Toe lift-off test (Houston test)

- Range of motion, extensor lag, fixed flexion deformity.
- Ligamentous laxity.
- Always examine the hips in patients with knee arthritis.

The foot

History

- Age, sex, occupation.
- Problems with shoe wear.
- Diabetes, rheumatoid disease, endocrine disease, gout, pseudogout, vasculitis.
- Swelling around the ankles represents cardiac, renal or hepatic disease.
- Unilateral swelling indicates venous or lymphatic obstruction.
- Ankle pain – degenerate joint pain is usually felt anteriorly.
- Instability – recurrent sprains or apprehension on walking on uneven surfaces.
- Instability may also be due to tarsal coalition.

A painful foot can be due to the following:

- Gout, pseudogout or seronegative arthritis.
- Pain of the subtalar joint around the sinus tarsi due to valgus deformity in rheumatoid disease.
- Heel pain – insufficiency fracture of the calcaneus or Paget's disease.
- Plantar fasciitis – plantar pain anteromedial to a calcaneal tuberosity.
- Retrocalcaneal pain – Achilles tendonitis is worse with resisted plantar flexion.
- Posterior tibial tendonitis – pain posterior to the medial malleolus.
- Flexor hallucis longus tendonitis – made worse with movement of the hallux.
- Lateral ankle pain – peroneal tendonitis.
- Midfoot pain – trauma, degeneration, inflammation or diabetic Charcot's neuroarthropathy.
- Forefoot pain with callosity:
  - hallux valgus;
  - bunionette;
  - claw toe, hammer toes or mallet toe;
  - intractable plantar keratosis.
- Forefoot pain without callosity and with neuritic symptoms:
  - Morton's neuroma;
  - tarsal tunnel syndrome;
  - prolapsed intervertebral disc.
- Forefoot pain without callosity and without neuritic symptoms:
  - metatarsophalangeal joint (MTPJ) instability;
  - MTPJ capsulitis;
  - stress fracture;
  - rheumatoid disease – synovitis leads to extension of the MTPJ, which causes rupture of the volar plate. This pulls the plantar fat pad distally causing pain (a sensation of walking on pebbles).

Intractable plantar keratosis is under the second or third metatarsal (MT) head and is caused by insufficiency of the first ray or long second MT (transfer lesion). The patient will exhibit localised plantar pain under the head of the second MT.

Morton's neuroma causes localised plantar burning pain.

Tarsal tunnel syndrome can be due to a ganglion, schwannoma, lipoma or myxoedema. Pain and tingling on the plantar aspect is worse with exercise. Pain radiating up the medial aspect of leg is known as the Valleix phenomenon.

In a cavovarus foot, patients have pain under the MT heads and lateral instability.

A flat foot may be due to tibialis posterior dysfunction, rheumatoid disease, trauma, osteoid osteoma or infection. Pain is present medially due to a prominent talar head and laterally due to impingement of the lateral talar process.

Examination

Examine the footwear of the patient, noting areas of wear.

Inspection in standing
- From behind:
  - spinal dysraphism in the lumbar spine;

- pelvic obliquity;
- leg-length inequality;
- asymmetry of the calves;
- swelling of the Achilles tendon;
- position of the heel (varus or valgus). Ask the patient to stand on their toes and check if the heel tilts into varus;
- 'too-many toes' sign – in tibialis posterior dysfunction or flat foot;
- knee deformity – genu varum or valgum.

- From the front – swelling around the ankle.
- From the medial side – a flat or high longitudinal arch.
- From the dorsum – skin and nail changes, toe deformities.
- On plantar aspect – keratosis, ulcers.
- Coleman block test – the heel should correct into valgus when the first ray is not supported. Correction implies a flexible cavus foot.

Gait

Antalgic or high-stepping (in foot drop).

Palpation

- Ankle – swelling, tenderness.
- Medial side – tibialis posterior rupture, irritation or compression of the tibial nerve. The notch of Harty is medial to the tibialis anterior tendon – feel for synovitis and effusion in this area.
- Tendons of the tibialis anterior, extensor digitorum longus and extensor hallucis longus are palpated for tenderness.
- Anterolateral aspect:
  - feel for effusion and swelling;
  - inferior tibiofibular syndesmosis – squeeze the calf at the mid-third. If there is injury to the syndesmosis then this will cause local pain. ER of the foot with the leg stabilised also stresses the syndesmosis.
- Anterior talofibular ligament:
  - sinus tarsi;
  - peroneal tendons;
  - calcaneofibular ligament.
- The peroneus brevis is normally tense in resisted eversion and lies anterior to the peroneus longus.
- The peroneus longus is tested by resisted plantar flexion of the first ray.

- Achilles tendon – check for tenderness, thickening of the tendon or sheath, nodules and Haglund's deformity.
- Calcaneus – tenderness over the tuberosity. Dorsiflexion of the great toe tenses the plantar fascia and produces pain. It also recreates a longitudinal arch if the patient has a flexible flat foot (windlass mechanism).
- Pain on side-to-side compression of the calcaneus may be present in fractures, infection or tumours.
- Chopart's joint and midfoot joints – check for tenderness, crepitus.
- Forefoot – hallux valgus. Tenderness over the second MT indicates a stress fracture.
- Tenderness over the head of the second MT indicates Freiberg's disease.
- Synovitis of the MTPJ is indicated by pain on passive movement.
- Toes pushed apart due to swelling of the MTPJ – 'daylight sign' in rheumatoid and psoriatic disease. Pain on the squeeze test (squeezing the metacarpal heads) indicates synovitis.
- Morton's sign:
  - tenderness between the MT heads in the third web space;
  - a click on pressure in the dorsal direction from the plantar side (Mulder's sign);
  - pain on squeezing the toes.
- Pain under the first MTPJ – sesamoiditis.

Movements

- The standing patient is asked to rise onto tiptoes:
  - the ability to do this confirms gastrosoleus function;
  - if the heels go into varus on tiptoeing, this indicates a functioning tibialis posterior.
- Ankle movements are checked with the patient seated and the knee flexed and extended:
  - 20° dorsiflexion and 40° plantar flexion is normal;
  - passive movements are checked with the forefoot supinated to lock the Chopart and midfoot joints.
- Inversion and eversion – 20° inversion and 10° eversion is the normal range of motion.

- Hallux (great toe):
  - 80° dorsiflexion and 40° plantar flexion is normal at the MTPJ;
  - impingement in dorsiflexion is checked;
  - grind test – the great toe is rotated. Pain on rotation indicates whole joint involvement.
- Pronation is the combined movement of abduction, eversion and dorsiflexion
- Supination is the combined movement of adduction, inversion and plantar flexion.

Neurovascular examination
- Lumbar spine and full neurologic examination.
- Distal pulses.
- Tinel's sign over the tarsal tunnel.
- Deep peroneal nerve entrapment under the inferior extensor retinaculum.
- Superficial peroneal nerve entrapment is 10cm proximal to the ankle as it emerges from the deep fascia.

Achilles tendon rupture

The patient is unable to perform a heel raise. There may be a palpable gap between the two ends of the Achilles tendon. On Thompson's test, squeezing the calf does not produce plantar flexion.

Peroneal tendon disruption

There is a snapping sensation lateral to the ankle. Moving from plantar flexion and inversion to dorsiflexion and eversion reproduces the symptoms. Local tenderness may be present.

Posterior tibial tendon rupture due to degenerative changes

- Pain and swelling on the medial aspect of the ankle.
- Loss of the medial arch.
- Hindfoot valgus.
- 'Too-many toes' sign.
- The heel does not go into varus on tiptoeing.
- The patient is unable to perform a single heel rise.

- Resisted inversion in plantar flexion and everted position.
- Assess the correctability of the deformity.

Ankle instability

- Perform an inversion stress test in slight plantar flexion to check ligament integrity.
- Anterior drawer test – pull the talus anteriorly in relation to the distal tibia. Increased anterior translation versus the opposite side indicates laxity.
- A positive suction sign anterior to the lateral malleolus on distraction of the ankle indicates instability.

Cavovarus foot

- This may be due to Charcot-Marie-Tooth disease or spinal dysraphism.
- Cavovarus foot is associated with hindfoot varus and pes cavus.
- Plantar flexion of the first ray is due to a functioning peroneus longus.
- A Coleman block test is performed to check the flexibility of a cavus foot.

Tarsal coalition

- Patients present with foot fatigue and hindfoot pain.
- They may have recurrent ankle sprains.
- There is tenderness in the sinus tarsi (in patients with calcaneonavicular bar) or medially near the sustentaculum (talocalcaneal bar).
- Peroneal spastic flat-foot patients have a fixed hindfoot valgus.

Rheumatoid foot

- Hindfoot valgus.
- Midfoot abduction.
- Flat medial arch.
- Clawing of lesser toes.
- Hallux valgus.
- Callosities over prominent MT heads.

Peripheral nerves

History

- Nature of injury, duration and course.
- Age, dominance and occupation.
- Previous injuries or operations.
- Medical illness – diabetes, thyroid disease.
- Smoking, alcohol intake.
- Numbness, pain or wasting.

Examination

- Colour.
- Sweating – ball-pen test (tactile adherence test), warm water immersion test.
- Swelling.
- Callosities.
- Scars.
- Deformities.
- Touch sensation.
- Tinel's sign.
- Static and moving two-point discrimination – assesses innervation density. Apply pressure just less than that required to blanch. Two-point discrimination is 4-5mm in the distal phalanx and 20-50mm in the forearm.
- A Semmes Weinstein monofilament is used to assess the threshold of slow-adopting fibres.
- Pin-prick test.

Median nerve at wrist

- Phalen's test – maximal wrist flexion for 30-60 seconds.
- Reverse Phalen's test – with wrist extended.
- Direct pressure over the carpal tunnel for 30-120 seconds reproduces symptoms.
- For abductor pollicis brevis – the patient lies the dorsum of the hand flat on the table and abducts the thumb against resistance.
- Thenar muscle wasting may be evident.
- Numbness over palm – indicates pronator teres syndrome.
- Tourniquet test.
- Straight-arm raising test – elevating the arm above the head reproduces symptoms.

Medial nerve in proximal forearm and elbow

- Sites of compression:
  - ligament of Struthers;
  - pronator syndrome due to lacertus fibrosus, pronator teres or FDS arch.
- Ache in proximal forearm.
- Thenar numbness.
- Supination against resistance with elbow flexed – biceps becomes tight.
- Pronate against resistance – pronator teres becomes tight.
- Tinel's sign.
- Forcible flexion of the PIPJ middle finger against resistance – FDS becomes tight.

Anterior interosseous syndrome

- The anterior interosseous nerve can be compressed by the band of the pronator teres or FDS.
- Loss of flexion of the DIPJ of the index finger and thumb IPJ.
- Tip-to-tip pinch of the index finger and thumb is lost in anterior interosseous nerve palsy.

Ulnar nerve at elbow

- Cubital tunnel syndrome caused by:
  - arcade of Struthers;
  - medial intermuscular septum;
  - exostosis from medial epicondyle;
  - cubital tunnel;
  - Osborne's fascia – a fascial band between the two heads of the flexor carpi ulnaris;
  - anconeus epitrochlearis (accessory muscle).
- Direct pressure on the nerve elicits paraesthesia along the distribution.
- Tinel's sign.
- Intrinsic weakness.
- Elbow flexion test – full flexion with supination. Dorsiflexion of the wrist for 3-5 minutes reproduces the symptoms.
- Clawing of the little and ring fingers.
- Froment's sign – ask the patient to grasp a card between the thumb and index finger. Because

of weakness in the adductor pollicis and the first dorsal interosseous muscle, the flexor pollicis longus comes into action and flexes the IPJ.

- Wartenberg's sign – the little finger is abducted due to a weak third palmar interosseous.
- 'Making a wish' sign – the ability to cross index and middle fingers depends on interosseous function.

Ulnar nerve at wrist

- Compression in Guyon's canal may be due to:
  - pisotriquetral arthritis;
  - fracture of the hook of hamate;
  - thrombosis of the ulnar artery due to repeated hypothenar trauma (hypothenar hammer syndrome).
- This may be a pure motor or pure sensory lesion.
- The dorsal sensory branch is spared. The patient has normal sensation on the dorsum of the fourth and fifth metacarpals.

Martin Gruber anastomosis

Martin Gruber anastomosis is caused by communication of the motor fibres of the median and ulnar nerve in the forearm. It occurs in 15-20% of people.

Communication of the sensory fibres in the wrist is known as Riche-Cannieu anastomosis.

Posterior interosseous nerve syndrome

The proximal border of the supinator in the arcade of Frohse can compress the posterior interosseous nerve.

Patients have pain on the lateral aspect of the elbow radiating into the forearm. There is also motor weakness, and radial deviation of the wrist on extension due to a weak extensor carpi ulnaris. Resisted active supination with the elbow extended will tighten the arcade of Frohse.

Brachial plexus

History

Brachial plexus injuries are commonly traction injuries sustained in high-energy accidents.

Examination

- General – head injury, cervical injury, Horner's syndrome, Tinel's sign.
- Sensory – pinwheel for pain, light touch with the examiner's fingers.
- Neurapraxia – pain sensation may be preserved despite dense motor loss. Grading of sensory recovery is described in Chapter 14.
- Autonomic – sweating.
- Motor – MRC grading (see Chapter 14).
- Rhomboids.
- Trapezius – unable to sustain abduction of shoulder at 90°.
- Deltoid.
- Supraspinatus.
- Scapular winging due to rhomboids, serratus and trapezius.
- Elbow flexion – C6 (and C5) nerve roots.
- Elbow extension – C7 nerve root.
- Wrist extension – C7 (and C8) nerve roots.
- Finger and thumb extension – C7 and C8 nerve roots.
- Extension of IPJ – C7, C8 and T1 nerve roots.
- Finger and thumb flexion – C8 nerve root.
- Finger and thumb abduction – T1 nerve root.
- C5, C6 lesion – arm is adducted, internally rotated and cannot be flexed at the elbow.
- C5, C6, C7 lesion – as above, with weak elbow extension and weak wrist extension.
- C8, T1 lesion – clawing, Horner's syndrome.

Chapter 17 Surgical approaches

Shoulder

Deltopectoral approach

- Indications – shoulder arthroplasty, open stabilisation, cuff repair, fixation of proximal humeral fractures.
- Position of patient – beach-chair position.
- Incision – starts at the coracoid and extends distally along the deltopectoral groove (Figure 17.1). The cephalic vein can be retracted medially or laterally. The proximal end can be curved laterally along the anterior border of the lateral third of the clavicle.
- Plane – between the deltoid and pectoralis major.
- Extension:
  - the deltoid can be elevated from the lateral third of the clavicle. The superficial and deep fascia of the deltoid should be preserved and can be used to reattach the deltoid to the clavicle. The tip of the coracoid process can be removed and retracted medially with the conjoint tendon for added exposure;
  - distally, the deltoid insertion on the deltoid tuberosity can be released and will reattach to bone spontaneously. The brachialis can be split to expose the humeral shaft.
- Structures at risk – the cephalic vein, musculocutaneous nerve, brachial plexus and axillary vessels. The musculocutaneous nerve is at risk of neurapraxia from retraction of the conjoint tendon, especially when the tip of the coracoid has been removed.

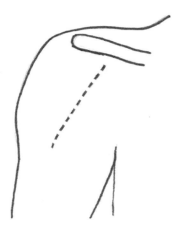

Figure 17.1. Incision for the deltopectoral approach to the shoulder.

Anterosuperior approach

- Indications – rotator cuff repairs, fracture of greater tuberosity.
- Position of patient – beach-chair position.
- Incision – from the anterolateral margin of the acromion towards the coracoid process.
- Plane – there is no true internervous plane. The deltoid fibres are split.

Posterior approach

- Indication – fixation of posterior rim fractures of the glenoid.

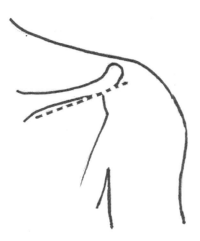

Figure 17.2. Incision for the posterior approach to the shoulder.

- Position of patient – lateral position.
- Incision – along the spine of the scapula, extending to the posterolateral border of the acromion (Figure 17.2).
- Plane – the deltoid fibres are split or detached from the spine of the scapula. The plane is between the teres minor and infraspinatus.
- Structures at risk – the axillary nerve runs in the quadrilateral space inferior to the teres minor. The suprascapular nerve is at risk of traction injury on the infraspinatus.

Humerus

Anterior approach

- Indications – internal fixation of fractures, treatment of tumours or humerus infections.
- Position of patient – supine with the arm abducted.
- Incision – the incision runs along the line from the coracoid tip to the deltoid insertion. Distally, it can be extended along the lateral border of the biceps brachii.
- Plane – proximally, the plane is between the deltoid and the pectoralis major. Distally, it lies between the medial and the lateral half of the brachialis.

- Structures at risk – the radial nerve and axillary nerve. The anterior humeral circumflex artery may have to be ligated as it crosses the operative field.

Posterior approach

- Indications – fractures of the lower half of the humerus, treatment of tumours or humerus infections, exploration of radial nerve.
- Position of patient – lateral with the arm across the chest, or prone.
- Incision – a longitudinal incision along the midline posteriorly.
- Plane – the triceps is split in line with fibres. The radial nerve must be identified in the spiral groove and protected throughout the procedure.
- Structures at risk – radial nerve, profunda brachii artery, ulnar nerve.

An olecranon osteotomy can be combined with this approach to expose the distal humerus for fixation of intercondylar fractures. The osteotomy is predrilled, with the chevron shaped and aimed at the bare area on the olecranon surface.

Lateral approach to the distal humerus

- Indication – exposure of the lateral condyle humerus.
- Position of patient – supine with the arm across the chest.
- Incision – a curved incision overlying the lateral epicondyle.
- Plane – between the triceps and brachioradialis.
- Structure at risk – the radial nerve is at risk proximally.

Elbow

Posterior approach – transolecranon

- Indication – intercondylar fracture of the humerus.

- Position of patient – prone or lateral, with the arm across the chest.
- Incision – a posterior midline incision, avoiding the tip of the olecranon.
- Plane – the ulnar nerve is identified and protected. An olecranon osteotomy is performed to elevate the triceps from the distal humerus and expose the joint.
- Structures at risk – ulnar, median and radial nerve, brachial artery.

Medial approach

- Indications – fixation of a coronoid fracture, removal of loose bodies.
- Position of patient – supine with the arm abducted and externally rotated.
- Incision – medial aspect of the elbow, centred on the medial epicondyle.
- Plane – proximally, the plane lies between the brachialis and triceps. Distally, it is between the brachialis and pronator teres.
- Structures at risk – median nerve, ulnar nerve.

Posterolateral approach

- Indication – excision/replacement of the radial head.
- Position of patient – supine with the arm across the chest.
- Incision – a curved incision centred on the lateral epicondyle.
- Plane – between the anconeus and extensor carpi ulnaris. The forearm is pronated to protect the posterior interosseous nerve.
- Structures at risk – posterior interosseous nerve, radial nerve.

Forearm

Anterior approach to the radius

- Indications – fixation of fractures of the radius, radial osteotomy, tumour excision.

- Position of patient – supine with the arm on an arm board.
- Incision – along a line from the lateral border of the bicipital aponeurosis to the radial styloid.
- Plane – the brachioradialis lies on the lateral side of the approach, with the pronator teres on the medial side in the proximal part. Distally, the approach is between the brachioradialis and flexor carpi radialis.
- Structures at risk – superficial radial nerve (on the deep surface of the brachioradialis), radial nerve (in the proximal end of the approach), radial artery.

Posterior approach to the radius

- Indications – reduction and fixation of fractures, osteotomy, approach to the posterior interosseous nerve.
- Position of patient – supine with the arm on an arm board.
- Incision – along a line joining the lateral epicondyle of the humerus to Lister's tubercle on the dorsum of the distal radius.
- Plane – in the proximal part of the approach, the plane is between the extensor carpi radialis brevis and the extensor digitorum. Distally, it lies between the extensor carpi radialis brevis and the extensor pollicis longus.
- Structure at risk – the posterior interosseous nerve at the proximal end of the approach.

Approach to the ulna

- Indications – reduction and fixation of fractures of the ulna, ulnar osteotomy.
- Position of patient – supine with the arm across the chest.
- Incision – along the subcutaneous border of the ulna.
- Plane – between the extensor carpi ulnaris and the flexor carpi ulnaris.
- Structure at risk – ulnar artery.

Wrist

Dorsal approach to the wrist

- Indications – extensor tendon repair, wrist fusion, fixation of distal radius fractures, proximal row carpectomy, wrist synovectomy.
- Position of patient – supine with the forearm pronated.
- Incision – a longitudinal incision on the dorsum of the wrist in the midline.
- Plane – the approach is made between the extensor carpi radialis longus and the extensor carpi radialis brevis.
- Structures at risk – superficial branches of the radial nerve.

Volar approach to the wrist

- Indications – fixation of distal radius fractures, access to the medial nerve and flexor tendons in the wrist, infection of the midpalmar space.
- Position of patient – supine with an arm board.
- Incision – the incision runs from the ulnar to the thenar crease in the palm. At the level of the flexor crease, the incision curves toward the ulna to avoid crossing the crease at a right angle. The incision in the carpal tunnel is made on the ulnar side of the median nerve to protect the motor branch of the median nerve to the thenar muscles.
- Plane – there is no true internervous plane.
- Structures at risk – palmar cutaneous branch of the median nerve, ulnar vessels and nerve, radial vessels, medial nerve.

Volar approach to the scaphoid

- Indications – scaphoid non-union, bone grafting, excision of radial styloid.
- Position of patient – supine with the forearm supinated.
- Incision – a curved incision lateral to the flexor carpi radialis towards the scaphoid tuberosity.
- Plane – there is no true internervous plane.
- Structure at risk – radial artery.

Dorsal approach to the scaphoid

- Indications – scaphoid fractures and non-union, excision of radial styloid.
- Position of patient – supine with the arm pronated.
- Incision – a curved incision on the dorsolateral aspect of the scaphoid centred on the snuff box.
- Plane – there is no true internervous plane.
- Structures at risk – branches of the superficial radial nerve.

Pelvis

Ilioinguinal approach

- Indication – anterior column exposure for fracture fixation.
- Position of patient – supine, with a urinary catheter inserted.
- Incision – a curved incision along the inguinal ligament.
- Plane – there is no true internervous plane:
  - the external oblique muscle is divided in line with the fibres protecting the spermatic cord/round ligament in a sling at the medial extent. The transversus abdominis and the internal oblique muscles are divided on exposing the posterior wall of the inguinal canal;
  - the inferior epigastric artery runs medial to the deep inguinal ring and should be identified and ligated. The lateral cutaneous nerve is often divided in the lateral part of the incision;
  - three slings are passed. The first goes round the spermatic cord (in males) or the round ligament (in females). The second sling goes around the femoral vessels. The third sling goes around the iliopsoas tendon and femoral nerve. Access to the pelvis is obtained by retraction of these slings.
- Structures at risk – femoral nerve, femoral vessels, inferior epigastric artery, lateral cutaneous nerve, spermatic cord, bladder.

Hip

Anterior (iliofemoral or Smith-Petersen) approach

- Indications – congenital dislocation of the hip, hip arthrodesis, rarely hip arthroplasty.
- Position of patient – supine with a sandbag under the ipsilateral buttock.
- Incision – along a line from the anterior superior iliac spine to the lateral border of the patella.
- Plane – between the sartorius and tensor fascia lata and then between the rectus femoris and glutei – medius and minimus. The rectus can be detached from the ilium for access.
- Advantages – good access to the anterior acetabulum.
- Limitations – poor access to the posterior acetabulum.
- Structures at risk – ascending branch of the lateral circumflex femoral artery and branches of the lateral cutaneous nerve of the thigh.

Anterolateral (Watson-Jones) approach

- Indications – hip arthroplasty, washout of hip infections.
- Position of patient – supine with a sandbag under the ipsilateral buttock.
- Incision – centred over the tip of the greater trochanter, curving posteriorly.
- Plane – between the tensor fascia lata and gluteus medius. The anterior third of the gluteus is reflected off the greater trochanter.
- Advantages – minimal bleeding, no significant structures at risk.
- Limitation – limited access to the posterior acetabulum.
- Structures at risk – ascending branch of the lateral circumflex femoral artery.

Direct lateral (Hardinge) approach

- Indications – hemiarthroplasty and total hip replacement, hip revision surgery, rarely hip resurfacing.
- Position of patient – supine with a sandbag under the ipsilateral buttock, or lateral position.
- Incision – centred on the tip of the trochanter, curving posteriorly in the proximal part.
- Plane – the abductors are split, and the anterior third is reflected anteriorly along with the vastus lateralis.
- Advantages – low dislocation rate (0.3%).
- Disadvantages and limitations – a postoperative limp in up to 10% of patients because of injury to the superior gluteal nerve or gluteal muscle weakness. Exposure of the acetabulum is often limited.
- Structures at risk – abductor muscle weakness postoperatively.

> **Note**
>
> Hardinge K. The direct lateral approach to the hip. *J Bone Joint Surg Br* 1982; 64: 17-9.

Posterior (Moore or Southern) approach

- Indications – this approach can be used for most hip operations, including replacements, resurfacing, tumour surgery and revisions.
- Position of patient – lateral.
- Incision – centred about 2cm distal to the tip of the trochanter. The proximal half is parallel to the fibres of the gluteus maximus, while the distal half is parallel to the femur.
- Plane – split the gluteus maximus, detach short external rotators and capsule from the femur.
- Advantages – preserves abductors. Lower heterotopic ossification.
- Disadvantages – a higher dislocation rate if the capsule is not adequately repaired. With an enhanced repair of capsule to bone, the dislocation rate is comparable with that of the direct lateral approach. Pellicci and colleagues reported a reduction in the dislocation rate from 6.2% to 0.8% if the capsule is repaired to bone.

Note

Pellicci PM, Bostrom M, Poss R. Posterior approach to total hip replacement using enhanced posterior soft tissue repair. *Clin Orthop Relat Res* 1998; 355: 224-8.

- Structures at risk – superior gluteal vessels, sciatic nerve.

For fixation of posterior column fractures of the acetabulum, the same approach can be extended proximally to expose the posterior column. The gluteus medius is elevated by blunt dissection from the outer aspect of the ilium.

Trochanteric slide

- Indications – hip replacement, hip infection.
- Position of patient – supine or lateral.
- Incision – centred on the tip of the greater trochanter.
- Plane – the abductors and the vastus are not detached but a flake of bone is taken off from the greater trochanter.
- Advantages – avoids damage to abductors and injury to superior gluteal nerve.
- Limitations – exposure can be limited.
- Structures at risk – trochanteric anastomosis.

Trochanteric osteotomy (Charnley)

- Indication – hip replacement.
- Position of patient – supine or lateral.
- Incision – centred on the tip of the greater trochanter.
- Plane – the abductors are not detached. Osteotomy is performed in line with the superior border of the neck of the femur using a Steinman pin inserted in line with the superior border of the neck to create a chevron (Figure 17.3).

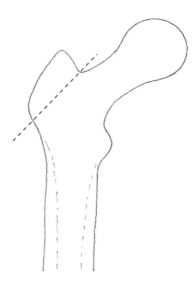

Figure 17.3. Osteotomy of the greater trochanter.

Note

Wroblewski BM, Shelley P. Reattachment of the greater trochanter after hip replacement. *J Bone Joint Surg Br* 1985; 67: 736-40.

- Advantages – avoids damage to the abductors. Excellent exposure.
- Disadvantages – trochanteric non-union with resultant pain or a limp.
- Structure at risk – superior gluteal nerve due to retraction.

Extended trochanteric osteotomy

- Indications – extensile exposure for hip replacement, revision surgery.
- Position of patient – supine or lateral.
- Plane – the abductors are not detached. The length of the osteotomy is planned preoperatively and the lateral third of the proximal femur is osteotomised. The osteotomy

narrows distally to avoid a stress fracture at the end of the osteotomy (Figure 17.4). The lateral fragment is reattached using cerclage wiring.

- Advantages – avoids damage to the abductors and injury to the superior gluteal nerve. Good exposure of the femoral canal makes it easier to remove components and cement from the femur. Acetabular exposure is also improved with extended trochanteric osteotomy.
- Disadvantages – non-union of the fragment is rare. Eccentric reaming and femoral fracture have been reported.
- Structures at risk – none.

> **Note**
>
> Younger TI, Bradford MS, Magnus RE, Paprosky WG. Extended proximal femoral osteotomy. A new technique for femoral revision arthroplasty. *J Arthroplasty* 1995; 10: 329-38.

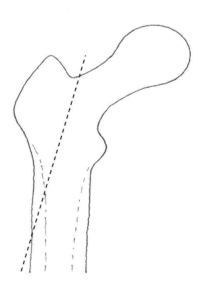

Figure 17.4. Extended trochanteric osteotomy.

Minimally invasive hip replacement

- Indication – hip replacement.
- Various approaches have been described, which essentially use a part of conventional approaches to perform the arthroplasty. The approach can be posterior, direct lateral or through a Smith-Peterson approach.
- Advantages – potentially faster recovery and shorter hospital stay.
- Disadvantages – limited access, long learning curve for surgeons.
- Structures at risk – depends on posterior or direct lateral approach, as described above.

Two-incision hip replacement

This approach is based on making two separate incisions: one to insert the acetabular component and the other to insert the femoral component. Each incision is around 5cm in size and does not involve cutting any muscles. The intermuscular plane is used for access.

Despite widespread enthusiasm, there has been some concern about the benefits of minimally invasive surgery in terms of early results. In a study by Ogonda and colleagues, 219 patients were randomised to surgery through a short (≤10cm) or standard (16cm) incision. The short-incision approach offered no postoperative benefit in terms of blood loss, pain score, walking ability, cement mantle quality, component placement or hospital stay.

> **Note**
>
> Ogonda L, Wilson R, Archbold P, *et al*. A minimal-incision technique in total hip arthroplasty does not improve early postoperative outcomes. A prospective, randomized, controlled trial. *J Bone Joint Surg Am* 2005; 87: 701-10.

Knee

Medial parapatellar approach

This is the most commonly used approach to the knee. It allows full and extensile access.

- Indications – total knee replacement, fixation of proximal tibial and patellar fractures, patellectomy, synovectomy.
- Position of patient – supine. Using a lateral support and foot rest, the knee can be maintained in a flexed position with minimal assistance.
- Incision – a longitudinal, straight midline incision.
- Plane – there is no internervous plane. Deep dissection involves a medial parapatellar arthrotomy dividing the quadriceps tendon. The patella can be everted if required.
- Extension – proximally, the quadriceps tendon can be divided transversely to aid exposure (quadriceps snip). Distally, the tibial tubercle can be divided and reflected laterally.
- Structures at risk – the infrapatellar branch of the saphenous nerve is often divided. This can lead to neuroma formation along the scar.

Posterior approach

- Indications – repair of bony avulsion of the posterior cruciate ligament, access to the posterior capsule, excision of cyst or tumour from the posterior aspect of the knee.
- Position of patient – prone.
- Incision – a curved incision starting from the superolateral aspect over the biceps femoris tendon, curving across the popliteal fossa and downwards medially and inferiorly (Figure 17.5).
- Plane – there is no internervous plane. The fascia of the popliteal fossa is divided medial to the short saphenous vein. The muscles forming the boundary of the popliteal fossa are retracted for access. The popliteal artery gives off five genicular arteries. One of these may have to be divided to enable retraction of the neurovascular bundle.

- Structures at risk – medial sural cutaneous nerve, peroneal vessels, tibial and common peroneal nerve.

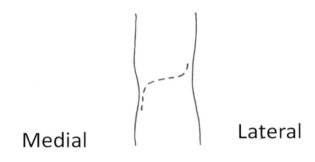

Figure 17.5. Incision for the posterior approach to the knee.

Medial approach

- Indications – access to the medial collateral ligament, fixation of medial tibial plateau fractures.
- Position of patient – supine. The hip is externally rotated and abducted and the affected knee is flexed.
- Incision – begins proximal to the adductor tubercle and curves anteriorly and distally.
- Plane – there is no internervous plane. Deep dissection can be carried out anterior or posterior to the medial collateral ligament.
- Structures at risk – infrapatellar branch of the saphenous nerve, medial inferior genicular artery, saphenous vein.

Lateral approach

- Indication – lateral ligament repair.
- Position of patient – supine with a sandbag under the ipsilateral buttock. The knee is flexed to 90°.
- Incision – a curved incision on the lateral aspect with the proximal part parallel to the femur and the distal part parallel to the tibia.
- Plane – the plane lies between the iliotibial band and the biceps femoris. The fascia between these can be incised to gain access to the joint. The arthrotomy can be made anterior or posterior to the lateral collateral ligament.
- Structures at risk – lateral popliteal nerve, lateral meniscus, popliteus tendon, lateral superior genicular artery.

Tibia

Posterolateral approach

- Indications – internal fixation of fractures, posterolateral bone grafting of delayed union or non-union.
- Position of patient – lateral with the operated leg up.
- Incision – along the lateral border of the gastrocnemius.
- Plane – between the posterior and lateral compartments. The plane lies between the gastrosoleus and the flexor hallucis longus on the medial side and the peroneal muscles on the lateral side.
- Structures at risk – the branches of the peroneal artery may need to be ligated. The posterior tibial artery and tibial nerve are separated from the plane of dissection by the flexor hallucis longus.

Ankle

Anterior approach

- Indications – ankle arthrodesis or replacement, drainage of septic arthritis, fixation of pilon fractures.

- Position of patient – supine.
- Incision – a longitudinal incision between the two malleoli. An alternative approach is along the tibialis anterior tendon.
- Plane – the tendon of the extensor hallucis longus is retracted medially along with the neurovascular bundle.
- Structures at risk – branches of the superficial peroneal nerve, the deep peroneal nerve and the anterior tibial artery.

Posteromedial approach

- Indication – access to the medial malleolus.
- Position of patient – supine with the hip externally rotated or lateral with the non-operated leg up.
- Incision – midway between the medial malleolus and the Achilles tendon.
- Plane – the dissection can be performed between the flexor hallucis longus and the peronei, or the flexor hallucis longus and the flexor digitorum longus.
- Structures at risk – posterior tibial artery, tibial nerve.

Posterolateral approach

- Indications – fixation of the posterior malleolus, fusion of the subtalar joint.
- Position of patient – prone.
- Incision – midway between the lateral border of the Achilles tendon and the lateral malleolus.
- Plane – between the peroneus brevis and the flexor hallucis longus.
- Structures at risk – short saphenous nerve, sural nerve.

Lateral approach for triple arthrodesis

- Indications – approach to the talocalcaneal joint, calcaneocuboid joint and talonavicular joint.
- Position of patient – supine with a sandbag under the ipsilateral hip.

- Incision – from the tip of the lateral malleolus, over the sinus tarsi and curving medially.
- Plane – between the peroneus tertius and the peroneal tendons.
- Structures at risk – dorsalis pedis artery, deep peroneal nerve.

Index